Palliative Care in Nephrology

INTEGRATING PALLIATIVE CARE
Published and Forthcoming Books in the *Integrating Palliative Care* Series

Surgical Palliative Care
Anne C. Mosenthal and Geoffrey P. Dunn

Palliative Care in Nephrology
Alvin H. Moss, Dale E. Lupu, Nancy C. Armistead, and Louis H. Diamond

Palliative Care in Nephrology

Edited by

Alvin H. Moss, MD
*Professor of Medicine, Sections of Nephrology
and Palliative Medicine, Department of Medicine
West Virginia University School of Medicine
Morgantown, WV, USA*

Dale E. Lupu, MPH, PhD
*Associate Research Professor, Center for Aging,
Health and Humanities, George Washington University
Washington, DC, USA*

Nancy C. Armistead, MPA
*Executive Director (Retired), Mid-Atlantic Renal Coalition
Polson, MT, USA*

Louis H. Diamond, MD, FCP
*Consultant
Rockville, MD, USA*

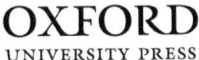

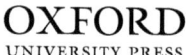

Oxford University Press is a department of the University of Oxford. It furthers the University's objective of excellence in research, scholarship, and education by publishing worldwide. Oxford is a registered trade mark of Oxford University Press in the UK and certain other countries.

Published in the United States of America by Oxford University Press
198 Madison Avenue, New York, NY 10016, United States of America.

© Oxford University Press 2020

All rights reserved. No part of this publication may be reproduced, stored in a retrieval system, or transmitted, in any form or by any means, without the prior permission in writing of Oxford University Press, or as expressly permitted by law, by license, or under terms agreed with the appropriate reproduction rights organization. Inquiries concerning reproduction outside the scope of the above should be sent to the Rights Department, Oxford University Press, at the address above.

You must not circulate this work in any other form
and you must impose this same condition on any acquirer.

Library of Congress Cataloging-in-Publication Data
Names: Moss, Alvin H., editor. | Lupu, Dale E., editor. | Armistead, Nancy C., editor. | Diamond, Louis H., editor.
Title: Palliative Care in Nephrology / edited by Alvin H. Moss, Dale E. Lupu, Nancy C. Armistead, and Louis H. Diamond.
Other titles: Integrating palliative care (Series).
Description: New York, NY : Oxford University Press, [2020] |
Series: Integrating palliative care |
Includes bibliographical references and index.
Identifiers: LCCN 2020005781 (print) | LCCN 2020005782 (ebook) |
ISBN 9780190945527 (paperback) | ISBN 9780190945541 (epub) |
ISBN 9780190945558 (electronic)
Subjects: MESH: Kidney Diseases | Palliative Care—methods
Classification: LCC RC903 (print) | LCC RC903 (ebook) | NLM WJ 300 |
DDC 616.6/1029—dc23
LC record available at https://lccn.loc.gov/2020005781
LC ebook record available at https://lccn.loc.gov/2020005782

This material is not intended to be, and should not be considered, a substitute for medical or other professional advice. Treatment for the conditions described in this material is highly dependent on the individual circumstances. And, while this material is designed to offer accurate information with respect to the subject matter covered and to be current as of the time it was written, research and knowledge about medical and health issues is constantly evolving and dose schedules for medications are being revised continually, with new side effects recognized and accounted for regularly. Readers must therefore always check the product information and clinical procedures with the most up-to-date published product information and data sheets provided by the manufacturers and the most recent codes of conduct and safety regulation. The publisher and the authors make no representations or warranties to readers, express or implied, as to the accuracy or completeness of this material. Without limiting the foregoing, the publisher and the authors make no representations or warranties as to the accuracy or efficacy of the drug dosages mentioned in the material. The authors and the publisher do not accept, and expressly disclaim, any responsibility for any liability, loss, or risk that may be claimed or incurred as a consequence of the use and/or application of any of the contents of this material.

Contents

Contributors — ix

1. Overview — 1

SECTION I — Why We Need This Book—Unmet Supportive Care Needs of Patients With Kidney Disease

2. Birth of a Benefit—Brief History of the ESRD Program — 13
   Nancy C. Armistead and Jeffrey A. Perlmutter

3. Unmet Palliative Care Needs of Patients With Kidney Disease and Consequences — 21
   Kate Schueller and Dale E. Lupu

4. Models for Operationalizing Supportive Care in Kidney Care — 36
   Dale E. Lupu and Emma Murphy

SECTION II — Supportive Care Capacity—Creating the Infrastructure to Provide Kidney Supportive Care

5. Assessing Patients' Unmet Palliative Care Needs With Tools for Assessment — 49
   Chandra Thomas and Amanda Halpin

6. Primary Palliative Care Education for the Multidisciplinary Nephrology Team — 58
   J. Pedro Teixeira and Sara A. Combs

7. Establishing Relationships With Specialty Palliative Care for More Complex Patient Needs — 67
   Kate Schueller and Joseph D. Rotella

8. Physician Wellness in Nephrology and Palliative Care ... 76
   Sarah Ramer and Holly Koncicki

SECTION III   Patient-Centered Care—Values Guide Care

9. The Shared Decision-Making Process as the Recommended Standard for Treatment Decisions in Kidney Disease and Requisite Communication Skills to Implement the Process ... 87
   Ernest I. Mandel, Jane O. Schell, and Robert A. Cohen

10. Advance Care Planning to Elicit and Respect Patient Values and Preferences ... 98
    Jean L. Holley and J. April Yasunaga

11. Involving Family and Friends in Palliative Care for Persons With Kidney Disease ... 108
    Elizabeth Anderson and David M. White

12. The System to Implement Advance Care Planning and Make Proxies, Advance Directives, and Portable Medical Orders Available and Actionable Across Care Settings ... 116
    Valerie Satkoske and Alvin H. Moss

SECTION IV   Just Right Care—The Right Care to the Right Person at the Right Time

13. The Role of Estimating and Communicating Prognosis in Kidney Supportive Care ... 127
    Bjorg Thorsteinsdottir and Michael J. Germain

14. Active Medical Management Without Dialysis for Patients With Advanced Chronic Kidney Disease ... 136
    Kelly Li and Mark Brown

15. Systematic Pain Assessment and Management ... 148
    Sara N. Davison

16. Systematic Nonpain Symptom Assessment and Management ... 167
    Hana Yu and Jennifer S. Scherer

17. Systematic Psychosocial and Spiritual Needs Assessment and Management ... 178
    Daniel Cukor and Elissa Kozlov

18. Geriatric Nephrology Syndromes and Assessment and Management of Cognitive Impairment ... 188
    Edwina A. Brown and Osasuyi Iyasere

19. Palliative Considerations for the Patient With Acute Kidney Injury in the Intensive Care Unit   197
Tamara Rubenzik and Alvin H. Moss

SECTION V   Throughout the Continuum—Enhanced Support at the End of Life

20. Coordination of Care and Care Transitions With Primary Care Clinicians, Specialty Palliative Care, and Hospice   211
Areeba Jawed and Joseph D. Rotella

21. Palliative Dialysis   220
Vanessa Grubbs

22. Process of Dialysis Withdrawal for Patients Failing to Thrive on Dialysis   227
Daniel Lam and Rebecca J. Schmidt

SECTION VI   The Future of Palliative Care Nephrology

23. Ethical Issues in the Supportive Care of Patients With Advanced Kidney Disease   239
Catherine R. Butler and Alvin H. Moss

24. Transforming Practice to Support Person-Centered Care for Patients With Advanced Kidney Disease   248
Ann M. O'Hare and Nancy C. Armistead

Index   261

Contributors

Elizabeth Anderson, DSW, LCSW
Assistant Professor of Social Work
Western Carolina University
Asheville, NC, USA

Edwina A. Brown, DM (Oxon), FRCP
Consultant Nephrologist
Imperial College Renal and
  Transplant Centre
Hammersmith Hospital
London, UK

Mark Brown, MB, FRACP, MD
Senior Staff Specialist and Professor
  of Renal Medicine
Department of Renal Medicine
St George Hospital and St George and
  Sutherland Clinical School
Sydney, Australia

Catherine R. Butler, MD
Acting Instructor of Medicine
University of Washington
Seattle, WA, USA

Robert A. Cohen, MD, MSc
Director of Education, Nephrology Division,
  Beth Israel Deaconess Medical Center
Harvard Medical School
Boston, MA, USA

Sara A. Combs, MD, MSCS
Assistant Professor
Department of Internal Medicine, Divisions
  of Nephrology and Palliative Care
University of New Mexico School of
  Medicine
Albuquerque, NM, USA

Daniel Cukor, PhD
Director of Behavioral Health
The Rogosin Institute
New York, NY, USA

Sara N. Davison, MD, MSc
Professor of Medicine
Department of Medicine
University of Alberta
Edmonton, AB, Canada

Michael J. Germain, MD
Professor of Nephrology
University of Massachusetts Medical School–Baystate Campus
Springfield, MA, USA

Vanessa Grubbs, MD, MPH
Associate Professor of Nephrology
University of California–San Fransico
San Francisco, CA, USA

Amanda Halpin, MD, FRCPC
Adult Nephrologist
Department of Medicine, Division of Nephrology
University of Saskatchewan
Saskatoon, SK, Canada

Jean L. Holley, MD
Clinical Professor of Medicine, Internal Medicine, Carle Illinois College of Medicine
University of Illinois, Urbana–Champaign
Urbana, IL, USA

Osasuyi Iyasere, MBBS, MD MRCP (UK)
John Walls Renal Unit
Leicester General Hospital
Leicester, UK

Areeba Jawed, MD
Assistant Professor, Internal Medicine–Nephrology
Wayne State University School of Medicine
Detroit, MI, USA

Holly Koncicki, MD, MS
Assistant Professor
Division of Nephrology, Department of Internal Medicine, Brookdale Department of Geriatrics and Palliative Care
Icahn School of Medicine at Mount Sinai
Woodcliff Lake, NJ, USA

Elissa Kozlov, PhD
Instructor of Psychology in Medicine, Weill Cornell Medicine, Division of Geriatric and Palliative Medicine
New York Presbyterian Hospital
New York, NY, USA

Daniel Lam, MD
Clinical Assistant Professor
Department of Medicine, Division of Nephrology
University of Washington
Seattle, WA, USA

Kelly Li, MBBS, FRACP, MBioethics
Staff Nephrologist, Renal Medicine
St George Hospital
Sydney, Australia

Ernest I. Mandel, MD, SM
Associate Physician/Instructor in Medicine
Brigham and Women's Hospital/Harvard Medical School
Boston, MA, USA

Emma Murphy, PhD
Clinical Lecturer, School of Health Sciences
University of Southampton
Southampton, UK

Ann M. O'Hare, MA, MD
Professor of Medicine
Department of Medicine
University of Washington
Seattle, WA, USA

Jeffrey A. Perlmutter, MD
Nephrologist, Nephrology Associates of Montgomery County
Rockville, MD, USA

Sarah Ramer, MD, MS
Instructor in Medicine
Division of Geriatrics and Palliative Medicine
Weill Cornell Medical College
Hackensack, NJ, USA

Joseph D. Rotella, MD, MBA, HMDC, FAAHPM
Chief Medical Officer, American Academy of Hospice and Palliative Medicine; Clinical Assistant Professor of Medicine
Department of General Internal Medicine, Palliative Medicine and Medical Education
University of Louisville School of Medicine
Louisville, KY, USA

Tamara Rubenzik, MD
Physician, Nephrology and Hypertension, Palliative Medicine
University of California–San Diego
San Diego, CA, USA

Valerie Satkoske, PhD
Assistant Professor
School of Medicine
West Virginia University
Wheeling, WV, USA

Jane O. Schell, MD, MHS
Associate Professor
Medicine, Palliative Care and Medical Ethics, Renal–Electrolyte
University of Pittsburgh
Pittsburgh, PA, USA

Jennifer S. Scherer, MD
Assistant Professor, Internal Medicine
NYU School of Medicine
New York, NY, USA

Rebecca J. Schmidt, DO, FACP, FASN
Assistant Dean for Outreach and Community Engagement, Department of Medicine, Section of Nephrology
West Virginia University School of Medicine
Morgantown, WV, USA

Kate Schueller, MD
Clinical Assistant Professor, Director of Ambulatory Palliative Care
Department of Medicine
University of Wisconsin
Madison, WI, USA

J. Pedro Teixeira, MD
Assistant Professor
Department of Internal Medicine, Divisions of Nephrology and Pulmonary, Critical Care, and Sleep Medicine
University of New Mexico School of Medicine
Albuquerque, NM, USA

Chandra Thomas, MSc, MD
Clinical Associate Professor of Medicine
University of Calgary
Calgary, AB, Canada

Bjorg Thorsteinsdottir, MD
Physician, Internal Medicine and Program in Bioethics
Mayo Clinic
Rochester, MN, USA

David M. White
Community Outreach Coordinator, Jack J. Dreyfus Center for Health Action and Policy
The Rogosin Institute
Hillcrest Heights, MD, USA

J. April Yasunaga, MD
Physician, Palliative Medicine
Carle Foundation Hospital
Urbana, IL, USA

Hana Yu, DO
Assistant Professor in Internal Medicine/Palliative Medicine, General Internal Medicine
University of Texas at Southwestern Medical Center
Irving, TX, USA

1

Overview

The need to improve provision of supportive care to patients with kidney disease has been well documented and international guidelines point the way forward to improvement. Yet integration of supportive care into kidney care in the United States lags far behind the guidelines. This book is intended to help practitioners understand the evidence base in supportive (also called palliative) kidney care and apply it to their practice. This chapter defines supportive kidney care in relation to primary and specialty palliative care and provides an overview of the emergence of supportive kidney care, including its essential components.

There is an urgent unmet need for the provision of supportive care to patients with kidney disease. Many have a high symptom burden that impairs their quality of life, multiple co-morbid conditions, a shortened life expectancy, and significant cognitive and functional impairments. Those treating them have not been trained to address these needs.

Kidney palliative (supportive) care is a field that has been in existence since at least 2000 but has yet to gain solid traction in terms of integration into nephrology practice or consistent visibility in publications and professional meetings. This is beginning to change. A search of PubMed for "kidney AND palliative care" reveals over 1,300 articles with the majority having been written in the last 10 years with a particular upsurge in the last 5 years (Figure 1.1).

Internationally, two global summits have outlined the critical role that supportive care plays in a comprehensive kidney care system. In 2013 Kidney Disease: Improving Global Outcomes (KDIGO) held an international controversies conference on supportive care that articulated the

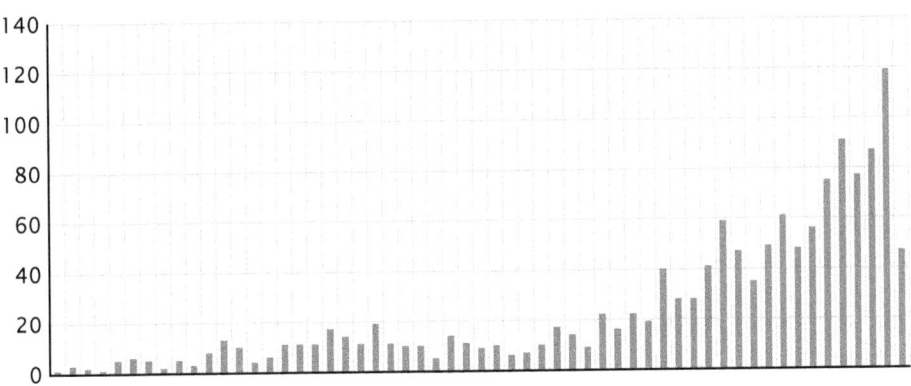

FIGURE 1.1. PubMed search—kidney supportive care citations per year.

Care Recommendations: the 2013 KDIGO Controversies Conference on Supportive Care in Chronic Kidney Disease

Symptom assessment and management
- Symptom assessment and management is an integral component of quality care for patients with advanced CKD. Regular global symptom screening using validated tools such as the ESAS-r:Renal and POS-renal should be incorporated into routine clinical practice.
- Symptom management requires a stepwise approach. First-line treatment includes nonpharmacological interventions and then advancing to more complex therapies. Second-line treatment is pharmacologic therapy. Consideration should be given to low-dose pharmacological therapy that may have efficacy across several symptoms.
- Current evidence is sufficient to support the development of clinical guidelines to aid in the stepwise approach to uremic pruritus, sleep disturbances, restless legs syndrome, pain, and depression in CKD.

Estimating prognosis
- Estimate and communicate prognosis to patients and family, balancing biomedical facts with relevant emotional, social, cultural, and spiritual issues. Such communication should be viewed as an integral component of shared decision-making to align treatment goals with patient preferences. It will aid in the timely identification of patients who are most likely to benefit from supportive care and is essential for quality care.

Shared decision making and advance care planning
- Shared decision making is recommended to align treatment with patient and family goals, values, and preferences. Because patients' health status, preferences, and treatment options may change over time, shared decision making requires a flexible approach of reevaluation and redirection to ensure that the goals of care and treatment plans remain aligned with patients' values and preferences.
- The treatment care team should engage in ACP. These discussions should start early in the illness trajectory and should include discussions about health states in which patients would want to withhold or withdraw dialysis.

Withdrawal from dialysis

- Withdrawal from dialysis is ethically and clinically acceptable after a process of shared decision making. It is incumbent upon all providers caring for a patient contemplating stopping dialysis to address potentially remedial factors contributing to the decision such as depression or other symptoms such as pain as well as potentially reversible social factors.
- Situations in which it is appropriate to withdraw dialysis include the following:
  - Patients with decision-making capacity, who being fully informed and making voluntary choices, refuse dialysis or request that dialysis be discontinued.
  - Patients who no longer possess decision-making capacity who have previously indicated refusal of dialysis through appropriate ACP.
  - Patients who no longer possess decision-making capacity and whose properly appointed legal agents/surrogates refuse dialysis or request that it be discontinued.
  - Patients with irreversible, profound neurological impairment such that they lack signs of thought, sensation, purposeful behavior, and awareness of self and environment.
- Ensuring access to appropriate supportive and/or hospice care is an integral part of the care following a decision to withdraw dialysis.

Medical Management without Dialysis*

Medical management without dialysis* is planned holistic patient-centered care for patients with G5 CKD that includes the following:

- Interventions to delay progression of kidney disease and minimize risk of adverse events or complications
- Shared decision making
- Active symptom management
- Detailed communication including advance care planning
- Psychological support
- Social and family support
- Cultural and spiritual domains of care
- Comprehensive conservative care does not include dialysis

*KDIGO uses the term "Conservative Care" or "Comprehensive Conservative Care." We substitute the term medical management without dialysis because patients advising the Pathways project preferred this term.

elements of supportive kidney care that should be broadly available.[1] (See call out box.) In 2018, the International Society of Nephrology's Second Global Kidney Health Summit recommended the integration of supportive care as a necessary component of comprehensive kidney care.[2]

Momentum Builds in the United States

The scope and evidence for palliative care across all populations and diseases in the United States has been well articulated in the Clinical Practice Guidelines for Quality Palliative Care,[3] a series of Institute of Medicine reports[4,5] and National Institutes of Health,[6] and Agency for Health Care Research and Quality evidence reviews.[7] Applying those broad findings to the specific needs of patients with kidney disease began in earnest in the United States with the publication in 2000 of the clinical practice guideline *Shared Decision-Making in the Appropriate Initiation of and Withdrawal from Dialysis* by the American Society of Nephrology and the Renal Physicians Association.[8] This guideline and its 2010 revision have explicit palliative care recommendations for patients for whom dialysis was to be withheld or withdrawn. In 2003 as part of the Robert Wood Johnson Foundation's national program, Promoting Excellence in End-of-Life Care, the End-Stage Renal Disease[i] Peer Work Group was established and released a report, *Completing the Continuum of Nephrology Care: Recommendations to the Field*, which noted among other things that lack of knowledge about palliative care is a key barrier to change in the dialysis community and that the culture of "death denial" in dialysis units needs to be addressed.[9]

In 2004 the Kidney End-of-Life Care Coalition (now the Coalition for Supportive Care of Kidney Patients) held its first national conference. There has been gradual uptake of interest in the topic since then, but the signs have been even more promising recently. In 2017 the Gordon and Betty Moore Foundation funded the Coalition for Supportive Care of Kidney Patients to plan and implement a kidney supportive care intervention for advanced chronic kidney disease (CKD) and ESKD patients, called the Pathways Project. In 2017 the American Academy of Hospice and Palliative Medicine launched a Kidney Forum for palliative care clinicians interested in the care of kidney patients. However, while interest in the topic is growing, implementation of supportive care practices in the United States lags behind that in other developed countries.

Definition of Supportive Care

Most definitions of supportive care echo the World Health Organization definition of palliative care, as shown in Box 1.1. The KDIGO Controversies Conference on Supportive Care in CKD defined supportive care as:

> Services that are aimed at **improving the health related QOL** for patients with established CKD, at any age, and can be **provided together with therapies intended**

---

i. Where the title of the organization or article explicitly uses ESRD, the name will be preserved. This book will use the more modern term *end-stage kidney disease* (ESKD) otherwise.

BOX 1.1. Definitions of Key Terms

Palliative care
— Defined by the World Health Organization as an approach that improves the health-related quality of life (HRQoL) of patients and their families facing problems associated with life-threatening illness through the prevention and relief of suffering by means of early identification and impeccable assessment and treatment of pain and other physical, psychosocial, and spiritual problems.[14]
— Encompasses both "specialty palliative care" provided by specialists trained and certified in palliative care and "generalist palliative care" provided by the nephrology team and primary care providers.

Supportive care
— Involves services aimed at improving the health-related quality of life of patients with established chronic kidney disease.
— Applies the principles of palliative care throughout the continuum of care for chronic kidney disease and end-stage kidney disease, regardless of setting.
— Usually refers to "generalist palliative care" provided by the nephrology team, who may then consult or refer to specialty palliative care teams as needed.

Medical management without dialysis
— Also known as "comprehensive conservative care"
— Delivered as alternative to dialysis where nondialytic care is either chosen or medically advised
— Is planned, holistic, person-centered care that includes the following:
  Interventions to delay progression of kidney disease and minimize risk of adverse events or complications
  Shared decision-making
  Active symptom management
  Detailed communication including advance care planning
  Psychological support
  Social and family support
  Cultural and spiritual domains of care

Hospice
— Hospice/terminal care focuses on end-of-life needs and is typically limited to patients who are expected to be within months of death. Most hospice care is provided in the patient's place of residence, either the home or a nursing home.
— Inpatient hospice care in a hospital or freestanding hospice house is used by a minority of hospice patients

Adapted from Harris DCH, Davies SJ, Finkelstein FO, et al. Increasing access to integrated ESKD care as part of universal health coverage. *Kidney Int.* 2019;95(4):S1–S33.

to prolong life, such as dialysis. Supportive care helps patients cope with living, as well as dying, regardless of life expectancy.[1]

Supportive care is often used as a synonym for *palliative care*. In this book, we use the term *supportive care* because patients and healthcare professionals prefer it.[1,10] At times, we also distinguish supportive care from palliative care. *Supportive care* generally refers to the care that the nephrology team provides, while *palliative care* refers to the care provided by specialists in palliative care. Supportive care (also called *generalist palliative care* or *primary palliative care*) encompasses skills that all clinicians should have: management of uncomplicated pain and symptoms including anxiety and depression and essential discussions about prognosis, goals of treatment, code status, quality of life, and suffering. *Primary supportive care* is delivered to patients with kidney disease by both primary care providers and the kidney care team, who usually is in closest and most frequent contact with patients. *Specialist palliative care* refers to the specialist role of physicians with board certification in hospice and palliative medicine, and to other clinicians with specialist-level expertise and/or certification in palliative care, usually working as part of interdisciplinary teams specializing in palliative care.

In *Dying in America*, the IOM proposed the following definitions for specialty and primary palliative care:[5]

Specialty palliative care: Palliative care that is delivered by healthcare professionals who are palliative care specialists, such as physicians who are board certified in this specialty, palliative-certified nurses, and palliative care–certified social workers, pharmacists, and chaplains.

Primary palliative care (also known as generalist palliative care): Palliative care that is delivered by healthcare professionals who are not palliative care specialists, such as primary care clinicians; physicians who are disease-oriented specialists (such as oncologists and cardiologists); and nurses, social workers, pharmacists, chaplains, and others who care for this population but are not certified in palliative care.[3]

Ideally, specialty palliative care should be available to help with managing more complex and difficult cases. In this ideal coordinated care model, the primary care physician or nephrologist manages many (if not most) palliative care problems, initiating a palliative care consultation for more complex or refractory problems including difficult goals of care conversations[11] (Figure 1.2). However, primary supportive care skills have not yet been incorporated into most nephrology training programs, leaving most experienced and new nephrologists without the expertise to manage these needs.[12] Chapter 7 further describes the collaboration between the specialty level of palliative care and the nephrologist providing a generalist level of supportive care.

Hospice/terminal care falls under the larger umbrella of specialty palliative care but focuses on end-of-life needs and is typically limited to patients who are expected to be within six months of death (Figure 1.2).[1]

Supportive care for patients with kidney disease and medical management without dialysis are sometimes conflated, but it is worth noting the distinction between the two. Supportive care is both the philosophy and the services that are provided throughout the entire continuum of kidney care to improve health-related quality of life and make care more

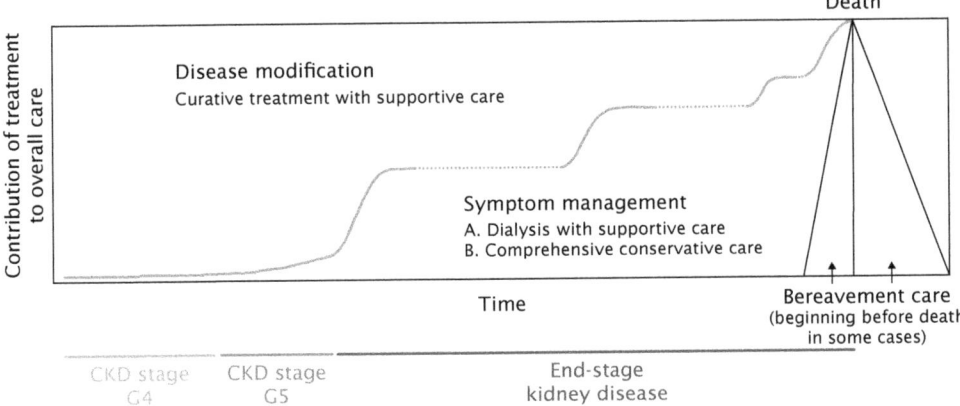

FIGURE 1.2. Overview of the contribution of kidney supportive care to overall care in end-stage kidney disease. Dashed gray lines represent a period of stability, which may be short or long. Supportive care should be offered at each stage of the disease, including information, education, relief of pain and associated symptoms, nutritional support, and psycho-social and spiritual care. Source: Used with permission. © Kidney International, Harris 2019.

Abbreviation: CKD, chronic kidney disease.

patient-centered. In contrast, medical management without dialysis is a specific management approach or pathway for patients with advanced kidney disease choosing not to undergo dialysis. To fully implement the patient-centered aspect of supportive care, the medical management without dialysis pathway needs to be available as a viable choice for patients. As described in chapter 14, this approach includes active management of symptoms, managing and trying to forestall the progression and metabolic complications of CKD, and proactive planning for end of life; it is far more comprehensive than simply "not starting dialysis."

Components of Supportive Care for Patients With Kidney Disease

The 2013 KDIGO Controversies Conference on Supportive Care in CKD urged making supportive care available to patients with kidney disease based on need, not prognosis, at any stage of kidney disease.[13] To do this, the KDIGO conferees recommended actions to enhance:

- symptom management
- provision of prognostic information
- shared decision-making and advance care planning
- withdrawal from dialysis
- provision of medical management without dialysis.[ii]

Building on the components outlined by KDIGO, the Pathways Project of the Coalition for Supportive Care of Kidney patients developed a change package of 14 best practice

---

ii. Based on input from patients and experts, the authors of this volume use the term *medical management without dialysis* rather than *comprehensive conservative care,* which is the term KDIGO used.

recommendations to implement supportive care for patients with kidney disease (http://go.gwu.edu/pathwaysprojectchangepackage).[15]

This change package was created through a focused literature review and collaboration with a Technical Expert Panel (TEP) composed of a physician, nurse practitioner, nurse, social worker, chaplain, and large dialysis organization administrator members in the fields of nephrology and palliative care. Two patient representatives also participated in the TEP. The best practice recommendations provide the framework for this book, with chapters organized to help practitioners understand the evidence base and then apply it to their practice.

Putting This Book to Use

The purpose of this book is to enhance the palliative care knowledge and skills of clinicians caring for patients with kidney disease and to improve the delivery of high-value quality supportive care to them. The book is written by experts in supportive care, and their disciplines and expertise include nephrology, palliative medicine, geriatrics, nephrology nursing, nephrology social work, psychonephrology, public health, implementation science, and health policy. Each chapter is written by authors with special expertise in the subject with the goal of providing practical, immediately useful primary palliative care knowledge and skills to those caring for patients with kidney disease.

Chapter formats include a case to illustrate the application of the knowledge and skills, a summary, practice pointers, and practice improvement opportunities. The expectation is that those who integrate the primary palliative care content in this book into their practices will be leaders in transforming the care of patients with CKD and ESKD from a disease-oriented approach to one that is truly patient centered. The patient and family experience and satisfaction with care should skyrocket as patients receive treatment that is respectful of and responsive to their values, preferences, and goals.

References

1. Davison SN, Levin A, Moss AH, et al. Executive summary of the KDIGO Controversies Conference on Supportive Care in Chronic Kidney Disease: developing a roadmap to improving quality care. *Kidney Int*. 2015;88(3):446–459. doi:10.1038/ki.2015.110
2. Harris DCH, Davies SJ, Finkelstein FO, et al. Increasing access to integrated ESKD care as part of universal health coverage. *Kidney Int*. 2019;95(4):S1–S33. doi:10.1016/j.kint.2018.12.005
3. National Consensus Project for Quality Palliative Care. *Clinical Practice Guidelines for Quality Palliative Care*. 4th ed. Richmond, VA: National Coalition for Hospice and Palliative Care; 2018. https://www.nationalcoalitionhpc.org/ncp. Accessed April 9, 2020.
4. Field M, Cassel C. *Approaching Death: Improving Care at the End of Life*. (Committee on Care at the End of Life, Institute of Medicine, eds.). Washington, DC: National Academy of Sciences; 1997.
5. Institute of Medicine. *Dying in America: Improving Quality and Honoring Individual Preferences Near the End of Life*. Washington, DC: National Academies Press; 2014.
6. National Institute for Health NI for NR. *Building Momentum: The Science of End-of-Life and Palliative Care. A Review of Research Trends and Funding, 1997–2010*. Bethesda, MD: NIH; 2013.
7. Dy S, Aslakson R, Wilson R. Improving health care and palliative care for advanced and serious illness: Closing the quality gap. *Evid Rep Technol Assess (Full Rep)*. 2012;208(8):1–249.
8. Fine A, Fontaine B, Kraushar MM, Rich BR. Nephrologists should voluntarily divulge survival data to potential dialysis patients: a questionnaire study. *Perit Dial Int J Int Soc Perit Dial*. 2005;25(3):269–273.

9. Moss, AH; End Stage Renal Disease Workgroup Promoting Excellence in End-of-Life Care. End-stage renal disease workgroup final report summary: recommendations to the field. Report. 2002:1–7.2011. https://www.promotingexcellence.org/downloads/esrd_report_summary.pdf. Accessed April 9, 2020.
10. Public Opinion Research on Palliative Care: A Report Based on Research by Public Opinion Strategies; https://media.capc.org/filer_public/18/ab/18ab708c-f835-4380-921d-fbf729702e36/2011-public-opinion-research-on-palliative-care.pdf Published 2011. Accessed April 9, 2020.
11. Quill T, Abernethy AP. Generalist plus specialist palliative care—creating a more sustainable model. *N Engl J Med*. 2013;368(13):1173–1175. doi:10.1056/NEJMp1302093
12. Combs SA, Culp S, Matlock DD, Kutner JS, Holley JL, Moss AH. Update on end-of-life care training during nephrology fellowship: a cross-sectional national survey of fellows. *Am J Kidney Dis*. 2014;65(2):233–239. doi:10.1053/j.ajkd.2014.07.018
13. KDIGO concludes landmark controversies conference on supportive care—KDIGO. http://kdigo.org/kdigo-concludes-landmark-controversies-conference-on-supportive-care/. Published 2013. Accessed November 29, 2017.
14. World Health Organization. Palliative care. http://www.who.int/cancer/palliative/en/. Accessed December 24, 2015.
15. Coalition for Supportive Care of Kidney Patients. Pathways Project Change Package. http://go.gwu.edu/pathwaysprojectchangepackage. Accessed April 22, 2020.

SECTION I

Why We Need This Book—Unmet Supportive Care Needs of Patients With Kidney Disease

2

Birth of a Benefit—Brief History of the ESRD Program

Nancy C. Armistead and Jeffrey A. Perlmutter

The story of the end-stage renal disease (ESRD) entitlement program is told through progressive scientific and technological advances, selection committees, and exploration of public policy values. The legislative history shows a program thought to accommodate a limited number of patients who, returning to work, would contribute to the social security program paying for their benefits. The reality has been different. Treatment is offered to virtually all patients with ESRD, often with little regard to the individual's likelihood of benefit from dialysis and quality of life. The program's next chapter will tell whether patient-centered care becomes a focal point in the program's history.

In 1962 *Life* magazine was delivered weekly to millions of American homes. Known for iconic photographs and timely stories, it appealed to both the greatest generation and their upcoming baby boomers. The cover of the November 9 issue was entitled "Dealing with the Deadly Crisis. The US and Its People Withstand the Nuclear Threat." But the real bombshell wasn't the cover story, but Shana Alexander's inside article titled "They Decide Who Lives, Who Dies."[1]

This article displays a 2-page black-and-white photograph of 5 men and 1 woman around a table in what might be a medical library. Their faces are not revealed, but their hands are crossed as if in prayer. And indeed, divine guidance is needed, for their task is to determine who among the many with kidney failure should be offered the life-extending technology known as dialysis, a treatment being offered at Seattle's new Artificial Kidney Center.

The anonymous group consisted of a lawyer, minister, banker, housewife, official from state government, labor leader, and a surgeon. Provided with some guidance from the Center's nephrologists, the committee was not asked to make medical decisions as patient suitability was prescreened. The criteria that they used in their deliberations were patient age and sex, marital status and number of dependents, income, net worth, emotional stability, education, occupation, past performance and future potential, and the names of individuals who could serve as references.[1]

The medical technology that brought Seattle to this point was built on years of research and experimentation. The medical history of dialysis dates back to the 1820s when Rene Joachim Henri Dutrochet first described osmosis, the diffusion of fluids through membranes or porous partitions. It was Scottish chemist Thomas Graham who defined this as "the conversion of chemical affinity into mechanical power."[2] As early as 1913, members of a research team from Johns Hopkins (John Jacob Abel, Leonard Rowntree, J. J. Turner) were experimenting with a process of purifying blood which they called vividiffusion. In 1924, George Hass, a German scientist, performed dialysis on the first human. Using a tubular devise made of collodion immersed in dialysate solution in a glass cylinder, he showed that some uremic substances in the dialysate and water could be removed from the blood.[3]

However, it was Willem Kolff who laid the foundation that made hemodialysis a practical application. Kolff, from the Netherlands, developed an interest in an artificial kidney in the 1940s. Working in Nazi-occupied Netherlands, he learned the properties of cellophane and how it could be applied to his research. Cellophane was an ideal substance as it was permeable to small molecular weight metabolites such as urea and creatinine, but relatively impermeable to proteins and intermediate size molecules such as peptides.[3]

In a memorial to Kolff, Denton Cooley states that Kolff invented the first artificial kidney "using orange-juice cans, used auto parts, and sausage casings."[4] Kolff's machine consisted of a varnished wood drum with its lower portion rotating in an enamel tub. The "rinsing solution" was in this tub, which was wrapped in cellophane in a special pattern. When blood was put into the cellophane, it moved to the lowest level so as the drum turned, gravity would force the blood from one of the wet cellophane sheets to the other. A rotating coupling, obtained from a Ford automobile dealer, allowed the cellophane to be inserted in a hollow axle and remain stationary as the drum turned. Initially using this machine on patients resulted in 16 deaths, but Kolff was able to keep the 17th patient alive.[3]

This patient was Sophia Schafstat, a Nazi collaborator. While the irony of this was not lost on Kolff, who not only supported the Dutch resistance but had helped save upwards of 800 people from the Nazi concentration camps, he successfully treated her acute kidney disease and she lived for another 7 years.[5]

While Kolff "perfected" the dialysis machine, it was Belding Scribner who made the application viable for patients by resolving the complex limiting issue of repeated blood access. Christopher Blagg notes that Scribner "transformed clinical nephrology with what came to be called the Scribner shunt." Prior to this, it was necessary to "fresh cut down an artery and vein for each treatment."[6] Over a brief period of time, a patient would run out of potential blood access sites. Scribner and his team developed the concept of connecting the arterial and venous cannulas by a short shunt thereby preserving the blood access. Working with Wayne Quinton, a bioengineer from the University of Washington, and using the inert polymer polytetrafluoroethylene (PTFE) called "Teflon," they created the "Scribner shunt."

Their findings were presented in the 1960 edition of *Transactions of the American Society of Artificial Internal Organs*. This article reads like a do-it-yourself guide to cannulation of long-term dialysis, complete with graphics and specifics such as "Teflon pulls best when it is heated gently until it turns slightly opaque or white. If it turns clear, it has heated too much." Or "a special fixture has been developed to cut the Teflon tubing square on the ends. The fixture consists of a pair of pliers with holes drilled in the ends which are slightly smaller than the tubing."[7]

The pieces were starting to fall into place for the ESRD program as it exists today (Table 2.1). The technology was available to care for patients, the ability to continuously

TABLE 2.1. Timeline of Key Events in Development of End-Stage Kidney Disease Care System in the United States

Date	Event/Publication
1960	Scribner shunt
1962	Shana Alexander's *Life* article
1972	Public Law 92-603, establishing ESRD entitlement
1976	Final program regulations issued
1981	NIDDK National Cooperative Dialysis Study
1993	USRDS Dialysis Morbidity Study
1997	NKF Kidney Dialysis Outcomes Quality Initiative
2000	RPA/ASN Shared Decision-Making Guideline
2010	RPA Revision to Shared Decision-Making Guideline
2012	ESRD Quality Incentive Program

Abbreviations: ASN, American Society of Nephrology. American Society of Nephrology. ESRD, end-stage renal disease. NIDDK, Institute of Diabetes and Digestive and Kidney Disease. NKF, National Kidney Foundation. RPA, Renal Physicians Association. USRDS, US Renal Disease Service.

access blood vessels was in place, and awareness was increasing, not only among the general public, but within the medical community. For example, between 1941 and 1950, PubMed references 94 English articles on the search term "uremia." By 1971 to 1980, this had increased to 3,423. What was missing was the ability to pay for this expensive treatment that was estimated to cost between $15,000 and $20,000 annually per patient. At the time, the US census reports the median family income at $11,120.

After his election in 1964, President Lyndon Johnson confirmed through his 1965 State of the Union address his agenda for hospital insurance for the aged, a Social Security benefit increase, and improvements in medical assistance. Johnson's 3-part proposal was introduced in January, and by July reconciliation was complete. The Medicare program to provide healthcare for individuals 65 and over became law in July 1965. The legislation originally proposed to extend Medicare coverage to the disabled, but this provision was removed before its passage. The debate focused, in part, on whether to have a National Health Insurance Partnership as favored later by Republican President Richard Nixon and Democratic Senator Ted Kennedy. However, these provisions failed to make it into the original legislation.

In 1967, the US Bureau of the Budget sponsored a committee chaired by Carl Gottschalk who recommended government support for kidney dialysis and transplantation. There is debate on whether this report was influential in Congress, but it was distributed among the medical community and provided endorsement for the treatment modalities as established therapies.

Congressional champions of this included Henry "Scoop" Jackson, a Democratic senator from Washington State whose support was motivated by a childhood friendship with a dialysis patient. Russell Long, senator from Louisiana and chair of the powerful Senate Finance Committee had a long-standing interest in insuring people, especially working individuals, from the costs of catastrophic health problems.[8]

Nephrology champions of the program were many, but one notable individual who spearheaded legislative efforts was George Schreiner, chief of nephrology at Washington, DC, Georgetown University. Schreiner helped found the American Society of Internal Artificial Organs and later the American Society of Nephrology. Partnering with Charles Plante, a Washington lobbyist for the National Kidney Foundation (NKF), they began a course of lobbying and saw the introduction of numerous, albeit, unsuccessful bills in Congress between 1965 and 1970. It was Vance Hartke, an Indiana senator, who would add a last-minute amendment to the 1972 Social Security Act that extended Medicare to individuals with end-stage kidney disease who required dialysis or transplantation to sustain life.

Richard Rettig, a historian of the ESRD program, has written a comprehensive examination of the origins of the Medicare program. He cites this compelling excerpt from the US Congress Finance Committee by Hartke:

> In what must be the most tragic irony of the twentieth century, people are dying because they cannot get access to proper medical care. More than 8,000 Americans will die this year from kidney disease who could have been saved if they had been able to afford an artificial kidney machine or transplantation. These will be needless deaths—deaths which should shock our conscience and shame our sensibilities. We have the opportunity now to begin a national program of kidney disease treatment assistance administered through the Social Security Administration, and I propose that we take that opportunity so that more lives are not lost needlessly.[8]

Hartke estimated, from figures supplied by the NKF, that up to 25,000 patients would benefit from dialysis and that the first-year cost would be about $75 million. The Senate backed Hartke's amendment by a vote of 52 to 3, and the provision was adopted.[8]

The tipping point that assured passage of the amendment providing coverage for end-stage kidney disease care in the Social Security Act was the appearance of Shep Glazer at the House Ways and Means Committee hearing on November 4, 1971. According to Rettig, "the most dramatic moment of the hearing, however, came when Glazer briefly dialyzed before the Committee. This event was widely publicized afterwards and was believed by many to have been decisive in the decision of Congress to enact the kidney disease entitlement."[8]

Glazer, a patient representing the National Association of Patients on Hemodialysis, testified before the House Committee:

> I am 43 years old, married for 20 years, with two children age 14 and 10. I was a salesman until a couple of months ago until it became necessary for me to supplement my income to pay for the dialysis supplies. I tried to sell a non-competitive line, was found out, and was fired. Gentlemen, what should I do? End it all and die? Sell my house for which I worked so hard, and go on welfare? Should I go into the hospital under my hospitalization policy, then I cannot work? Please tell me. If your kidneys failed tomorrow, wouldn't you want the opportunity to live? Wouldn't you want to see your children grow up?

Public Law 92-603 (Social Security Amendments of 1972), effective October 30, 1972, was legislation that was 165 pages long. Section 299I, the small portion of the law establishing the ESRD entitlement, took up less than 1 page.

After the passage of legislation, the hard work of promulgating regulations and program implementation began. The Medicare ESRD program became effective on July 1, 1973, and operated under interim regulations that provided for reimbursement to facilities that were furnishing care on or before June 1, 1973. In June 1976, final regulations were issued for the implementation of coverage of suppliers of end-stage kidney disease services as well as the designation of 32 network organizations (consolidated over the years to the current 18).[9]

Throughout the late 1970s and early 1980s, a consistent string of regulatory requirements and clarifications were published in the Federal Register. While networks were designed to assure quality of care through their Medical Review Boards, in the early years they played a coordination role to assure the community was aware of proposed and final regulations and was alerted to submit community responses. Since networks were also collecting and analyzing data and had, through their membership, an understanding of utilization and operational aspects of the program they engaged in establishing the need for new services. This led to relationships with state organizations responsible for Certificate of Public Need.

As series of national studies impacted the ESRD networks' role in quality improvement. In 1981 the National Cooperative Dialysis Study supported by the National Institute of Arthritis, Metabolism, and Digestive Disease was the first randomized trial of hemodialysis adequacy in the practice of dialysis medicine and influenced the networks' quality improvement activities. Between 1993 and 1998, the United State Renal Disease Service (USRDS) funded by the National Institute of Health's National Institute of Diabetes and Digestive and Kidney Disease conducted the Dialysis Morbidity Study. This was an observational study collecting demographic, comorbidity, laboratory, treatment, socioeconomic, and insurance data on a large random sample of dialysis patients. In 1997 the NKF supported by Amgen, led the Kidney Disease Outcomes Initiative and developed evidence-based clinical practice guidelines on a variety of topics including anemia, bone metabolism, diabetes, glomerulonephritis, adequacy, and vascular access. Using these studies, networks eventually settled into a quality improvement role and lead initiatives to improve dialysis adequacy, anemia management, arteriovenous fistula usage, immunization rates, and recently reducing unnecessary hospitalizations and infection rates.

Before the Medicare entitlement, the number of reported dialysis patients alive in July 1970 was 2,874. These patients were supported in centers such as the one described in Seattle, through programs funded by state Regional Medical Programs, Public Health Service program, and the Veterans Administration. By September 1977, there were approximately 39,000 Medicare beneficiaries receiving care in 840 dialysis/transplant centers, and roughly $700 million was spent in that fiscal year. In a 1977 policy publication, it was noted that the program was estimated to cost between $1 to $1.7 billion annually.[10] As of December 2016, 511,270 patients were being treated in 7,140 dialysis centers, and 215,061 patients had functioning transplants with an annual expenditure exceeding $35.4 billion. In 1982, 60% of dialysis patient received treatment in free-standing nonprofit centers (11%) or hospital-based centers (49%). The remaining 40% were treated in free-standing for-profit dialysis centers.[11] This model changed over the years with 2 free-standing for-profit corporations, Fresenius

Medical Services and DaVita, treating 69% of patients in 2014.[12] As an indication of the program's significance, it is noted that the 2016 Medicare fee for services spending accounts for 7.2% of the overall Medicare claims for a population that represents 1.2% of Medicare beneficiaries.[13] Figure 2.1 shows program growth from 1982 to 2012.

In 1993, John Iglehart wrote a series in the *New England Journal of Medicine* on the American healthcare system. No discussion of the system is complete without an examination of the nation's first national healthcare program—the ESRD program. While explaining the financial implications of the program Inglehart states "physicians are also using dialysis to treat an increasing number of older, sicker patients whose life expectancy is short and whose quality of life is relatively poor. This trend has increased program expenditures and the number of beneficiaries served and has sharpened the debate about the ethics of patient selection."[14] The proportion of patients greater than 65 years of age had increased from 5% in 1973 to 40.7% in 2016.[11]

The ESRD program is an excellent case study for bioethics as it addresses the ethical questions that arise in the relationship between life sciences, biotechnology, medicine, politics, laws, and philosophy. While the ESRD program has extended the lives and provided quality of life to untold numbers of individuals and families, the fact remains that many have come to expect dialysis as a "right" because there is a federal program designed specifically to pay for services and to which they have contributed through their Social Security taxes. In 1991, the Institute of Medicine Committee for the Study of the Medicare ESRD Program noted:

> Physicians should recognize that the existence of a public entitlement does not mean that they are obligated to treat all patients who present with kidney failure. Clinical judgement and patient-family preferences will sometimes indicate terminal palliative care rather than life- extending care. Thus, the choice is not between treatment and abandonment, but rather between different goals of treatment.[15]

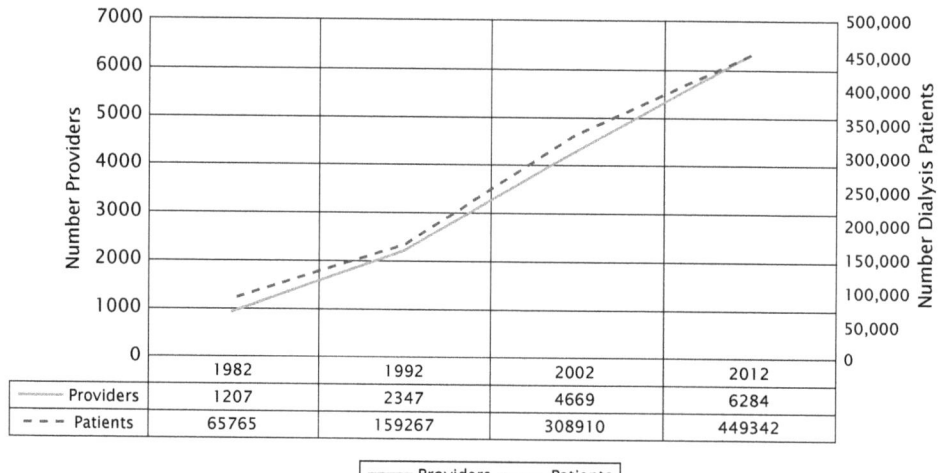

FIGURE 2.1. Dialysis providers and patients, 1982–2012. Source: USRDS Annual Reports 2004–2014.

In 2000, the Renal Physicians Association and the American Society of Nephrology oversaw the development of *Clinical Practice Guideline on Shared Decision-Making in the Appropriate Initiation of and Withdrawal from Dialysis*. This document addressed for the first time recommendations concerning withholding or withdrawing dialysis in adult patients. The Renal Physicians Association revised this document in 2010 with new recommendations and a toolkit for shared decision-making.

In many respects the ESRD program has traveled from one end of the spectrum to the other since Shana Alexander's article in 1962, from limiting the number of patients who receive dialysis to providing treatment to all patients who have renal failure and choose dialysis or transplantation with little discussion as to treatment modality or quality of life. Medicine has traditionally taken a disease-oriented approach to care, focusing on outcomes important to practitioners and supported by evidence-based medicine. Patient-centered care requires a re-examination of the practitioner–patient relationship with a focus on what is important to the individual patient. Patients, rather than disease processes, and shared, rather than paternalistic, approaches to decision-making are the tenants of patient-centered care.[16] The Medicare program has fully embraced patient-centeredness as evidenced by the ESRD Quality Incentive Program. This first-of-its-kind program links reimbursement directly to the facilities' performance on quality improvement measures, one of which is patient experience of care.

The program is moving toward more patient-centered care—that which is respectful of and responsive to individual patient preferences, needs, and values and consideration to the patient's quality of life. To this end, the national Coalition of Supportive Care of Kidney Patients is leading the effort to help nephrology healthcare providers understand and implement primary palliative care skills in their practices and assist patients with kidney disease and families make informed decisions about treatment options in accordance with their values, preferences and goals. The next chapter in the history of this important and impactful program will tell the extent to which care for patients with kidney disease successfully made this transition.

References

1. Alexander S. They decide who lives, who dies. *Life*. Nov 9 1962:102–125.
2. Cameron S. Thomas Graham (1805–1869) the father of dialysis. In: Ing T, Rahman MA, Kjellstrand CM, eds. *Dialysis History, Development and Promises*. Hackensack, NJ: World Scientific; 2012:19–25.
3. Tracy Kathleen. *Unlocking the Secrets of Science: Willhem Kolff and the Invention of the Dialysis Machine*. Bear, DE: Mitchell Lane; 2003.
4. Cooley DA. In Memoriam Willem Johan Kolff. *Tex Heart Inst J*. 2009;36(2):83–84.
5. Davison P. Dutchman who turned Nazi debris into a dialysis machine. *Financial Times*. https://www.ft.com/content/023560b4-ff84-11dd-b3f8-000077b07658. Published 2009. Accessed January 8, 2019.
6. Blagg C. Belding Scribner-better known as Scrib. *J Am Soc Nephrol*. 2010; 5:2146–2149.
7. Quinton W, Dillard D, Scribner BH. Cannulation of blood vessels for prolonged hemodialysis. *Trans Am Soc Artif Intern Organs*. 1960;6:104–113.
8. Rettig R. Origins of the Medicare kidney disease entitlement: the social security amendments of 1972. In: Institute of Medicine. *Biomedical Politics*. Washington, DC: The National Academies Press; 1991:176–214.

9. Department of Health, Education, and Welfare, Social Security Administration. Renal disease implementation of coverage of suppliers of end stage services. *Federal Register*. Jun 3 1976:22502–22522.
10. Baydin LD. The end-stage renal disease networks: an attempt through federal regulation to regionalize health care delivery. *Med Care*. 1977;15(7):586–98.
11. United States Renal Data System. *1994 USRDS Annual Data Report: Epidemiology of Kidney Disease in the United States*. Bethesda, MD, National Institutes of Health, National Institute of Diabetes and Digestive and Kidney Diseases 1994.
12. United States Renal Data System. *2016 USRDS Annual Data Report: Epidemiology of Kidney Disease in the United States*. Bethesda, MD, National Institutes of Health, National Institute of Diabetes and Digestive and Kidney Diseases 2016.
13. United States Renal Data System. *2018 USRDS Annual Data Report: Epidemiology of Kidney Disease in the United States*. Bethesda, MD, National Institutes of Health, National Institute of Diabetes and Digestive and Kidney Diseases 2018.
14. Inglehart J. The American healthcare system—the end stage renal disease program. *NEJM*. 1993;328:366–371.
15. Rettig RA, Levinsky NG ed. *Summary Kidney Failure and the Federal Government*. Washington DC: National Academy Press; 1991.
16. O'Hare A, Armistead N, Schrag W, Diamond L, Moss A. Patient centered care: an opportunity to accomplish the "three aims" of the national quality strategy in the Medicare ESRD program. *Clin J Am Nephrol*. 2014;9:2189–2194.

Unmet Palliative Care Needs of Patients With Kidney Disease and Consequences

Kate Schueller and Dale E. Lupu

This chapter enumerates the evidence for unmet supportive care needs at numerous points along the continuum of kidney care. Gaps in the following areas are described: shared decision-making, advance care planning, symptom management, specialty palliative care consultation, kidney supportive dialysis, medical management without dialysis, end-of-life planning, end-of-life care, and hospice care. Providers can use the Kidney Supportive Care Implementation Quotient survey with their own staff as an initial step to assess gaps in supportive care in their own practice. Understanding the scope of these gaps is key to building a kidney care system that is more patient centered and better meets the supportive care needs of seriously ill patients.

Case

Mr. P was a 76-year-old living at home with his wife, independent in his activities of daily living and enjoying getting together with his friends for a breakfast roll and coffee each day at the local café. He was looking forward to golfing again in the spring, although he noted it was getting more challenging physically. He had been followed as an outpatient for the past few years by both nephrology and cardiology with history of cardiomyopathy with implantable cardioverter–defibrillator, diabetes mellitus, and chronic kidney disease (CKD) stage 4. In that time, dialysis was brought up by both cardiology and nephrology as it was clear cardiac and renal functioning were worsening. Cardiology note indicated he would be a poor candidate for dialysis given his diminished cardiac function. Nephrology recommended attending an education session on his dialysis options. Documentation in the record was unclear as to what, if any, prognostic information had been shared with the patient.

Mr. P attended the educational session on dialysis where peritoneal and hemodialysis were the only 2 options discussed. He had several questions about the impact of dialysis on his quality of life and was hoping to talk to his doctors about it. However, he was unable to get these answered before developing acute kidney injury due to dehydration from a viral gastroenteritis. A catheter was placed urgently, and he was started on in-center hemodialysis. The first month on hemodialysis was very difficult. It seemed like he spent most of his time on dialysis or feeling wiped out after the treatments. He recalls his primary care physicians mentioning he should complete a healthcare power of attorney document but never felt like he had enough energy to do it. He kept hoping life on dialysis would get easier but feared this may be as good as he'd feel. He struggled with the fluid and dietary restrictions, and his blood pressure became so low that they often had to pause his dialysis treatments, making the treatments even longer. His mood plummeted and fatigue worsened, and he was no longer able to meet up with his friends. In addition, he worried about the toll this was taking on his wife.

This ups and downs of dialysis continued for another month until one day while at home he developed fever, chills, and confusion. Mrs. P called emergency medical services, and he was transported to the hospital. He was admitted to the intensive care unit (ICU) for sepsis (likely due to his indwelling catheter) requiring vasopressors. He was started on IV antibiotics and eventually continuous veno-venous hemofiltration. Despite these efforts, he became more obtunded and was unable to protect his airway. His wife was asked about intubation, and she pleaded with the team to "save him." Despite the efforts of the ICU team, he died later that day when he had a cardiac arrest from asystole for which his implantable cardioverter–defibrillator did not shock him, and resuscitative measures were unsuccessful. His wife expressed disbelief, saying his death "came as a complete shock."

The Gap Between the Ideal State of Patient-Centered Care for Seriously Ill Patients With Kidney Disease and the Current State

The ideal care system for patients with kidney disease would be one that guides patients and their families to navigate the challenges of their situation to maximize quality of life according to their own values and preferences. It should offer a true array of customizable options, not one-size-fits-all care. As we see from the previous case, care often falls short of this ideal. The gaps in the case that could be addressed with better supportive kidney care include the following.

- Lack of shared decision-making: patient and wife were not given prognostic information, not helped to understand prognostic implications, and not given information about other treatment options (medical management without dialysis).
- Clinicians did not elicit patient goals: no documentation that the patient's ambivalence about dialysis was explored. No goals-of-care discussion held. No sense of what mattered most to patient given his worsening overall health (ie, how/where he wanted to spend his time, preferred place of death).
- Patient symptoms not managed well: difficulty coping, depressed mood, fatigue.
- No documentation of patient wishes for end of life: no healthcare power of attorney noted in chart, and no code discussion noted, so presumption was full code.
- No involvement or preparation of family: no sense that the family was involved in decisions, traumatic end-of-life experience for patient that likely did not align with his preferences, resulting in wife at higher risk for complicated grief.

Figure 3.1 shows these gaps, and others, in the current kidney care system in the United States that tends to compartmentalize care into silos based on setting and that rarely offers the choice of medical management without dialysis.

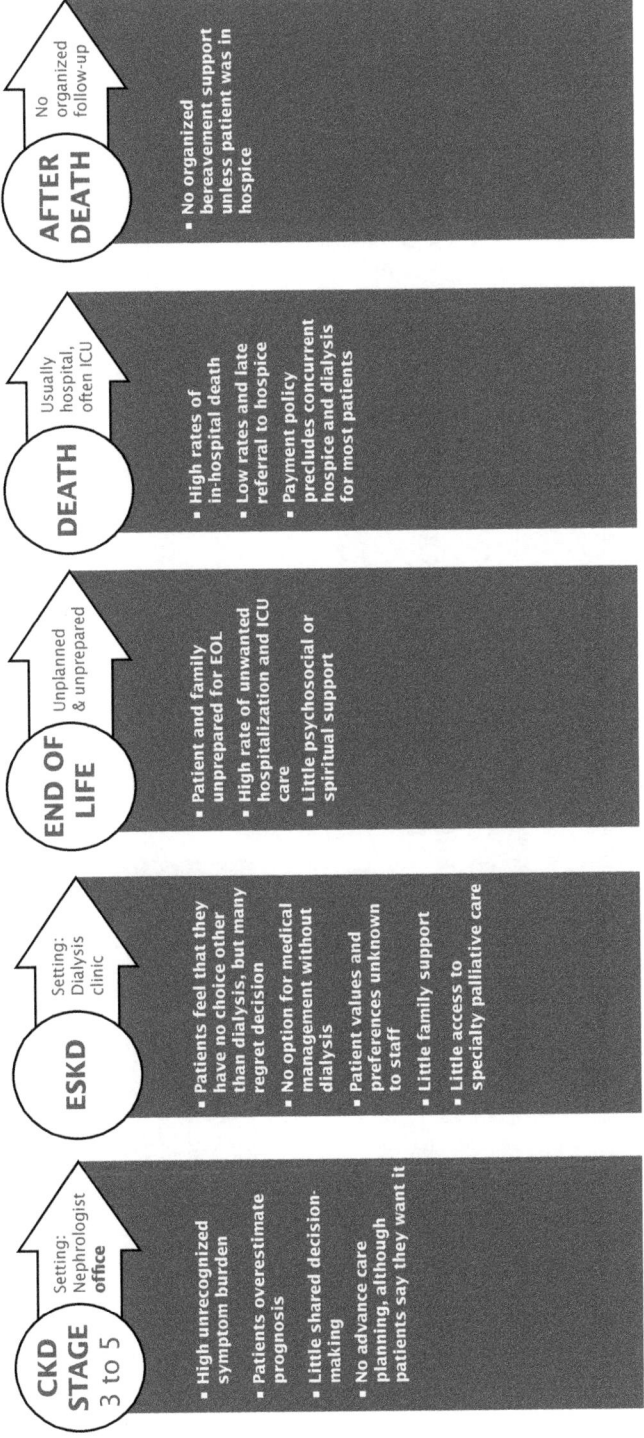

FIGURE 3.1. Problems with current typical pathway for frail, elderly patients with chronic kidney disease. Abbreviations: CKD, chronic kidney disease; EOL, end of life; ESKD, end-stage kidney disease; ICU, intensive care unit; QoL, quality of life.

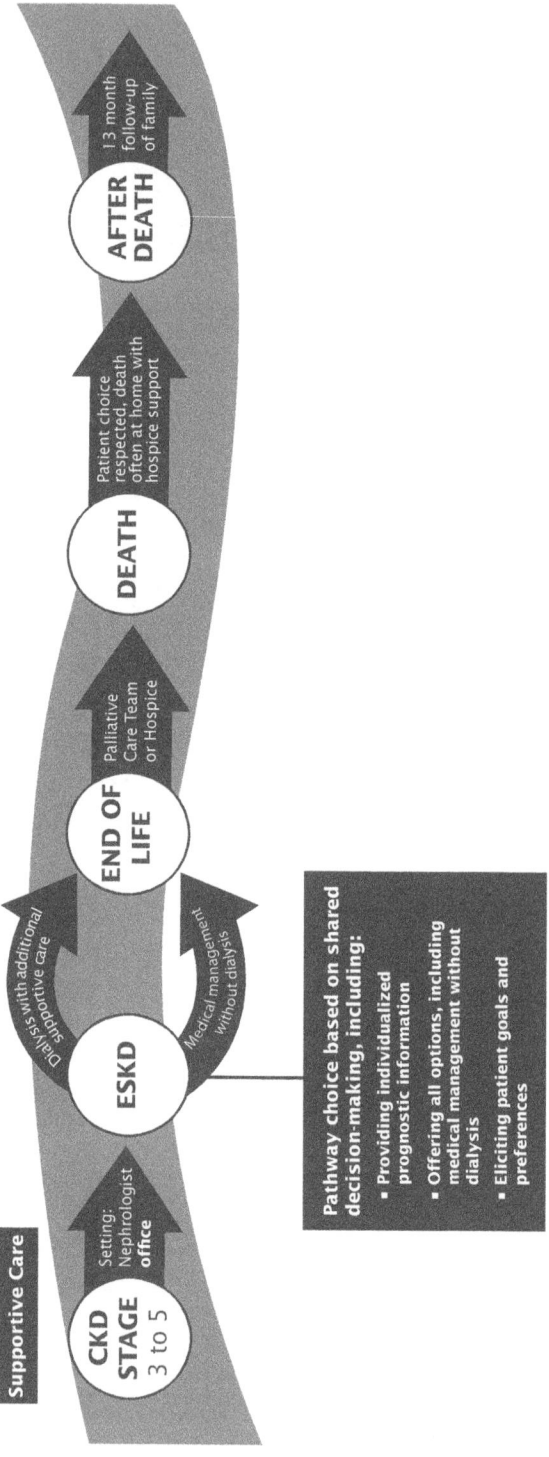

FIGURE 3.2. Improved chronic kidney disease pathway for frail, elderly patients: integration of supportive care practices and kidney supportive care pathway.

Supportive care is a delivery model that can help fill these gaps through a patient-centered approach to the treatment of people with kidney disease. Figure 3.2 shows the ideal care pathway for frail patients with serious kidney disease. The International Society of Nephrology's 2018 Global Kidney Health Summit called supportive care an "essential component of an integrated ESKD care program" and strongly recommended the inclusion of both supportive care and medical management without dialysis (which they termed "comprehensive conservative care").[1]

Supportive Kidney Care Gap in the United States—An Overview

The absence in the United States of supportive care for patients with kidney disease is a major deficit in US kidney care.[2,3] Of all patients with chronic disease, patients with end-stage kidney disease (ESKD) are arguably among the sickest, with a high symptom burden rivaling the symptom burden of patients with cancer[4] and with incident 5-year life expectancy half that of cancer patients.[5] Older patients, if also frail with multiple comorbid conditions, may not experience a survival benefit or even a quality-of-life benefit from dialysis.[6] Yet alternatives such as medical management without dialysis, which may align better with patient goals, are not widely available. Even when dialysis is desired by and beneficial for patients, appropriate symptom management, support to caregivers, and preparation for end of life is lacking.

Opportunities to improve supportive care exist at multiple points along the continuum of kidney care. We enumerate the evidence at each of these points in the care continuum, but it is helpful to remember that each is just one of the multiple, interrelated components needed to create a culture of person-centered care. Figure 3.3 illustrates the interrelated nature of these components, leading toward the goal of providing person-centered, goal-concordant care that supports quality of life. We can only deliver person-centered care when we know what the individual person values and prefers. We can only know that if we ask the person explicitly, instead of assuming we know what they want because of education level, age, or frailty level. If they can

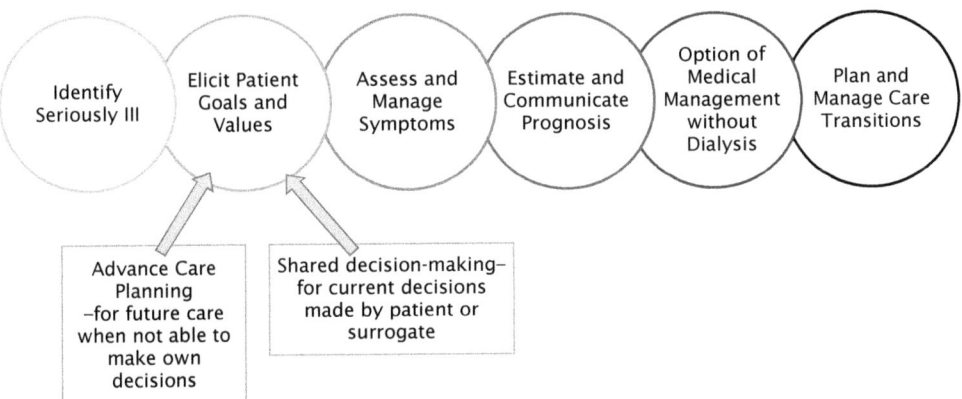

FIGURE 3.3. Supportive care elements. Adapted from KDIGO recommendations in Davison SN, Levin A, Moss AH, et al. Executive summary of the KDIGO Controversies Conference on Supportive Care in Chronic Kidney Disease: developing a roadmap to improving quality care. *Kidney Int.* 2015;88(3):446–459.

no longer speak for themselves, we can only provide person-centered care if the patient had the foresight to tell us who their surrogate decision maker should be and if that decision maker is prepared and understands the patient's wishes. It can only be person-centered when we share enough information (such as prognosis) with the person through shared decision-making, so that they are well informed. It can only be person-centered if we offer a full array of choices, such as medical management without dialysis, and help the patient and family understand the pros and cons of those choices according to their own preferences. Finally, it can only be person centered when we recognize that end of life is an especially vulnerable and precious time and that "the way the story ends" matters deeply to patients and their surviving family members.

Progress on providing patient-centered supportive kidney care has been made in other countries but has lagged in the United States. This chapter outlines the gaps in care that result in unnecessary suffering for patients and families, moral distress for providers, and inefficiency and higher costs for the system. We present evidence for shortcomings at each step in the kidney care continuum.

Unmet Needs for Supportive Kidney Care: The Specifics

Epidemiology of ESKD Population in the United States

At the end of 2016, there were 726,331 people living with ESKD in the United States; an increase of 86% since 2000. Of these, 124,675 were new incident cases, with patients older than 75 years the fastest growing segment of the dialysis population.[7] In 2016, 50,046 people died of kidney disease, more than died of breast or prostate cancer.[8] Mortality rates, although dropping impressively over the past 2 decades, are still much higher for older people with ESKD than for older people with cancer, congestive heart failure, or the general Medicare population

TABLE 3.1. Adjusted Mortality (Deaths per 1, 000 Patient Years) by age, Sex, Treatment Modality, and Comorbidity Among ESRD Patients and the General Medicare Population, 2015

Age (Yrs)	Dialysis	Transplant	All Medicare	Cancer	Diabetes	CHF	CVA/TIA	AMI
65–74								
Male	225	65	28	72	41	111	74	90
Female	211	54	18	65	30	97	58	100
75+								
Male	345	129	88	131	106	223	156	182
Female	316	111	81	131	99	221	184	187

Data source: Special analyses, USRDS ESRD Database and Medicare 5% sample. Adjusted for race. Medicare data limited to patients with at least 1 month of Medicare eligibility in 2015. Reference population: Medicare patients, 2015.
Source: United States Renal Data System. Incidence, prevalence, patient characteristics, and treatment modalities In USRDS Annual Data Report. Vol. 2, Chapter 5. United States Renal Data System; 2018:411–426. https://www.usrds.org/2018/view/v2_05.aspx.
Abbreviations: AMI, acute myocardial infarction; CHF, heart failure; CMS, Centers for Medicare & Medicaid Services; CVA/TIA, cerebrovascular accident/transient ischemic attack; ESRD, end-stage renal disease.

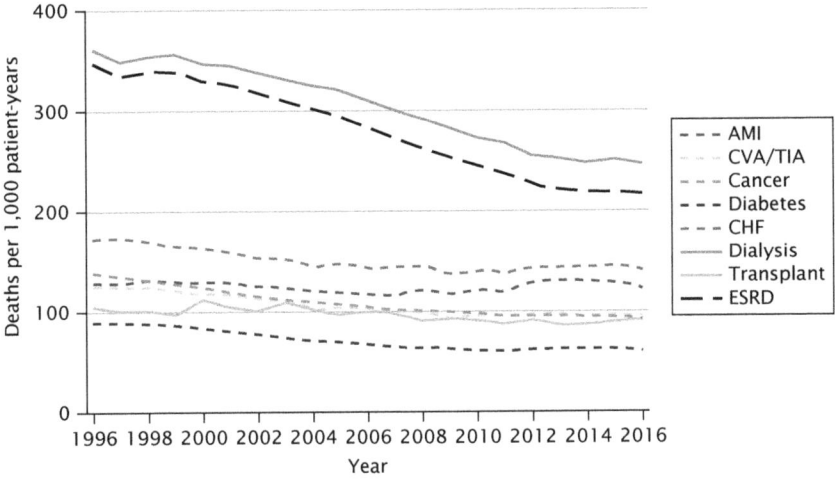

FIGURE 3.4. Supportive care elements.

(Tables 3.1; Figure 3.4). For patients with significant comorbidities, risk of death within a year of starting dialysis is stark. Of patients who had 4 or more comorbidities, 26% died within 30 days of dialysis initiation, 49% died within 180 days, and 60% died within a year.[9]

Lack of Shared Decision-Making

Shared decision-making is a necessary component to informed consent for patients with advanced CKD. The Renal Physician's Association recommended shared decision-making prior to the initiation of dialysis.[10] Despite Renal Physician's Association's recommendation, shared decision-making—the process in which patients and their families collaborate with healthcare providers to develop a care plan and make decisions about treatments based on patient preferences and values as well as the clinical risks and advantages[11,12]—is poorly integrated into the care of patients with kidney disease. Most nephrologists express lack of comfort in discussing end-of-life issues.[13] Consequently, most patients with CKD and those on dialysis have little awareness of their prognosis and may make treatment decisions based on unrealistic expectations.[14]

Furthermore, physicians do not routinely elicit patient goals and preferences, which is a fundamental first step in shared decision-making. In specialty care encounters, physicians did *not* elicit patient concerns 80% of the time.[15] Specifically in nephrology, 90% of patients said it was extremely or somewhat important to talk about their prognosis, but only 10% of patients recall having done so.[16]

Without such discussions, it is unlikely that the healthcare team will have a clear understanding of the patient's goals and preferences, as providers and patients often prioritize very different aspects of care. In a study of the health priorities of stage 4 and 5 CKD patients, providers' perceptions about patients' top health outcome priorities were incorrect 65% of the time.[17] Forty-nine percent of patients ranked maintaining independence as their top health priority, with only 35% ranking staying alive as their top priority. Other studies in CKD and ESKD find similar discordance about patient values for their care, making it essential that providers elicit, record, and honor as much as possible the preferences of patients.[18]

Lack of Advance Care Planning

Advance care planning is a process of communication that supports adults at any age or stage of health in understanding and sharing their personal values, life goals, and preferences regarding *future* medical care.[i] The goal of advance care planning is to help ensure that people experiencing serious and chronic illness receive medical care that is consistent with their values, goals, and preferences even when they become unable to make decisions for themselves. Few patients with CKD engage in advance care planning, and the vast majority lack a written advance directive or surrogate decision maker, leaving them unprepared to make medical decisions in a crisis.[20-23] Because the risk of cognitive decline is very high for patients on dialysis, many are unable to speak for themselves as their condition worsens. The lack of advance care planning plunges patients, families, and providers into avoidable crises that often lead families to choose aggressive and burdensome care that the patient may not have wanted.

Lack of Symptom Management

The symptom burden of patients on dialysis rivals that of patients with cancer.[4,24,25] Investigators have found that the symptoms of patients with CKD and ESKD are underrecognized, their severity is underestimated, and treatment is largely lacking.[26-29] Particularly severe and troubling symptoms include uremic pruritus (itching), sleep disturbances, restless legs syndrome, pain, and depression.[27] Dry skin, fatigue, itching, anorexia, and bone/joint pain each have been reported by more than 50% of patients.[30] Regular symptom assessment using validated tools helps redirect treatment toward a patient-centered care model, yet is not a common practice in nephrology practices.[2,31] This tremendous suffering may be one reason withdrawal rates are as high as 35% in the oldest groups.[32]

Patients with advanced CKD have identified symptom assessment and management as a top priority, yet few nephrologists have incorporated validated symptom assessments into care workflows. Studies show that nephrologists, nurse practitioners, physician assistants, and nurses are largely unaware of the presence and severity of symptoms in patients who are on maintenance hemodialysis.[33] The inattention to psychosocial symptoms, including depression and anxiety, adds to the burden of this disease.[34]

Lack of Specialty Kidney Supportive Care Consultation

The early introduction of kidney supportive care along with usual disease-modifying treatment has been shown to be beneficial for cancer patients and heart failure patients.[36-38] However, neither robust supportive care nor specialty palliative care consultation is routinely available to US patients with kidney disease. In the period 2012–2013, fewer than 1% of hospitalizations longer than 2 days for ESKD patients on dialysis more than 90 days included an inpatient palliative care consultation, even though such consultations were associated with

---

i. Shared decision making refers to the process whereby patients (or their proxy decision makers) make decisions about current care. Advance care planning refers to the process for helping patients express what they would want IN THE FUTURE if they were no longer able to make decisions for themselves—and who they would want to make those decisions on their behalf.

lower costs for patients who died during the index hospitalization and lower readmission rates and higher hospice use for the patients who were discharged.[38] In a single center study at Mayo Clinic, 26% of hemodialysis patients who died between 2001 and 2013 received at least 1 palliative care consultation within 6 months of death. The rate was slightly higher for patients who chose to withdraw from dialysis, but was still only 34%.[39] It is highly likely that the Mayo Clinic rates are an upper bound rather than representative of usual care in typical kidney care settings.

While inpatient palliative care is now widely available (although not well used for kidney patients), outpatient palliative care is still scarce for all patients. In a 2013 survey of dialysis center staff, only 4.5% of 487 respondents believed they were presently providing high-quality supportive care and end-of-life care. These respondents felt that specialty palliative care consultation was 1 of the 2 most important changes needed to improve supportive care in their setting.[40]

Lack of Patient-Centered Care Options, Including Palliative Dialysis and Medical Management Without Dialysis

Patients older than 75 years are the fastest growing segment of the dialysis population, but these patients, especially if they are frail or have comorbidities, may not experience a survival benefit from standard dialysis treatment.[25,41] The current default is to start elderly patients with advanced kidney disease and multiple comorbid conditions on a standard dialysis schedule, irrespective of their prognosis, likelihood of benefit, or goals. In multiple studies, many dialysis patients have indicated that they prefer to avoid pain and suffering even if they live for a shorter period of time.[16,17] The high dialysis discontinuation rate may reflect these value preferences. United States Renal Data System data shows that 25% of dialysis patient deaths are due to dialysis discontinuation, although other studies report rates as high as 49%.[39] The most common reason for discontinuation is an unacceptable quality of life secondary to failing to thrive on dialysis. Patients with kidney disease have also reported that they would be willing to make trade-offs in which they live a shorter period of time and forgo dialysis to have more independence and not be restricted to a 3-times-per-week dialysis schedule.

Two qualitative studies of American nephrologist attitudes revealed significant concerns about foregoing dialysis, with many equating medical management without dialysis as "no care."[42,43] In one study, only one-third of participants routinely discussed medical management without dialysis. Most nephrologists opted not to present medical management without dialysis neutrally as a legitimate alternative to dialysis therapy.[42] Both payment mechanisms and quality measurement requirements were reported as barriers to discussing medical management without dialysis. These same barriers have also likely impeded innovation in developing flexible palliative dialysis options.

Lack of End-of-Life Planning and Unwanted High-Intensity End-of-Life Care

Patients on dialysis are subjected to more aggressive treatment at the end of life than patients with other serious illnesses.[28,29,44] This appears to be unwanted, as families of deceased

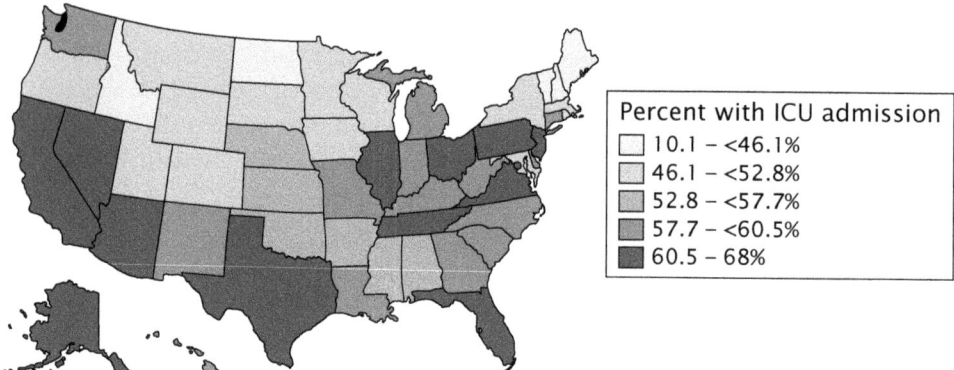

FIGURE 3.5. Intensive care unit admission during the last 90 days of life among Medicare beneficiaries with end-stage kidney disease by state of residence, 2000–2015. Source: USRDS Chapter 12, 2018 https://www.usrds.org/2018/view/v2_12.aspx.

dialysis patients rate the quality of their loved ones' end-of-life care worse than families of those with cancer and other chronic conditions.[28] Families of veterans with CKD or ESKD rated end-of-life care better if the veteran had received a palliative care consult or hospice care and worse if they spent 2 or more weeks in the hospital during the last 90 days of life, received intensive procedures in the last 30 days of life, or died in the ICU.[45] There also appear to be substantial race- and ethnicity-based disparities in end-of-life care practices for US patients receiving dialysis.[46]

The trajectory of ESKD is usually characterized by a sharp escalation in symptoms and decline in functional status 2 to 3 months before death.[47,48] If this escalation is not anticipated and planned for, it leads to missed opportunities to control symptoms, support patients and families, and avoid unwanted hospitalizations.[49] More than 4 out of 5 ESKD patients are admitted to the hospital in the last 90 days of life; 63% were admitted to the ICU, although this varies widely by state (Figure 3.5).[50p12] In 2016, 27% of Medicare ESRD patients had a hospital admission or discharge within 3 days of death. The use of intensive procedures in the last 90 days of life has risen over the last 15 years, with mechanical ventilation now used by 30% of patients who died in 2015 (Figure 3.6). Use of intensive procedures was lower for older patients, with only 20% of the oldest (85+ years) using intensive procedures compared to 50% of the youngest group, aged 20 to 44 years.

Hospice Care

Use of hospice care among ESKD patients has risen from 11% in 2000 to 26% in 2015 (Figure 3.7). However, it is still just half of the 50.4% rate for all regular Medicare beneficiary decedents in 2015.[50,51] Rates of both end-of-life hospitalization and hospice use vary widely by state, suggesting that it is not just patient preference, but possibly also system capacity and practice patterns that are driving utilization. Hospice use was much higher for those who discontinued dialysis than for those who did not discontinue in 2015 (62% vs. 16%).[50p12] The large difference in hospice use between those who discontinued dialysis and those who did not discontinue most likely reflects the intertwined nature of these 2 treatment decisions. Financial

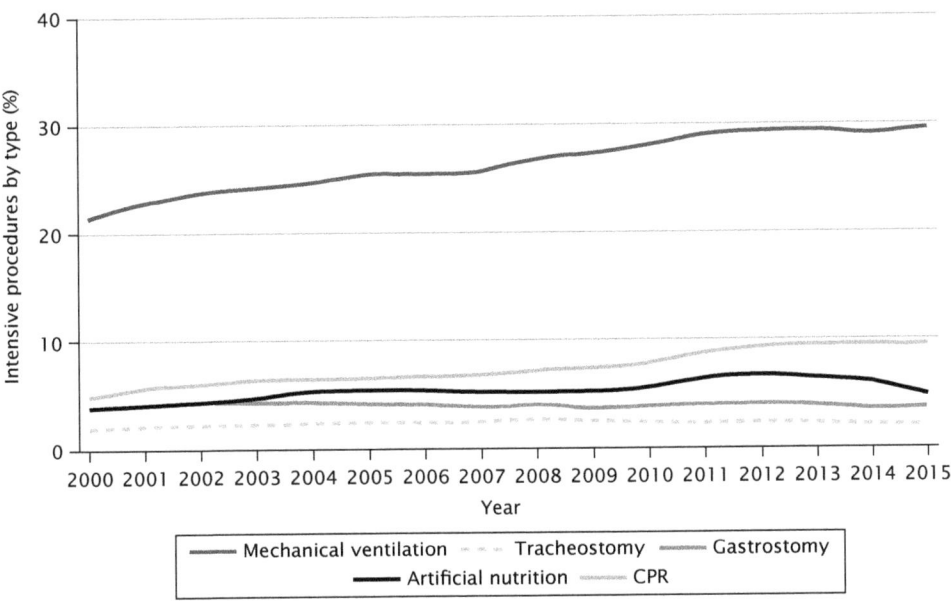

FIGURE 3.6. Intensive procedures during the last 90 days of life among Medicare beneficiaries with end-stage kidney disease, 2000–2015. Source: USRDS Chapter 12, 2018 https://www.usrds.org/2018/view/v2_12.aspx.

and regulatory barriers to concurrent receipt of dialysis and hospice services makes transition to hospice care particularly difficult for patients on dialysis.[52] Specifically, the Medicare regulations require hospices to pay for all care and treatment related to the terminal diagnosis. This means that the hospice is required to pay for dialysis treatments if kidney disease is the

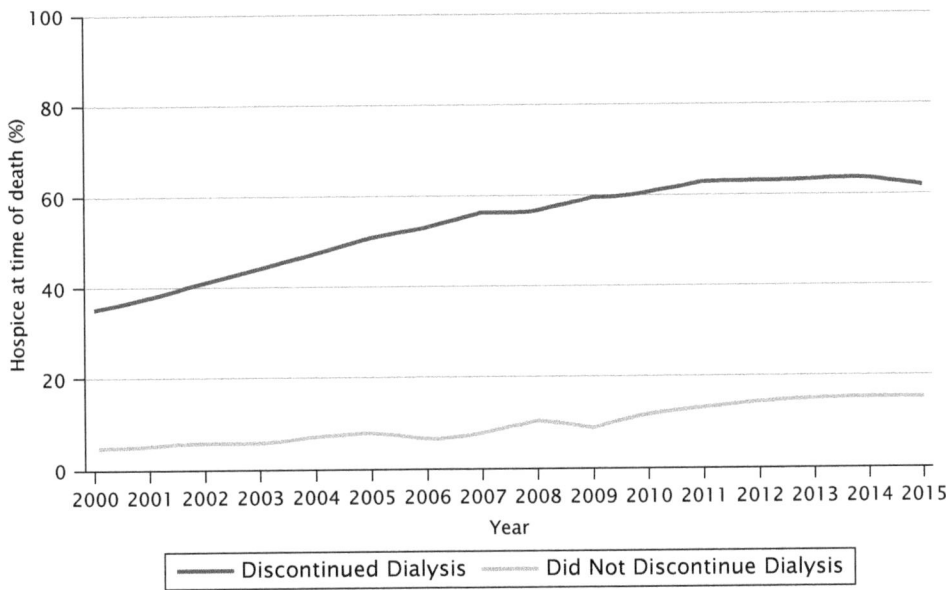

FIGURE 3.7. Hospice utilization by whether patients discontinued dialysis before death. Source: USRDS 2018. https://www.usrds.org/2018/view/v2_12.aspx.

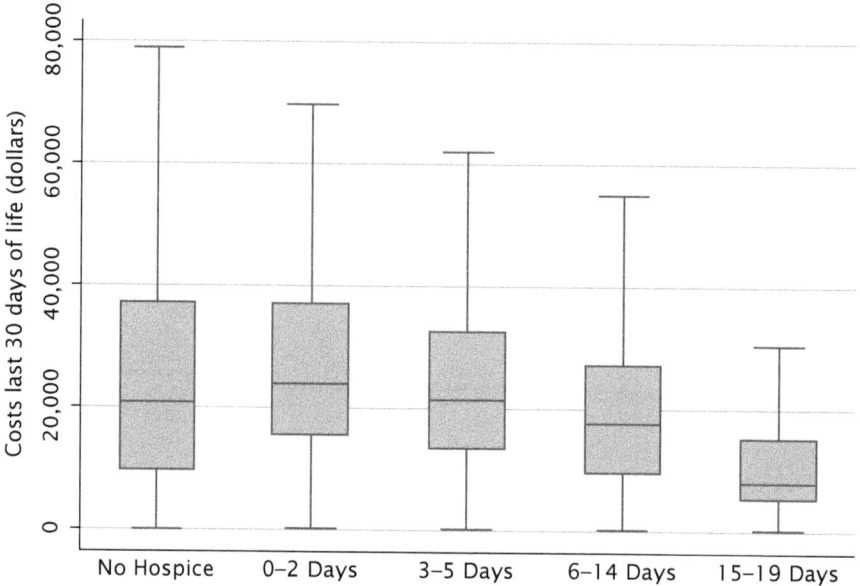

FIGURE 3.8. Costs in the last 30 days of life in relation to timing of hospice care, 2000–2015. Source: USRDS 2018, https://www.usrds.org/2018/view/v2_12.aspx.

terminal diagnosis. With hospices receiving approximately $154 per day to cover all care costs for routine home care, including medications, equipment, and staffing, only hospices that have additional financial resources are able to take on the costs of dialysis care.

Cost in Last Month of Life

For ESKD patients, the median cost of care in the last month of life was $19,734 (interquartile range $9,217–$34,979), with costs lower the earlier the person entered hospice care prior to death (Figure 3.8). For patients who did not use hospice, median costs in the last 30 days of life were $20,766. Patients who used hospice for 15 to 19 days had median costs of $7,790.59.[50]

Conclusion

There exists a tremendous gap between the ideal state and current state of care for people seriously ill with kidney disease. The number of people impacted by disease and treatment burdens is increasing yearly. To address their unmet supportive care needs, it is imperative that we move away from disease-focused care and toward patient-centered care, in particular for our older, medically complex patients.

Practice Pointer

- The end of life experience for patients with kidney disease is markedly worse than for patients with cancer or heart disease. Patients are far more likely to die in the ICU and/or receive other high-intensity treatments toward the end of life, but this is likely unwanted, as families rate the death experience worse than for patients with other diseases.

Practice Improvement Opportunity

- Assess how well supportive care practices are integrated into your kidney care using the Kidney Supportive Care Implementation Quotient https://nursing.gwu.edu/pathways-phase-2

References

1. Harris DCH, Davies SJ, Finkelstein FO, et al. Increasing access to integrated ESKD care as part of universal health coverage. *Kidney Int.* 2019;95(4):S1–S33. doi:10.1016/j.kint.2018.12.005
2. Tamura MKM, Meier DED. Five policies to promote palliative care for patients with ESRD. *Clin J Am Soc Nephrol.* 2013;8(10):1783–90. doi:10.2215/CJN.02180213
3. Tamura MK, O'Hare AM, Lin E, Holdsworth LM, Malcolm E, Moss AH. Palliative care disincentives in CKD: changing policy to improve CKD care. *Am J Kidney Dis.* 2018;71(6):866–873. doi:10.1053/j.ajkd.2017.12.017
4. Wachterman MW, Lipsitz SR, Lorenz KA, Marcantonio ER, Li Z, Keating NL. End-of-life experience of older adults dying of end-stage renal disease: a comparison with cancer. *J Pain Symptom Manage.* 2017;54(6):789–797. doi:10.1016/j.jpainsymman.2017.08.013
5. Moss AH. Palliative care in patients with kidney disease and cancer. In: *Online Curricula: Onco-Nephrology.* Chapter 19. American Society of Nephrology. https://www.asn-online.org/education/distancelearning/curricula/onco/Chapter19.pdf. Published 2016.
6. Brown L, Gardner G, Bonner A. A comparison of treatment options for management of end stage kidney disease in elderly patients: a systematic review. *JBI Database Syst Rev Implement Rep.* 2014;12(7):374–404. doi:10.11124/jbisrir-2014-1152
7. United States Renal Data System. Incidence, prevalence, patient characteristics, and treatment modalities. In *USRDS Annual Data Report.* Vol. 2, Chapter 1. United States Renal Data System; 2018:291–332. https://www.usrds.org/2018/download/v2_c01_IncPrev_18_usrds.pdf.
8. Kochanek KD, Murphy SL, Xu JQ, Arias E. Mortality in the United States, 2016. NCHS Data Brief, no 293. Hyattsville, MD: National Center for Health Statistics 2017;(293):8.
9. Wachterman MW, O'Hare AM, Rahman O-K, et al. One-year mortality after dialysis initiation among older adults. *JAMA Intern Med.* 2019;179(7):987–990. doi:10.1001/jamainternmed.2019.0125
10. Renal Physicians Association. *Shared Decision Making in the Appropriate Initiation of and Withdrawal From Dialysis.* 2nd ed. Rockville, Maryland, Renal Physicians Association, 2010. https://cdn.ymaws.com/www.renalmd.org/resource/resmgr/Store/Shared_Decision_Making_Recom.pdf
11. Informed Medical Decisions Foundation. What is shared decision making? http://www.informedmedicaldecisions.org/what-is-shared-decision-making/. Accessed July 3, 2015.
12. Sudore RL, Lum HD, You JJ, et al. Defining advance care planning for adults: a consensus definition from a multidisciplinary Delphi panel. *J Pain Symptom Manage.* 2016;53(5):821–832. doi:10.1016/j.jpainsymman.2016.12.331
13. Davison SN, Jhangri G, Holley JL, Moss AH. Nephrologists' reported preparedness for end-of-life decision-making. *Clin J Am Soc Nephrol.* 2006;1:1256–1262.
14. Wachterman MW, Marcantonio ER, Davis RB, et al. Relationship between the prognostic expectations of seriously ill patients undergoing hemodialysis and their nephrologists. *JAMA Intern Med.* 2013;173(13):1206–14. doi:10.1001/jamainternmed.2013.6036
15. Singh Ospina N, Phillips KA, Rodriguez-Gutierrez R, et al. Eliciting the patient's agenda- secondary analysis of recorded clinical encounters. *J Gen Intern Med.* 2018;34(1):36–40. doi:10.1007/s11606-018-4540-5

16. Davison SN. End-of-life care preferences and needs: perceptions of patients with chronic kidney disease. *Clin J Am Soc Nephrol.* 2010;5(2):195–204. doi:10.2215/CJN.05960809
17. Ramer SJ, McCall NN, Robinson-Cohen C, et al. Health outcome priorities of older adults with advanced CKD and concordance with their nephrology providers' perceptions. *J Am Soc Nephrol.* 2018;29(12):2870–2878. doi:10.1681/ASN.2018060657
18. Saeed F, Lupu D, Moss AH. The donut or the hole? Prioritizing patient and caregiver values in the delivery of high-quality medical management without dialysis. *Am J Kidney Dis.* 2019;73(2):153–155. doi:10.1053/j.ajkd.2018.10.003
19. Carson RC, Bernacki R. Is the end in sight for the "don't ask, don't tell" approach to advance care planning? *Clin J Am Soc Nephrol.* 2017;12(3):380–381. doi:10.2215/CJN.00980117
20. Lim C, Ng R, Cheng N, Cigolini M, Kwok C, Brennan F. Advance care planning for haemodialysis patients (review). *Cochrane Database Syst Rev.* 2016;7: CD010737. doi:10.1002/14651858.CD010737.pub2.
21. Kurella Tamura M, Goldstein MK, Pérez-Stable EJ. Preferences for dialysis withdrawal and engagement in advance care planning within a diverse sample of dialysis patients. *Nephrol Dial Transplant Off Publ Eur Dial Transpl Assoc—Eur Ren Assoc.* 2010;25(1):237–42. doi:10.1093/ndt/gfp430
22. Kurella Tamura M, Montez-Rath ME, Hall YN, Katz R, O'Hare AM. Advance directives and end-of-life care among nursing home residents receiving maintenance dialysis. *Clin J Am Soc Nephrol CJASN.* 2017;12(3):435–442. doi:10.2215/CJN.07510716
23. Feely MA, Hildebrandt D, Varayil JE, Mueller PS. Prevalence and contents of advance directives of patients with ESRD receiving dialysis. *Clin J Am Soc Nephrol.* 2016;11:2204–2209. doi:10.2215/CJN.12131115
24. Da Silva-Gane M, Wellsted D, Greenshields H, Norton S, Chandna SM, Farrington K. Quality of life and survival in patients with advanced kidney failure managed conservatively or by dialysis. *Clin J Am Soc Nephrol.* 2012;7(12):2002–2009. doi:10.2215/CJN.01130112
25. Verberne WR, Geers ABMT, Jellema WT, et al. Comparative survival among older adults with advanced kidney disease managed conservatively versus with dialysis. *Clin J Am Soc Nephrol.* 2016;(18):1–8. doi:10.2215/CJN.07510715
26. Feldman R, Berman N, Reid MC, et al. Improving symptom management in hemodialysis patients: identifying barriers and future directions. *J Palliat Med.* 2013;16(12):1528–1533. doi:10.1089/jpm.2013.0176
27. Scherer JS, Combs SA, Brennan F. Sleep disorders, restless legs syndrome, and uremic pruritus: diagnosis and treatment of common symptoms in dialysis patients. *Am J Kidney Dis.* 2016:1–12. doi:10.1053/j.ajkd.2016.07.031
28. Wachterman MW, Pilver C, Smith D, Ersek M, Lipsitz SR, Keating NL. Quality of end-of-life care provided to patients with different serious illnesses. *JAMA Intern Med.* 2016;176(8):1095–102. doi:10.1001/jamainternmed.2016.1200
29. Wachterman MW, Lipsitz SR, Lorenz KA, Marcantonio ER, Li Z, Keating NL. End-of-life experience of older adults dying of end-stage renal disease: a comparison with cancer. *J Pain Symptom Manage.* 2017;54(6):789–797. doi:10.1016/j.jpainsymman.2017.08.013
30. Davison SN, Jhangri GS. Impact of pain and symptom burden on the health-related quality of life of hemodialysis patients. *J Pain Symptom Manage.* 2010;39(3):477–485. doi:10.1016/j.jpainsymman.2009.08.008, doi:10.1001/jamainternmed.2018.0256
31. Weisbord SD, Fried LF, Arnold RM, et al. Prevalence, severity, and importance of physical and emotional symptoms in chronic hemodialysis patients. *J Am Soc Nephrol JASN.* 2005;16(8):2487–94. doi:10.1681/ASN.2005020157
32. United States Renal Data System. *2015 USRDS Annual Data Report: Epidemiology of Kidney Disease in the United States. CH12 End-of-Life Care for Patients with End-Stage Renal Disease: 2000-2012.* Bethesda, MD: National Institutes of Health, National Institute of Diabetes and Digestive and Kidney Diseases http://www.usrds.org/2015/view/v2_14.aspx.
33. Weisbord SD, Fried LF, Mor MK, et al. Renal Provider Recognition of Symptoms in Patients on Maintenance Hemodialysis. *Clin J Am Soc Nephrol.* 2007;2(5):960–967. doi:10.2215/CJN.00990207

34. Cukor D, Ver Halen N, Asher DR, et al. Psychosocial Intervention Improves Depression, Quality of Life, and Fluid Adherence in Hemodialysis. *J Am Soc Nephrol JASN*. 2014;25(1):196–206. doi:10.1681/ASN.2012111134
35. Temel JS, Greer J a, Muzikansky A, et al. Early palliative care for patients with metastatic non-small-cell lung cancer. *N Engl J Med*. 2010;363(8):733–742. doi:10.1056/NEJMoa1000678
36. Yoong J, Park ER, Greer JA, et al. Early Palliative Care in Advanced Lung Cancer. *JAMA Intern Med*. 2013;173(4):283. doi:10.1001/jamainternmed.2013.1874. https://www.usrds.org/2017/download/v2_c12_SS_EndLifeCare_17.pdf.
37. Gelfman LP, Bakitas M, Warner Stevenson L, Kirkpatrick JN, Goldstein NE. The State of the Science on Integrating Palliative Care in Heart Failure. *J Palliat Med*. 2017;20(6):592–603. doi:10.1089/jpm.2017.0178
38. Chettiar A, Montez-Rath M, Liu S, Hall YN, O'Hare AM, Kurella Tamura M. Association of Inpatient Palliative Care with Health Care Utilization and Postdischarge Outcomes among Medicare Beneficiaries with End Stage Kidney Disease. *Clin J Am Soc Nephrol*. 2018:CJN.00180118. doi:10.2215/CJN.00180118
39. Chen JC-Y, Thorsteinsdottir B, Vaughan LE, et al. End of Life, Withdrawal, and Palliative Care Utilization among Patients Receiving Maintenance Hemodialysis Therapy. *Clin J Am Soc Nephrol*. 2018;13:CJN.00590118. doi:10.2215/CJN.00590118
40. Culp S, Lupu D, Arenella C, Armistead N, Moss AH. Unmet Supportive Care Needs in U.S. Dialysis Centers and Lack of Knowledge of Available Resources to Address Them. *J Pain Symptom Manage*. 2016;51(4):756–761. doi:10.1016/j.jpainsymman.2015.11.017
41. Murtagh FEM, Burns A, Moranne O, Morton RL, Naicker S. Supportive Care: Comprehensive Conservative Care in End-Stage Kidney Disease. *Clin J Am Soc Nephrol*. 2016:1909–1914. doi:10.2215/CJN.04840516
42. Ladin K, Pandya R, Kannam A, et al. Discussing Conservative Management With Older Patients With CKD: An Interview Study of Nephrologists. *Am J Kidney Dis*. 2018;71(5):627–635. doi:10.1053/j.ajkd.2017.11.011
43. Grubbs V, Tuot DS, Powe NR, O'Donoghue D, Chesla CA. System-Level Barriers and Facilitators for Foregoing or Withdrawing Dialysis: A Qualitative Study of Nephrologists in the United States and England. *Am J Kidney Dis*. 2017;70(5):602–610. doi:10.1053/j.ajkd.2016.12.015
44. Wachterman MW, Hailpern SM, Keating NL, Kurella Tamura M, O'Hare AM. Association Between Hospice Length of Stay, Health Care Utilization, and Medicare Costs at the End of Life Among Patients Who Received Maintenance Hemodialysis. *JAMA Intern Med*. 2018;178(6):792–799. doi:10.1001/jamainternmed.2018.0256
45. Richards CA, Liu C-F, Hebert PL, et al. Family Perceptions of Quality of End-of-Life Care for Veterans with Advanced CKD. *Clin J Am Soc Nephrol*. August 2019:CJN.01560219. doi:10.2215/CJN.01560219
46. Foley RN, Sexton DJ, Drawz P, Ishani A, Reule S. Race, Ethnicity, and End-of-Life Care in Dialysis Patients in the United States. *J Am Soc Nephrol*. 2018;29(9):2387–2399. doi:10.1681/ASN.2017121297
47. Kilshaw L, Sammut H, Asher R, Williams P, Saxena R, Howse M. A study to describe the health trajectory of patients with advanced renal disease who choose not to receive dialysis. *Clin Kidney J*. 2016;9(3):470–475. doi:10.1093/ckj/sfw005
48. Murtagh FEM, Addington-Hall JM, Higginson IJ. End-stage renal disease: A new trajectory of functional decline in the last year of life. *J Am Geriatr Soc*. 2011;59(2):304–308. doi:10.1111/j.1532-5415.2010.03248.x
49. Schell J, Patel U, Steinhauser K, Ammarel N, Tulsky JA. Discussions of the Kidney Disease Trajectory by Elderly Patients and Nephrologists: A Qualitative Study. *Am J Kidney Dis*. 2012;59(4):495–503. doi:10.1053/J.AJKD.2011.11.023
50. United States Renal Data System. *Chapter 12: End-of-Life Care for Patients with End-Stage Renal Disease, 2000–2014*. Bethesda, MD: National Institutes of Health, National Institute of Diabetes and Digestive and Kidney Diseases; 2017. https://www.usrds.org/2017/download/v2_c12_SS_EndLifeCare_17.pdf.
51. Teno JM, Gozalo P, Trivedi AN, et al. Site of Death, Place of Care, and Health Care Transitions Among US Medicare Beneficiaries, 2000-2015. *JAMA*. 2018;320(3):264–271. doi:10.1001/jama.2018.8981
52. Grubbs V. ESRD and Hospice Care in the United States: Are Dialysis Patients Welcome? *Am J Kidney Dis*. 2018;72(3):429–432. doi:10.1053/j.ajkd.2018.04.008

4

Models for Operationalizing Supportive Care in Kidney Care

Dale E. Lupu and Emma Murphy

The field of kidney supportive care is in a period of innovation, with different models emerging from local efforts to improve care. We classify emerging models into six types: embedded, mobile/visiting, chronic kidney disease case management, medical management without dialysis, concurrent hospice/dialysis, and comprehensive regional or system-wide programs. Although individual programs have demonstrated positive impact on outcomes such as advance care planning and place of death, there is not yet systematic evidence comparing the impact of model type on effectiveness or cost effectiveness. Local considerations about need, resources, opportunities, and champions are key to planning a supportive kidney care strategy. Facilitators for program success include training for nephrology providers, active collaboration between nephrology and palliative care, local champions (often nurses), sensitive messaging about medical management without dialysis, and research to demonstrate program impact.

The Working Groups of the International Society of Nephrology's Second Global Kidney Health Summit called supportive care "an essential component of an integrated ESKD program."[1] To be a comprehensive program, a kidney supportive care program should cover 4 phases in the continuum of kidney care:

- Chronic kidney disease (CKD) care prior to making a decision about renal replacement therapy. This includes patient education about all care options, including medical management without dialysis.
- Medical management without dialysis.
- Supportive care concurrent with dialysis.
- End-of-life transition.

This chapter describes innovative kidney supportive care models that have emerged in the last decade, with emphasis on US programs. To the limited extent such information is available, the chapter covers the practical elements of program development, such as staffing models and specific services that are offered. There are not yet any comprehensive, regional programs in the United States, where most programs are limited to local initiatives that concentrate on only 1 or 2 of the 4 phases. For examples of fully comprehensive models spanning the continuum of care, we turn to Canada and Australia.

Literature Review

Published descriptions of models of kidney supportive care are scarce. Descriptions of the pragmatic details of running a supportive kidney care program are even scarcer, and comparisons of the efficacy of different models are almost nonexistent. To date, 2 papers have summarized the literature and have proposed classifications systems for the different types of programs that are developing.[2,3] Drawing on the classifications in those papers as well as a classification system for general palliative care programs,[4] we recognize 6 types of kidney supportive care programs:

1. Embedded programs, where the supportive care services and staff are integrated into the structure of existing dialysis centers or nephrology practices.
2. Mobile/visiting palliative care specialty teams, where specialty palliative cares teams provide services to nephrology patients.
3. CKD case management programs, which mostly emphasize case management of patients earlier in the disease state, but may also provide substantial input into shared-decision making and advance care planning.
4. Medical management without dialysis programs, which may or may not be part of CKD case management programs.
5. Concurrent hospice/dialysis programs.
6. Comprehensive regional or system wide programs integrated into kidney care.

Making comparisons across these models is difficult, because there are few specifics and little evidence about operational parameters such as staffing, admission criteria, or frequency of service, and outcomes to suggest which model is most effective or cost- efficient. Systematic comparisons across programs are needed to guide future practice.

Examples of Program Models
Embedded Programs

Embedded programs provide supportive care within the dialysis center or nephrology practice. This is a seamless integrated service provided by the patient's regular nephrology team in the context of usual care processes. The embedded program is commonly led by a nephrologist or nephrology nurse practitioner who has received extensive training in palliative care including communication skills, symptom management, and advance care planning. In the United States, it is common for programs to be led by nephrologists who are dually board certified in palliative care and nephrology. It is not clear that this is a necessary component of such programs.

Two examples of embedded models in the United States are the Kidney Comprehensive Advanced Renal Disease and ESKD Support (CARES) Program at New York University[5] and the Renal Supportive Care Clinic at the University of Pittsburgh.[3] both of which are led by nephrologists also board certified in palliative care. CARES is modeled after the embedded kidney–palliative care clinic first started in Australia,[6] modified after soliciting local institutional stakeholder feedback.[5] The CARES model home is the academic nephrology group practice. This nephrologist reviews patients with kidney-specific palliative care needs 1 half-day per week, supported by a registered nurse educated in advance care planning and a psychologist who focuses on patients with advanced illness. The Kidney CARES program works collaboratively with other nephrologists in the practice to address the kidney supportive care needs of patients regardless of CKD stage or treatment choice.[3] The clinic

- Manages physical and emotions symptoms of serious kidney disease;
- Facilitates shared decision-making concerning dialysis decision-making and end-of-life care planning;
- Collaborates with the primary nephrologist to care for patients choosing medical management without dialysis; and
- Works with community providers (hospice and home care) to promote smooth transitions, particularly at the end of life.[7]

The University of Pittsburgh Renal Supportive Care Clinic (also labeled Kidney Clinic) is one of several focused palliative care clinics operated by the UPMC Palliative and Supportive Institute.[8] The Kidney Clinic is physically located within the UPMC nephrology practice. Primary care physicians and nephrologists refer patients. Care may be collaborative or transitioned solely to the Renal Supportive Care Clinic. Nephrology nonphysician staff work alongside the nephrologists to obtain symptom scores, review and communicate about advance care planning documents, and coordinate referrals to home services such as hospice.[3] The clinic offers

- Symptom control;
- Psychosocial and spiritual support;
- Advance care planning and seamless transitions of care;
- Aid in treatment decision-making, particularly the decision to initiate or to withdraw renal replacement therapy; and
- Medical management without dialysis.[8]

Mobile/Visiting Specialty Palliative Care Teams

Visiting specialty palliative care teams provide services wherever the patient is, whether at a dialysis center, home, or nursing home. The key distinction between a visiting team and an embedded program is that the visiting palliative care team is not housed within a nephrology program. Although they are ideally well integrated and coordination of care is smooth between the nephrology team and the palliative care team, the two are functionally separate teams.

One US example is the mobile Renal Supportive Care (RSC) program at Northwest Kidney Centers.[9] RSC is a mobile/home-based kidney supportive care model developed to deliver supportive care to patients within the ESKD Seamless Care Organization (ESCO) program. The RSC program addresses barriers associated with access to outpatient supportive care, the burden of clinic visits, and the need to flexibly engage family members outside of a clinic setting. The interdisciplinary team comprises a nephrologist trained in palliative care (0.5 full-time employee [FTE]), a social worker (0.8 FTE), and a nurse (1.0 FTE). Team members engage patients and family members in the dialysis unit and in their residences, address kidney supportive care needs, and help coordinate care with the patients' primary nephrologists and dialysis interdisciplinary team.[3] Referrals come from electronic medical record trigger, the dialysis unit staff, primary nephrologist, and monthly "huddle" meetings with interdisciplinary teams from each dialysis center served. Referrals are cleared with the patient's primary nephrologist.[9]

In its first 18 months of operation, the team served 6 dialysis centers with 700 eligible patients. The service had an impact on advance care planning, with 96.6% of RSC patients engaging in advance care planning and 89.7% completing at least 1 key task of advance care planning. Of RSC patients who died, 33% used hospice at the time of death and 10% used concurrent hospice and dialysis. Because of the regulatory barriers and misunderstandings about hospice for dialysis patients, 100% of the patients requesting concurrent hospice and dialysis required escalation to the hospice medical director for approval of services.[9] Services provided include primary kidney supportive care education to dialysis staff at new employee orientations and in-service presentations at the dialysis center. One limitation is that it does not provide medical management without dialysis.

CKD Case Management Programs

CKD case management programs are another model of care. These programs cast a broader net and try to reach patients earlier in the course of their kidney disease. The goal is to slow down the progression of renal disease, enable shared decision-making of treatment options including dialysis and medical management without dialysis, and help patients prepare for end of life. One such program offered by Dialysis Clinics, Inc. (DCI) is entitled Real Engagement Achieving Complete Health (REACH) Kidney Care of Upstate South Carolina, which was created prior to the ESCO programs and was the progenitor of Palmetto Kidney Care Alliance ESCO based in Spartanburg, South Carolina. Since 2014, more than 10% of REACH program participants have chosen medical management without dialysis.[10]

The REACH program is staffed by a nurse care coordinator, a dietitian, and a social worker. The frequency of visits depends on the patient's clinical needs. At a minimum, the nurse care coordinator sees the patient between visits with the nephrologist, with the net effect that the patient is seen twice as frequently. If necessary, the nurse care coordinator reviews the patient weekly providing the nephrologist and other physicians with a progress note after every visit. DCI attributes substantial financial savings to the REACH program in that patients who would not benefit from dialysis are provided an alternative. The DCI ESCO whose patients are served by REACH saw substantial cost savings in its first year.[10]

Medical Management Without Dialysis

Well-articulated protocols for providing medical management without dialysis have been delineated in Canada, Britain, and Australia.[11-13] In the United States. there are few programs that explicitly offer medical management without dialysis, and the lack of a formal definition of the care pathway makes it difficult to track how often it is offered or chosen by patients.[14] Nephrologists—many of whom are reluctant to discuss medical management at all—often equate medical management with "no care,"[15-17] rather than with active management.

Through the work of a few early adopters, a standard of care for medical management in the United States is beginning to emerge. In addition to the DCI REACH, there is an emerging program at Truman Medical Centers in Kansas City, Missouri. This nurse practitioner-led clinic began in 2018 as a collaboration between nephrology and kidney supportive care. It assists patients with treatment decisions, advance care planning, symptom management, emotional support, and end-of-life care through referral to palliative care or hospice.[18] The University of Pittsburgh Renal Supportive Care Clinic also offers medical management without dialysis. Several CKD practices participating in the Pathways learning collaborative are currently working on jointly articulating a standard of care for medical management without dialysis patients.[19]

Concurrent Hospice/Dialysis Programs

In the United States, Medicare payment rules present formidable barriers to provision of concurrent hospice and dialysis to most patients on dialysis. (See chapter 24 for further explanation of the regulatory constraints.) Some hospice programs will accept dialysis patients on an occasional basis, agreeing ad hoc to limited dialysis. At least 3 programs have proactively developed guidelines and practices to make concurrent hospice and dialysis available to a wider group of patients. These are Chapters Health System Open Access hospice,[20] the open-access program at Holland Home in Michigan, and a partnership between Family Hospice in Pittsburgh and DCI. The latter program is called the ESRD Concurrent Care Program.

The ESRD Concurrent Care Program is a collaborative care program developed through a partnership between DCI, the Independence Kidney Care Alliance ESCO, and UPMC Family Hospice in Pittsburgh.[21] The program's aim is to promote timely hospice services for dialysis patients with limited prognosis by offering concurrent hospice and palliative dialysis (up to 10 sessions with weekly reassessment). Palliative dialysis includes adjustment in the timing and frequency of dialysis to address patient's comfort and quality of life. The program was initiated in December 2017 as a pilot. As of spring 2019, 8 patients had enrolled in hospice. Seven of these patients elected palliative dialysis (1 patient withdrew from dialysis). Of these 7 patients, 3 died before they could undergo the next planned dialysis treatment. There are plans to expand to additional cities where DCI has strong relationships with local hospices. Evaluation of the program will measure change in hospice utilization, duration of hospice care, percentage of deaths in the hospital and at home, and experience of the patient, family, and caregiver.

Comprehensive Regional or System-Wide Programs Integrated Into Kidney Care

To our knowledge, no regional or system-wide program has yet been established in the United States. The Pathways Project is an early effort to implement a consistent package of supportive kidney care practices across 11 dialysis centers and 3 CKD clinics.[19]

Two provinces in Canada have developed comprehensive supportive kidney care programs. Alberta's program, which is termed "conservative kidney management,[13] provides an extensive set of resources for patients and providers on the Conservative Kidney Management website (https://www.ckmcare.com/). The British Columbia Renal Agency has also developed standards for medical management without dialysis and has integrated those into an overall pathways for kidney care.[11]

In Australia, New South Wales (NSW) has developed a Renal Supportive Care Model, which includes both supportive care for patients on dialysis as well as medical management without dialysis.[22] This model was developed by the NSW Agency for Clinical Innovation Renal Network, in consultation with the NSW Ministry of Health, and other key stakeholders. The nurse-led, networked RSC model is aimed at 4 groups of patients with CKD or end-stage kidney disease:

- Patients deciding whether or not to pursue renal replacement therapies (including patients in the predialysis stage);
- Patients managed medically opting not to pursue renal replacement therapies;
- Patients receiving renal replacement therapies but experiencing symptoms that significantly reduce their quality of life; and
- Patients choosing to withdraw from dialysis.

The nurse is supported by other health professionals, such as a palliative care physician, dietitian, and social worker (where available). The model is based around the establishment of 3 hubs across the state, which provide education, mentoring, and long-term support to the affiliated renal units within their network. The model's report provides useful tools for others looking to build programs, including detailed job descriptions, suggested screening, and symptom assessment tools.[22]

Considerations for Choosing a Supportive Kidney Care Model

Given the current lack of evidence favoring any of these models over another, program leaders need a careful assessment of local conditions when planning a supportive kidney care program. The first decision is considering whether to start with adding supportive care to an existing dialysis program or to start by building a medical management without dialysis program. In the United States, the current divide between the CKD and the dialysis environment makes this an important consideration.

The second consideration is the staffing model. It is clear that some palliative care expertise is needed, but the question of whether to "skill up" the nephrology team, bring in specialist palliative care consultants, or some combination may rest entirely on local conditions and the inclinations and availability of local staff. Finally, the need to cultivate strong collaboration with local palliative care and hospice programs is universal, but the form it will take depends on local relationships and resources. Table 4.1 summarizes the authors' opinion about the pros and cons of each model.

TABLE 4.1. Pros and Cons of Alternative Care Models for Supportive Nephrology

Supportive Nephrology Care Model	Pros	Cons
Embedded within nephrology	- Seamless care from patient point of view - Likely will gain early acceptance from rest of nephrology team because providers are "one of us" - May impact practices and culture of whole nephrology team - May be fast, relatively easy way to start up a program - Provision of appropriate palliative alongside nephrology care	- Providers with sufficient expertise in both nephrology and palliative care are scarce - Investing the time for a nephrology provider to "skill up" with sufficient depth of palliative care skills may delay program, be expensive - Difficult to have entire inter-disciplinary team with palliative care skills (physician, nurse, social worker, chaplain) - Providing medical management and supportive care for dialysis patients is not a priority for many individual nephrologists
Mobile/visiting specialty palliative care team	- Brings depth of expertise in palliative care particularly for patients with multimorbidity with complex palliative care needs - Likely makes full interdisciplinary team available to patient - Provides a flexible responsive service to meet patient needs	- Patient may be burdened by having to see another provider/team - Palliative care team may need to "skill up" regarding particular needs of nephrology patients, especially for symptom management - Palliative care team may need to "skill up" in illness trajectories, renal disease, dialysis, and medical management without dialysis - Not always clear when the patient should transition from nephrology to palliative care
Chronic kidney disease case management	- Provides patients with early discussions about treatment modalities - Allows time to revisit discussions about goals of care upstream in the illness trajectory	- Does not extend to patients once they transition to dialysis
Medical management without dialysis	- Provides a coherent protocol for services to manage symptoms and to help patients prepare for end of life phase - Ideally, helps patients avoid unwanted hospitalizations and high intensity end of life care	- In United States, no clear payment source for additional services, such as case management, needed in this model
Concurrent hospice/dialytic care	- Provides care option that many patients want - Increases access to hospice - May improve end of life experience for dialysis patients - May reduce end of life costs for dialysis patients (evidence not yet available) - Palliative care alongside dialysis may improves quality of life upstream in the illness trajectory (no evidence in dialysis but in other populations)	- Need funding source, (usually charitable) to enable either hospice to cover cost of dialysis or dialysis organization to cover cost of hospice - Both dialysis team and hospice teams need to "skill up" in managing palliative dialysis during end-of-life phase because this is uncommon practice

TABLE 4.1. Continued

Supportive Nephrology Care Model	Pros	Cons
Comprehensive regional or systemic programs	- Comprehensive reform of system assures broadest access to patients to best care - Full array of supportive care services available - Lasting culture change possible - When robust evaluation and quality improvement included, can become a system that continues to evolve and improve based on incorporation of new evidence	- Time and resource intensive to establish - Needs visionary and dedicated leadership to accomplish - Long time window to establish

A white paper from the Coalition for Supportive Care of Kidney Patients described the experience of 16 programs around the world that had implemented supportive kidney care.[23] Program leaders identified facilitators of success as

- Providing training to the nephrology providers, especially on communication and symptom management;
- Creating active collaboration and exchange between nephrology and palliative care;
- Getting local champions, often nurses, to lead change;
- Using appropriate messages about medical management without dialysis;
- Fostering change to the entire culture of kidney care;
- Conducting research to advance the evidence base; and
- Having national guidelines to guide practice.

Barriers to success identified in the Coalition for Supportive Care of Kidney Patients white paper ranged from broad cultural attitudes toward death to specific economic and regulatory issues. General cultural reluctance to discuss death was mentioned as impeding open discussion. The particular culture of nephrology—centered on technology and dialysis—was mentioned numerous times as a significant barrier.

Economic incentives for dialysis were perceived as having a strong impact in the United States, whereas in other countries the economic incentive favoring dialysis was not as strong. Lack of resources to implement supportive care, lack of time to spend in family discussions, and a sense that staff assigned to supportive care might be diverted to the perceived "higher" priority of providing dialysis were all cited as impediments. Finally, the lack of a strong evidence base was cited many times as a barrier, both in convincing colleagues and in providing patients with information they need to make decisions. Further work is needed to build evidence for which program models are most effective.

Practice Pointers

- Six different innovative models have emerged for providing kidney supportive care: embedded, mobile/visiting, CKD case management, medical management without dialysis, concurrent hospice/dialysis, and comprehensive regional or system-wide programs.

- Ideally, a comprehensive supportive kidney care program covers all of these elements:
  - During CKD care, patient education that includes option of medical management without dialysis;
  - Medical management without dialysis;
  - Supportive care concurrent with dialysis; and
  - End-of-life transition.
- Individual programs have demonstrated positive impact on outcomes such as advance care planning and place of death, but there is not yet systematic evidence comparing impact of model type on effectiveness or cost-effectiveness.

Practice Improvement Opportunities.

- When selecting a model, assess whether local conditions favor starting by adding supportive care for patients receiving dialysis or starting by developing a medical management without dialysis pathways.
- Bring palliative care expertise into the nephrology setting by "skilling up" nephrology providers, and/or by developing strong clinical collaborations with palliative care specialists.
- Innovators in supportive kidney care identified these factors as facilitators for program success:
  - Training for the nephrology providers, especially on communication and symptom management;
  - Active collaboration and exchange between nephrology and palliative care;
  - Local champions, often nurses, to lead change;
  - Appropriate messages about medical management without dialysis;
  - Change to the entire culture of kidney care;
  - Research to advance the evidence base; and
  - National guidelines to guide practice.

References

1. Harris DCH, Davies SJ, Finkelstein FO, et al. Increasing access to integrated ESKD care as part of universal health coverage. *Kidney Int.* 2019;95(4):S1–S33. doi:10.1016/j.kint.2018.12.005
2. Purtell L, Sowa PM, Berquier I, et al. The Kidney Supportive Care programme: characteristics of patients referred to a new model of care. *BMJ Support Palliat Care.* December 2018. doi:10.1136/bmjspcare-2018-001630 [Epub ahead of print]
3. Lam DY, Scherer JS, Brown M, Grubbs V, Schell JO. A conceptual framework of palliative care across the continuum of advanced kidney disease. *Clin J Am Soc Nephrol.* 2019;14(4):635–641. doi:10.2215/CJN.09330818
4. Luckett T, Phillips J, Agar M, Virdun C, Green A, Davidson PM. Elements of effective palliative care models: a rapid review. *BMC Health Serv Res.* 2014;14(1):136. doi:10.1186/1472-6963-14-136
5. Scherer JS, Wright R, Blaum CS, Wall SP. Building an outpatient kidney palliative care clinical program. *J Pain Symptom Manage.* 2018;55(1):108–116.e2. doi:10.1016/j.jpainsymman.2017.08.005
6. Brown MA, Collett GK, Josland EA, Foote C, Li Q, Brennan FP. CKD in elderly patients managed without dialysis: survival, symptoms, and quality of life. *Clin J Am Soc Nephrol.* 2015;10(2):260–268. doi:10.2215/CJN.03330414

7. Kidney CARES (Comprehensive Advanced Renal Disease and End Stage Renal Disease Support) Program at NYU Langone Nephrology Associates, Division of Nephrology. https://med.nyu.edu/medicine/nephrology/research/kidney-cares-program. Accessed July 3, 2019.
8. Outpatient Clinics, Palliative and Supportive Institute, UPMC. https://www.upmc.com/services/palliative-and-supportive-institute/our-services/outpatient-clinics. Accessed July 3, 2019.
9. Meet them where they are: bringing palliative care to dialysis patients. *Center to Advance Palliative Care.* https://www.capc.org/seminar/poster-sessions/meet-them-where-they-are-bringing-palliative-care-to-dialysis-patients/. Accessed July 3, 2019.
10. Johnson DS, Meyer KB. Delaying and averting dialysis treatment: patient protection or moral hazard? *Am J Kidney Dis.* 2018;72(2):251–254. doi:10.1053/j.ajkd.2018.01.042
11. BC Provincial Renal Agency. Conservative care pathway. http://www.bcrenalagency.ca/resource-gallery/Documents/BCPRA Conservative Care Pathway Guideline.pdf. Published 2016.
12. Hoffman A, Tranter S, Josland E, Brennan F, Brown M. Renal supportive care in conservatively managed patients with advanced chronic kidney disease: a qualitative study of the experiences of patients and their carers/families. *Ren Soc Australas J.* 2017;13(3):100–106.
13. Davison SN, Tupala B, Wasylynuk BA, Siu V, Sinnarajah A, Triscott J. Recommendations for the care of patients receiving conservative kidney management: focus on management of CKD and symptoms. *Clin J Am Soc Nephrol.* 2019;14(4):626–634. doi:10.2215/CJN.10510917
14. Kurella Tamura M. Recognition for conservative care in kidney failure. *Am J Kidney Dis.* 2016;68(5):671–673. doi:10.1053/j.ajkd.2016.08.009
15. Ladin K, Pandya R, Kannam A, et al. Discussing conservative management with older patients with CKD: an interview study of nephrologists. *Am J Kidney Dis.* 2018;71(5):627–635. doi:10.1053/j.ajkd.2017.11.011
16. Wong SPY, McFarland LV, Liu C-F, Laundry RJ, Hebert PL, O'Hare AM. Care practices for patients with advanced kidney disease who forgo maintenance dialysis. *JAMA Intern Med.* 2019;179(3):305–313. doi:10.1001/jamainternmed.2018.6197
17. Ladin K, Smith AK. Active medical management for patients with advanced kidney disease. *JAMA Intern Med.* 2019;179(3):313. doi:10.1001/jamainternmed.2018.6195
18. Corbett CM. Effecting palliative care for patients with chronic kidney disease by increasing provider knowledge. *Nephrol Nurs J.* 2018;45(6):24.
19. Pathways Phase 2. School of Nursing, The George Washington University. https://nursing.gwu.edu/pathways-phase-2. Accessed November 17, 2019.
20. Expanding open access with dialysis. *Chapters Health System.* https://www.chaptershealth.org/dialysis-expanding-open-access-services/. Accessed July 3, 2019.
21. Lagnese K, Schell J. Partnerships in dialysis and palliative care and hospice: "innovative models for end-of-life care for end-stage renal disease patients" (TH315). *J Pain Symptom Manage.* 2019;57(2):372. doi:10.1016/j.jpainsymman.2018.12.047
22. ACI Renal Network. NSW renal supportive care service model. *Agency for Clinical Evaluation.* https://aci.health.nsw.gov.au/__data/assets/pdf_file/0020/443072/Renal-Supportive-Care-Service-Model.pdf. Published 2018.
23. Lupu D, Nyirenda J. Creating supportive nephrology programs: lessons learned around the world. *Coalition for Supportive Care of Kidney Patients*; https://www.kidneysupportivecare.org, 2018.

SECTION II

Supportive Care Capacity—Creating the Infrastructure to Provide Kidney Supportive Care

5

Assessing Patients' Unmet Palliative Care Needs With Tools for Assessment

Chandra Thomas and Amanda Halpin

High symptom burden of living with kidney disease negatively impacts patients' health-related quality of life, making it important to routinely screen for symptoms to identify their unmet needs. Research shows that clinicians are inaccurate at estimating symptoms of their patients; therefore, validated tools called patient-reported outcome measures have been developed to improve screening for and identification of troublesome symptoms patients are experiencing. Routinely incorporating patient-reported outcome measures will likely require some change to many current practices; utilizing a change management plan with appointed champion(s) and a supporting multidisciplinary team can help ensure the success of this practice transformation.

Case Example

Anne is a 73-year-old woman who has been treated with hemodialysis for 3 years for end-stage kidney disease (ESKD) due to autosomal dominant polycystic disease. She is mildly frail. She has excellent metabolic parameters and rarely has complaints for the nursing staff or nephrologists. Staff have noticed that Anne ambulates with more difficulty when coming into the unit with her walker.

A practice change is implemented, and the Integrated Palliative Outcome Scale–Renal (IPOS-R) is administered to all individuals in the unit who agree. Anne reports that she is overwhelmingly impacted by weakness or lack of energy and difficulty sleeping. Staff in the unit are quite surprised. Nursing staff sit with Anne and complete a sleep history noting very poor sleep hygiene. Education is provided, and Anne and the nurses work together to address napping during dialysis, replacing it with gentle seated cycling exercise. Two months later, the IPOS-R is repeated, and Anne now indicates that she is only slightly impacted by these symptoms.

Current Evidence

Palliative care, as defined by the World Health Organization and adopted by Kidney Disease: Improving Global Outcomes (KDIGO), "is an approach that improves the HRQL [health-related quality of life] of patients and their families facing the problem associated with life-threatening illness, through the prevention and relief of suffering by means of early identification and impeccable assessment and treatment of pain and other problems, physical, psychosocial, and spiritual."[1] The goal of providing quality kidney supportive care is to improve health-related quality of life and reduce suffering of patients living with established chronic kidney disease (CKD).

From the World Health Organization definition, clinicians need to be aware that supportive care needs of patients with kidney disease begin far before reaching ESKD. Consequently, they are obligated to begin assessing the needs of individual patients as early as CKD stage 4. Despite comprehensive predialysis care with multidisciplinary teams, patients living with advanced CKD still experience a high symptom burden, have numerous comorbidities, and a shortened life expectancy with significant physical, emotional, and spiritual suffering.[1-3] Once patients reach CKD stage 5, advance care planning should have ideally preidentified the care route the patient is wishing to pursue. Options to manage renal failure include both renal replacement therapy and medical management without dialysis. Since the mortality of dialysis patients remains quite high, patients selecting a renal replacement therapy have been increasingly recognized as appropriate candidates for continuous supportive care.[1,4,5] Utilizing the surprise question, dialysis mortality prediction equations, and symptom assessment tools, as was done for Anne with the IPOS-R, clinicians can identify the dialysis patients who are likely to benefit from supportive care, allowing them to receive treatment to better support their needs as they potentially near the end of their life.[6]

Providing quality supportive care requires an understanding of the potential diverse needs of the patient, which can range from physical effects of their disease (ie, shortness of breath), to psychological and psychosocial sequelae (ie, anxiety and depression). Needs that are not addressed and where additional support is required are deemed unmet needs. The goal of identifying unmet needs is to determine what is most important to the patient and address their needs to improve their health-related quality of life (HRQL).

Increased symptom burden in dialysis patients has been shown to negatively impact patients' HRQL. Additionally, it has been demonstrated that healthcare providers are inaccurate at estimating patients' symptoms and often only exhibit a "weak" agreement with the patient's rating of severity. Nephrologist sensitivity at estimating the severity of a patient's symptoms is often less than 50%, with nursing estimates only being slightly better.[7] The same study also found a higher patient-reported symptom burden was associated with a decrease in HRQL, showing that it is important to utilize a patient-reported assessment of symptoms.

Relying on unsystematic clinician assessment of symptoms would potentially miss opportunities to intervene and relieve suffering with a goal of improving HRQL. Given the importance of patient involvement in the symptom assessment, many symptom assessment tools have been created to help bridge this gap. These validated tools, known as patient-reported outcome measures (PROMs) help in the assessment of symptoms, functionality, and mental/social health and may also improve the quality of interactions between health professionals and the patient by redirecting care toward a patient-centered model of care. The benefits of using PROMs include better patient–physician communication, increased patient satisfaction, and improved quality of life.[8]

TABLE 5.1. Types of Patient-Reported Outcome Measures

	Benefits	Drawbacks	Example
Generic	Intended to be relevant to the widest range of patient conditions in the general population	• May lack condition specific items • Often difficult to complete regularly in clinical practice due to the length of the PROMs	SF-36
Preference-based	Broad in content, but also provide additional utility (ie, cost-analysis of intervention)	• May lack condition specific items	EQ-5D
Condition/Population Specific	Typically focused on a specific health condition	• Not applicable to all conditions • May not be able to identify unmet needs that result from comorbid conditions	Renal-specific measures: ESAS-R IPOS-R

Abbreviations: EQ-5D, European quality-of-life instrument; ESAS-R, Edmonton Symptom Assessment Scale–Renal; IPOS-R, Integrated Palliative Outcome Scale–Renal; PROMs, patient-reported outcome measures; SF-36, Medical Outcomes Study 36-Item Short-Form Health Survey.

There are several different types of PROMs that can be used to assess the unmet needs of patients living with kidney disease (Table 5.1). The 3 broad categories of PROMs include generic PROMs, preference-based PROMs, and condition/population-specific PROMs. Generic PROMs include items intended to be relevant to the widest range of patients' conditions in the general population and include tools like the 36-Item Short-Form Health Survey (SF-36). Preference-based measures are also broad in content, but additionally provide other utilities or values regarding health (like cost–utility analysis of intervention). Condition-specific instruments are often more focused on a particular health condition and provide greater clinical appeal due to inclusion of content specific to the condition and increased likelihood of responsiveness to interventions. Kidney-specific measures include Kidney Disease Quality-of-Life forms, the Edmonton Symptom Assessment Scale–Renal (ESAS-R), and the IPOS-R.[8]

There are numerous PROMs that have been studied for use in patients living with kidney disease (Table 5.2). The University of Oxford published in 2010 "A Structured Review of PROMs for Adults with Chronic Kidney Disease" and has recommended the use of the European quality-of-life instrument EQ-5D, the Medical Outcomes Study's SF-36, or the Kidney Disease Quality of Life (KDQOL).[8] The most studied generic and renal-specific PROMs are generic the SF-36 and the KDQOL—both the long form (LF) and short form (SF). The SF-36 is a generic health status instrument with 36-items assessing health across eight domains: bodily pain, general health perceptions, mental health, physical functioning, role limitations due to emotional health problems, role limitations due to physical health problems, social functioning, and vitality. All items on the SF-36 use categorical scoring with a range of 2 to 6 options. Scoring the SF-36 uses a weighted scoring algorithm, which typically needs computer programming, making it less appealing for wide-spread clinical use.[8]

The renal-specific KDQOL-LF is an additional PROM that has been well studied and actually includes the SF-36 items together with additional items assessing kidney-specific

TABLE 5.2. PROMs for Use in Patients with Kidney Disease

	Type of PROM		Scoring	Limitations
SF-36	Generic	Assesses health across eight domains: • Bodily pain • General health perceptions • Mental health • Physical functioning • Role limitations due to emotional health problems • Role limitations due to physical health problems • Social functioning • Vitality	All items are scored categorically with 2 to 6 options. Overall scoring via weighted scoring algorithm from computer program.	Requires computer programming for scoring. Longer than many of the renal specific PROMs. Lacks renal specific content.
KDQOL-LF and SF	Generic and Condition Specific	Includes the items in the SF-36, but adds in kidney-specific items SF contains 80 total items	All items are scored categorically with 2 to 6 options. Overall scoring is done by precoded numerical values to the categorical responses.	Often impractical for clinical use due the length of the PROM (the KDQOL-SF is 80 items long).
EQ-5D	Preference-based	Consists of 2 sections: • The EQ-5D, which assess health across five domains: anxiety/depression, mobility, pain, self-care, usual activities • EQ thermometer	Each domain has a 3-point categorical scale. EQ thermometer scored via a visual analogue of 0 to 100. From the 2 scores, an index score is then calculated.	Lacks renal specific content.
ESAS-R	Condition Specific	Has 10 items that cover physical and psychological symptoms. The last item is an optional spot for the patient to add an additional symptom.	Each symptom is scored on a visual analogue scale of 0 to 10. Individual symptom scores are tallied to make a combined symptom distress score.	Brevity of the questionnaire may not provide as robust of information as the longer PROMS.
IPOS-R	Condition Specific	Has ten items with 23 subitems and covers physical symptoms, psychological symptoms, and caregiver concerns.	Utilizes a 0 to 4 Likert scale with the tallied score representing total symptom burden.	Brevity of the questionnaire may not provide as robust of information as the longer PROMS.

Abbreviations: EQ-5D, European quality-of-life instrument; ESAS-R, Edmonton Symptom Assessment Scale–Renal; IPOS-R, Integrated Palliative Outcome Scale–Renal; KDQOL, Kidney Disease Quality of Life–Long Form; LF, long form; PROM, patient-reported outcome measure; SF, short form; SF-36, Medical Outcomes Study 36-Item Short-Form Health Survey.

issues. The KDQOL-SF is just a shorter version of the KDQOL-LF and includes the 36-items from the SF-36, plus 43 renal-specific items.[8] At 80-items included in the KDQOL-SF, both the long-form and short-form versions are impractical for inclusion in daily practice, but both remain important tools for researchers.

The EQ-5D is a preference-based PROM that consists of 2 sections: the EQ-5D and the EQ thermometer. The EQ-5D section assesses the health of the patient across 5 domains: anxiety/depression, mobility, pain/discomfort, self-care, and usual activities. Each domain has 1 item and a 3-point categorial scale: no problem, some problem, extreme problems. The EQ thermometer section is a single vertical 20 cm visual analogue scale with a range of 0 to 100, where 100 represents the best possible health. This information and weights based on societal valuations of health states are then used to calculate an index score. The EQ-5D is much shorter than the SF-36 and the KDQOL-LF/SF, making it more practical for wide-spread clinical use.[8]

Since the Oxford review has been published, additional kidney-specific PROMs have been validated for use in kidney disease. These condition specific measures include both the ESAS-R and the IPOS-R. These tools are highly focused on symptoms specifically related to patients with kidney disease and only take a few minutes at most to complete. Many supportive care programs have incorporated a condition-specific PROM into routine practice as a tool to identify patients' unmet needs and ongoing symptoms.

The ESAS-R has been adapted from the original version that was commonly used in palliative care and oncology settings to be specific for the symptoms of kidney disease. The ESAS-R is a simple and short tool that the patient completes independently to help avoid any bias from nurses or physicians. The ESAS-R has 10 items and covers physical and psychological symptoms, with the last item being an optional spot for the patient to add an additional symptom not covered in the survey. Each symptom is scored on a visual analogue scale from 0 (no symptom) to 10 (worst possible symptom). The individual symptom scores are tallied to make a combined symptom distress score that ranges from 0 to 100.[8] The ESAS-R has been validated in patients with kidney disease, and the overall symptom distress score strongly correlated with change in the KDQOL-SF subscales symptom/problem list, burden of kidney disease, effects of kidney disease, overall physical health composite, and overall mental health composite.[9,10]

The IPOS-R is also a short tool that has been tailored from the original Palliative Outcome Scale to be specific for the symptoms experienced by patients living with kidney disease. The IPOS-R has 10 items with 23-subitems and covers physical symptoms, psychological symptoms, and caregiver concerns (ie, caregiver anxiety). The patient scores their symptoms on a 0- to 4-point Likert scale with the tallied score representing the total symptom burden.[8] The IPOS-R has been studied in a variety of renal patients including hemodialysis, peritoneal dialysis, and medical management without dialysis patients. In the validation of the IPOS-R, increased symptom burden negatively correlated with the composite physical and mental health scores on the KDQOL-SF and was sensitive to change over time. Like the ESAS-R, the IPOS-R only takes a few minutes to complete, making it a good option for incorporation into routine practice.[11]

As condition-specific PROMs, the ESAS-R and the IPOS-R provide a good estimate of the concerns and symptoms most relevant to the patient. Both tools touch on psychological symptoms but only provide basic screening for depression or anxiety symptoms. The presence of depressive symptoms in CKD and ESKD are significantly higher when compared with the general population with up to 20% of CKD patients experiencing depression and up to 45% of patients at the onset of ESKD.[12] Given the high prevalence of depressive symptoms, PROMs specifically related to depression have been validated in patients with kidney disease and should be used when the ESAS-R or IPOS-R identify depression and anxiety as a potential concern for the patient. The Beck Depression Inventory is a 16-item screen for major depression that has been validated in CKD and ESKD with a score of 11 or greater being sensitive for detecting depression. It is important to be aware of the high rates of depression experienced by those living with kidney disease and screen for the symptoms as necessary.[12,13]

Routinely administering PROMs in clinical practice may require change in some centers, and adopting a change management strategy may help to ensure the success of implementing this change. When formulating a change management plan, it can be helpful to use the Plan–Do–Study–Act (PDSA) cycle to test a small-scale change to see if it results in improvement in the quality of care delivered to patients (see Figure 5.1).[14] Appointing a champion or champions, in addition to having a supporting interdisciplinary team can help implement the PDSA cycle and determine how to best incorporate the chosen PROM into routine practice. The interdisciplinary team should establish which care-provider role will be responsible for administering the PROM (ie, nurse, nephrologist, social worker, etc.) to standardize patient care at the facility. During the implementation phase, the interdisciplinary team should be available to meet and troubleshoot any logistical issues that arise with implementation of the PROM. Measuring the results of the new approach is a key element when testing and implementing changes; it is important for clinicians to establish the baseline quality of symptom assessment at their institution, so they have an initial measure to which to compare the results after implementation of the PROM.

Once a PDSA cycle has been implemented on a small scale (ie, a subset of patients), the results should be reviewed by the team to ensure there has been improvement in care delivery to the patients. Once the PROM has been successful on a small scale, the change should be routinely incorporated into all applicable clinical practices. Administering and

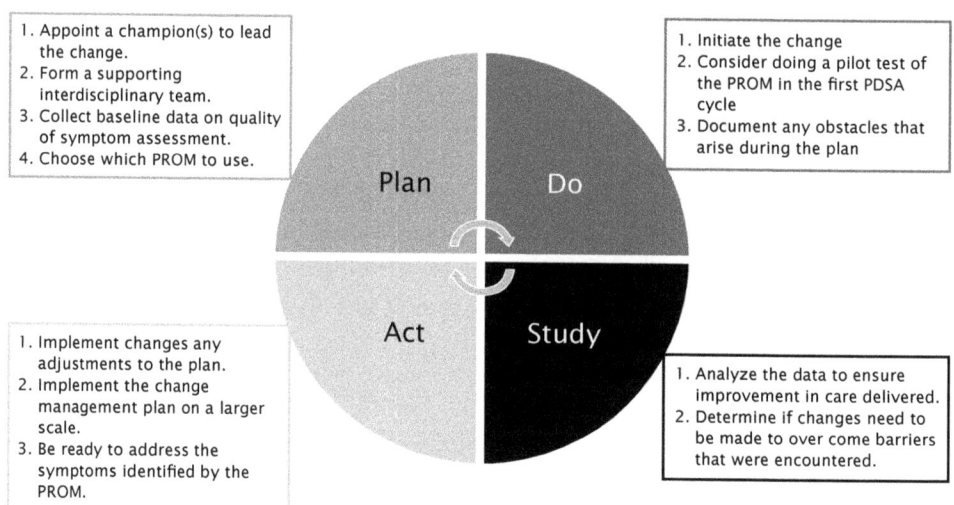

FIGURE 5.1. PDSA cycle for implementing PROMS. Abbreviations: PDSA, plan–do–study–act; PROMS, patient-reported outcome measures.

collecting the PROMs is not sufficient to improve patient HRQL; it will be important to have a plan to address the unmet needs of the patients identified by the PROM that the CKD clinic and the dialysis center choose to utilize.

Applicable Guidelines

Although there are not established guidelines on the use of patient-reported outcomes for use in kidney disease, there is an executive summary from KDIGO that states these validated PROMS are "appropriate for routine screening in renal programs to identify patients' common and troublesome symptoms, including patients who are in the last days of life."[1] This summary also states that symptom assessment is an integral component of quality care for patients with advanced CKD, and that regular global screening with a validated tool should be incorporated into routine clinical practice.

Summary

Supportive care needs are not limited to CKD stage 5 medical management without dialysis patients; clinicians need to remember to consider the needs of patients on the continuum of kidney disease, from CKD stage 4 through to those on dialysis.[1-3] Supportive care should be provided to all dialysis patients,[1,4,5] but utilizing a mortality risk prediction equation can help identify patients who have a higher priority for more intensive supportive care needs.[6] Delivering high-quality supportive care requires regular screening and management of patient symptoms and needs.[1] Patient symptoms should be self-reported as research has shown that healthcare providers are inaccurate when they try to estimate a patient's symptom burden.[7] High self-reported symptom burden negatively impacts HRQL, making it important to routinely screen for and manage symptoms of patients living with kidney disease.[2-5] PROMs are tools that have been developed to help in the assessment of symptoms, functionality, and mental/social health. The benefits of using PROMs include better patient–physician communication, increased patient satisfaction, and improved quality of life of the patient.[8] Routinely administering a validated PROM to all CKD and ESKD patients can help improve HRQL by identifying and facilitating treatment of unmet needs and bothersome symptoms patients are experiencing.

Implementing a PROM into routine clinical practice will likely require a change to practice at some centers, making it important to have a change management plan in place. An appointed champion or champions with a supporting multidisciplinary team can help develop a change management plan with a goal of incorporating these PROM tools into routine practice.[14] It will be important to determine which healthcare provider (ie, nurse, physician, etc.) will be responsible for administering the PROM to standardize patient care at your facility. Assessing symptom burden with validated tools is not sufficient to improve HRQL; it is necessary to intervene on the results to alleviate suffering and improve HRQL of CKD and ESKD patients.

Practice Pointers

- Symptom burden negatively impacts the HRQL of the patient.
- Healthcare providers are inaccurate at estimating symptom burden of the patient, so symptoms should always be self-reported by the patient.
- PROMs are tools that have been developed to help in the assessment of symptoms, functionality, and mental/social health.

Practice Improvement Opportunities

- Routinely administer a validated PROM to all CKD and ESKD patients to help improve HRQL by identifying and treating unmet needs and bothersome symptoms the patient is experiencing.
- When implementing change into routine clinical practice, a change management plan should be developed to ensure successful incorporation into practice.
- Appoint a champion or champions with a supporting multidisciplinary team to develop the implementation plan and measure success of the change by comparing it to the baseline practice.

References

1. Davison SN, Levin A, Moss, AH et al. Executive summary of the KDIGO Controversies Conference on Supportive Care in Chronic Kidney Disease: developing a roadmap to improving quality care. *Kidney Int.* 2015;88:447–459.
2. Almutary H, Bonner A, Douglas C. Symptom burden in chronic kidney disease: a review of recent literature. *J Ren Care.* 2013;39:140–150.
3. Pugh-Clarke K, Read SC, Sim J. Symptom experience in non-dialysis-dependent chronic kidney disease: a qualitative descriptive study. *J Ren Care.* 2017;43:197–208.
4. Kimmel PL, Emont SL, Newmann JM, Danko H, Moss AH. ESRD patient quality of life: symptoms, spiritual beliefs, psychosocial factors, and ethnicity. *Am J Kidney Dis.* 2003;42:713–721.
5. Culp S, Lupu D, Arenella C, Armistead N, Moss AH. Unmet supportive care needs in U.S. dialysis centers and lack of knowledge of available resources to address them. *J Pain Symptom Manag.* 2016;51:(4):756–761.
6. Cohen LM, Ruthazer R, Moss AH, Germain MJ. Predicting six-month mortality for patients who are on maintenance hemodialysis. *Clin J Am Soc Nephrol.* 2010;5:72–79.
7. Raj R, Ahuja KDK, Frandsen M, Jose M. Symptoms and their recognition in adult hemodialysis patients: interactions with quality of life. *Nephrology.* 2017;22:228–233.
8. Gibbons EJ, Fitzpatrick R. A structured review of patient-reported outcome measures (PROMs) for chronic kidney disease. Report to the Department of Health NHS Kidney Care 2010. *University of Oxford.* http://phi.uhce.ox.ac.uk/pdf/PROMS_Oxford_KidneyReview_24112010.pdf. Published 2010. Accessed January 28, 2019.
9. Davison SN, Jhangri GS, Johnson JA. Cross-sectional validity of a modified Edmonton symptom assessment system in dialysis patients: a simple assessment of symptom burden. *Kidney Int.* 2006;69(9):1621–1625.
10. Davison SN, Jhangri GS, Johnson JA. Longitudinal validation of a modified Edmonton symptom assessment system (ESAS) in haemodialysis patients. *Nephrol Dial Transplant.* 2006;21(11):3189–3195.

11. Raj R, Ahuja K, Frandsen M, Murtagh F, Jose M. Validation of the IPOS-Renal symptom survey in advanced kidney disease: a cross-sectional study. *J Pain Symptom Manag.* 2018;56(2):281–287.
12. Hedayati SS, Ninhajuddin AT, Toto RD, Morris DW, Rush AJ. Validation of depression screening scales in patients with CKD. *Am J Kidney Dis.* 2009;54(3):433–439.
13. Watnick S, Wang PL, Demadura T, Ganzini T. Validation of 2 depression screening tools in dialysis patients. *Am J Kidney Dis.* 2005;46(5):919–924.
14. Institute for Healthcare Improvement. Science of improvement: forming the team. http://www.ihi.org/resources/Pages/HowtoImprove/ScienceofImprovementFormingtheTeam.aspx. Accessed February 25, 2019.

6

Primary Palliative Care Education for the Multidisciplinary Nephrology Team

J. Pedro Teixeira and Sara A. Combs

Supportive care of patients with progressive kidney failure, like the care needed by all patients with chronic kidney disease and end-stage kidney disease, is most successfully provided through a multidisciplinary team. An effective kidney supportive care program requires that the multidisciplinary team be properly educated on the palliative needs of these patients and that team members develop primary palliative care skills to meet these needs. This chapter presents the case for why nephrology clinicians need to acquire primary palliative care knowledge and skills to better treat their patients. It reviews the existing state of supportive care for patients with kidney disease and of the training in primary palliative care currently provided to nephrology fellows and nephrologists. It recommends the development of a primary palliative care curriculum for members of the multidisciplinary kidney care team involved in patient care and makes suggestions on curriculum content for nephrology clinicians.

Case

Ms. V is an 81-year-old woman with stage 4 chronic kidney disease (CKD) with most recent estimated glomerular filtration rate of 18 mL per minute per 1.73 m². Her comorbidities include coronary disease status post stenting years ago, cerebrovascular disease with a history of transient ischemic attack but no residual neurologic deficit, localized breast cancer on anastrozole, and spinal stenosis with low back pain requiring her to use a wheelchair to get to clinic today. She presents with her daughter for routine nephrology follow-up and has been scheduled with a first-year nephrology fellow who is seeing her for the first time. The patient is upset when the appointment starts as the fellow arrived 15 minutes late after attending to a new consult in the intensive care unit. On review of symptoms, Ms. V states she is "fine" apart from her back pain, although the daughter does note some recent poor appetite and increasing forgetfulness. The fellow indicates that, due to worsening of her kidney function, she is going to order ultrasound vein mapping to prepare the patient for a fistula. However, Ms. V, after being explained what a fistula is, responds by indicating that she had a cousin who died after starting dialysis and that she'd "rather die than start dialysis." The fellow becomes frustrated when, after asking the patient and daughter if they would instead like a referral to palliative care clinic, the patient declines and states that she feels fine and "ain't dying yet."

Definition of Primary Palliative Care and Its Need in Nephrology

Despite the immense need for supportive care services among patients with kidney disease, it is unlikely that this need will be met simply through referral to palliative care specialists. Rather, nephrologists—despite the fact that nephrologists themselves are likely to be in shortage[1]—will likely need to carry much of the burden of providing supportive care to patients with CKD and end-stage kidney disease (ESKD).

The American Academy of Hospice and Palliative Medicine appointed a task force in 2008 to estimate the hospice and palliative medicine physician workforce shortage and concluded that another 6,000 to 18,000 individual physicians would be needed simply to meet the demands of 2008.[2] With the further projected aging of the US population, this demand is expected to continue to increase. A model of generalist-plus-specialist palliative care, in which the nonpalliative medicine specialist learns to provide "primary palliative care," has been proposed as a means to help address this shortage (see Figure 6.1).[3]

Primary palliative care refers to skills in palliative care that all providers, regardless of subspecialty, should feel comfortable in providing (see Table 6.1).[3] These skills include leading basic discussions about prognosis, assessing goals of treatment and aligning care with those goals, and basic symptom assessment and management specific to the population served.

Unfortunately, primary palliative care education is often lacking in trainee programs and these skills can be difficult to attain during practice without guided or intentional learning.

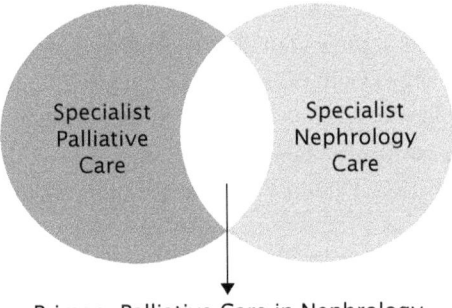

Primary Palliative Care in Nephrology

FIGURE 6.1. Conceptual model of primary kidney supportive care in nephrology. Adapted from Bickel KE, McNiff K, Buss MK, et al. Defining high-quality palliative care in oncology practice: an American Society of Clinical Oncology/American Academy of Hospice and Palliative Medicine guidance statement. *J Oncol Pract.* 2016;12(9):e828–e838.

TABLE 6.1. Primary and Specialty Palliative Care Skills

Primary Palliative Care	Specialty Palliative Care
• Basic management of pain and symptoms • Basic management of depression and anxiety • Basic discussions about 　• Prognosis 　• Goals of treatment 　• Suffering 　• Code status	• Management of refractory pain or other symptoms • Management of more complex depression, anxiety, grief, and existential distress • Assistance with conflict resolution regarding goals or methods of treatment 　• Within families 　• Between staff and families 　• Among treatment teams • Assistance in addressing cases of near futility

Adapted from Quill TE, Abernethy AP. Generalist plus specialist palliative care—creating a more sustainable model. *N Engl J Med.* 2013;368(13):1173–1175.

Current State of Palliative Care Education to Nephrology Trainees in North America

The program requirements outlined by the Accreditation Council for Graduate Medical Education for US nephrology fellowships assert that "clinical experience must include supervised involvement in dialysis therapy, including ... end-of-life care and pain management for patients undergoing chronic hemodialysis and peritoneal dialysis," but these requirements do not specify how this is to be accomplished.[4] Indeed, significant deficits in primary palliative care education appear to exist in nephrology training programs.

A 2013 survey of over 200 US nephrology fellows documented that quality of teaching of renal palliative care remains of poor quality and infrequent,[5] with no significant improvement in findings since a similar 2003 survey.[6] Interestingly, fellows in 2013 were overall *less accurate* in their ability to estimate mortality rates of ESKD patients than their 2003 counterparts.[5] In addition, fewer than half of fellows report receiving explicit teaching in the majority of palliative care nephrology content areas, despite the fact that the majority thought it was important to learn to provide care at the end of life, and nearly all believed physicians have a responsibility to help patients at the end of life.[5] When asked in an open-ended question, "In your opinion what one change would most improve end-of-life care education for fellows in Nephrology?" 29% of nephrology trainees suggested incorporation of a palliative medicine rotation and 14% requested formal didactics in palliative or end-of-life issues.[5] A similar survey of over 100 fellows in 2012 found that over 80% of the respondents' programs did not offer formal clinical training or a rotation in palliative medicine during their fellowship and that nearly 1 out of 5 fellows surveyed felt obligated to offer dialysis to every patient regardless of benefit. Similar to the 2013 study, over two-thirds of the respondents to this survey thought that a formal rotation in palliative medicine during fellowship would be helpful to them.[7]

Given these previous findings, it is not surprising that fewer than 40% of practicing nephrologists in the United States and Canada report that they feel very prepared to help their ESKD patients make end-of-life decisions.[8] The need for improved palliative care education among nephrologists is further underscored by a survey of dialysis professionals and administrators published in 2016.[9] Only 4.5% of the respondents believed their dialysis centers were presently providing high-quality supportive care, noting specific needs for bereavement support, spiritual support, and end-of-life care discussions.[9] Interestingly, the respondents identified that the "lack of a predictive algorithm for prognosis" and lack of "guidelines to help with decision-making in seriously ill patients" as major barriers to the provision of supportive care, but the majority were unaware that evidence-based validated prognostic models,[10,11] including an online calculator[12] and a clinical practice guideline to help with decision-making,[13] were already available.[9] Another recent survey of US nephrologists revealed that only one-third would even present the option of medical management without dialysis to their older patients with advanced CKD.[14]

Primary Palliative Care Education of the Multidisciplinary Team

It is largely accepted that supportive care is optimally provided via a multidisciplinary team, which may consist of physicians or advanced care practitioners (ie, nurse practitioners or physician assistants), nurses, social workers, pharmacists, psychologists, spiritual care providers, nutritionists, and volunteers. A team allows for a more holistic approach to the patient and their caregiver(s)' needs. Education in primary palliative care skills therefore lends itself well to multidisciplinary team-based learning. Studies have demonstrated that providing palliative care education in a multidisciplinary environment, rather than being oriented towards specific professions, can be very effective by helping to promote a team environment, establish common ground between disciplines, define boundaries and goals, and recognize mutual dependency.[15,16] Multidisciplinary palliative care education can help providers explore similarities and differences in skills, knowledge, and ideologies; allows them to begin to recognize their complementary skills and resources; and provides scope for greater opportunities for open communication.[16]

Of course, it is important that the variably skilled multidisciplinary audience be considered when developing or considering course curricula for the renal supportive care team. Choosing workshops or curricula that do not appropriately align with the audience members' backgrounds may result in the opposite of the intended effect, such as making the provider feel underappreciated or undervalued.

Certainly, developing relationships with palliative care colleagues can be instrumental to the success of a renal supportive care program; if they are able and willing to provide didactics to the multidisciplinary team, this not only improves primary palliative care knowledge but can contribute to development of team comradery and morale. Of course, many nephrology teams do not have ready access to palliative care or the teams' ability to provide didactics may be limited due to other restrictions; therefore, palliative education must be sought via other modalities. Table 6.2 lists useful nephrology-specific palliative, geriatric, or end-of-life education resources for all members of the multidisciplinary team.

TABLE 6.2. Palliative Care Resources in ESKD

Resource	Description (and website)
ASN Geriatric Nephrology Curriculum	An online curriculum addressing the most significant aspects of caring for aging patients with kidney disease (www.asn-online.org/education/distancelearning/curricula/geriatrics)
ASN Advances in Geriatric Nephrology Precourse	A 2-day precourse to the annual ASN meeting offered every few years, most recently in 2015 (https://www.asn-online.org/education/kidneyweek/)
ASN Improving Dialysis Rounds for Geriatric Patients	A series of videos conveying skills in geriatric nephrology (www.asn-online.org/kidneydisease/geriatrics/rounds)
RPA Clinical Practice Guideline and Toolkit on Shared Decision-Making in Dialysis	Recommendations for initiation, forgoing, and discontinuing dialysis and toolkit for estimating prognosis and assessing symptoms (www.renalmd.org/store/ViewProduct.aspx?id=7014408)
Coalition for Supportive Care of Kidney Patients	Formed by Renal Network 5, this website includes a variety of resources to support palliative and end-of-life care in ESKD (www.kidneysupportivecare.org)
Core Curriculum in Nephrology: Palliative Care[a]	Entry, published in 2004, in AJKD's Core Curriculum series of topic outlines directed towards renal fellows in training
NephroTalk[b]	A communication skills workshop for nephrology fellows adapted from oncology literature (OncoTalk)
Supportive Care for the Renal Patient[c]	Textbook in second edition (2010) reviewing palliative care management for patients with ESKD

Adapted from Kurella Tamura M, Meier DE. Five policies to promote palliative care for patients with ESRD. *Clin J Am Soc Nephrol.* 2013;8(10):1783–1790.
Abbreviations: AJKD, American Journal of Kidney Disease; ASN, American Society of Nephrology; ESKD, end-stage kidney disease; RPA, Renal Physicians Association.
[a] Moss AH, Holley JL, Davison SN, et al. Palliative care. *Am J Kidney Dis.* 2004;43(1):172–173.
[b] Schell JO, Cohen RA, Green JA, et al. NephroTalk: evaluation of a palliative care communication curriculum for nephrology fellows. *J Pain Symptom Manag.* 2018;56(5):767–773 e762.
[c] Chambers EJ, Germain M, Brown EA. *Supportive Care for the Renal Patient.* 2nd ed. Oxford: Oxford University Press; 2010.

Primary Palliative Care Education of Nephrology Providers: Communication Skills

As previously alluded to, specific deficits in communication skills may account in part for the discrepancy between care that patients with renal failure report they desire and the care they receive. Effective communication skills are a core feature of being able to successfully provide primary palliative care and achieve goal-concordant, patient-centered care in patients with serious life-limiting illness in general[17] and specifically kidney disease.[18] Unfortunately, as previously noted, communication skills training is frequently not emphasized in medical education (see Table 6.3).

TABLE 6.3. Educational Resources for Development of Communication Skills

Program Name	Target Audience	Website
Face-to-face workshops		
VitalTalk	Physicians	https://vitaltalk.org
Utah Certificate of Palliative Care Education	Mid-career healthcare providers	https://continue.utah.edu/proed/palliativecare
National Center for Ethics in Health Care Life Sustaining Treatments Initiative	Physicians, NPs, PAs, Nurses, Social Workers, spiritual care providers, psychologists, and pharmacists working in the US VA system	https://www.ethics.va.gov/LST.asp
Four Seasons Consulting Group Palliative Care Immersion Course	Physicians, NPs, PAs, social workers	https://www.fourseasonsconsultinggroup.com/education/palliative-care-immersion-course
Online modules		
California State University Primary Palliative Care Education	Physicians, NPs, PAs	https://csupalliativecare.org/programs/primary-pc/communication-and-acp
Center to Advance Palliative Care (CAPC)	Physicians, NPs, PAs	https://www.capc.org/providers/courses/
VitalTalk	Physicians	https://vitaltalk.org
Certificate/degree program		
University of Colorado Master of Science in Palliative Care degree or Interprofessional Palliative Care Certificate	Physicians, NPs, PAs, nurses, social workers, spiritual care providers, psychologists, pharmacists, ethicists	http://www.ucdenver.edu/academics/colleges/Graduate-School/academic-programs/Palliative%20Care/Pages/home.aspx
University of Washington Graduate Certificate in Palliative Care	Physicians, nurses, social workers, spiritual care providers, and others	http://uwpctc.org/
Penn State College of Nursing Primary Palliative Care Certificate	Nurses	https://bulletins.psu.edu/graduate/programs/certificates/primary-palliative-care-graduate-credit-certificate-program/#certificaterequirementstext
University of Maryland Online Master of Science and Graduate Certificates in Palliative Care	Physicians, nurses, social workers, NPs, PAs, spiritual care providers, psychologists, pharmacists, ethicists	https://graduate.umaryland.edu/palliative/About-the-Program/

Adapted from Carroll T, El-Sourady M, Karlekar M, Richeson A. Primary palliative care education programs: review and characterization. *Am J Hosp Palliat Care*. 2018:1049909118809947.
Abbreviations: NPs, nurse practitioners; PAs, physicians assistants; VA, Veterans Affairs.

Guidelines for Development of Palliative Care Education Programs and Practice Pointers

Although a variety of kidney-specific palliative care resources have been published or made available online, no guidelines on specifically how to best provide renal palliative care *education* have been published in the literature thus far. However, the most comprehensive renal palliative care education guidelines that have been proposed may be the recommendations set forth in the Pathways Project: Change Package.[19]

As part of their series of 14 best practices recommendations, the Pathways Project team identify "provid[ing] education to staff on the principles and practices of primary supportive care, including communication skills"[19] as a key step in creating a system that provides adequate supportive care capacity. They specifically outline a series of discrete improvement process innovations to be implemented in the development of local palliative care education programs. They also outline 3 specific strategies to overcome the potential challenges of implementing such a palliative care education program, including recruiting and training a local palliative care champion to overcome a lack of local supportive care knowledge and skills; seeking mentorship for the champion by networking with the Pathways Project team and local experts to overcome a lack of experience in palliative care education; and garnering institutional buy-in and using multiple formats geared toward learner-centered preferences to overcome the time constraints of CKD practice and dialysis center schedules.

If successful, the project may prove to be a useful model for implementation of supportive nephrology care at other sites across the United States.

Summary

Patients with CKD and ESKD have many supportive care needs. Unfortunately, data measuring quality of life, provision of care at the end of life, and utilization of hospice care in the ESKD population demonstrate that patients are not receiving the palliative care expertise that they require. This is largely due to 4 factors: (i) underrecognition of supportive care needs of patients with progressive kidney failure and ESKD; (ii) lack of access to palliative care outpatient services and the worldwide palliative care workforce shortage; and (iii) deficits in nephrology providers' palliative care knowledge and skills, which, in turn, stem from a (iv) lack of palliative care education in nephrology trainee curricula. Fortunately, primary palliative care skills can be successfully taught. Indeed, effectiveness in palliative care education specifically in nephrology has been best demonstrated with communication skills training for nephrology fellows. There are a variety of palliative care resources available that are applicable to all subspecialties, but they are likely to prove specifically useful to nephrologists and multidisciplinary renal supportive care teams. While validated guidelines on the development and implementation of kidney-specific palliative care education programs are still lacking in the nephrology literature, the educational practice recommendations proposed by the Pathways Project appear promising as an effective model for renal palliative care education in the United States. Regardless, successful education in primary palliative care skills is essential to optimal patient-centered care by any multidisciplinary renal supportive care team.

Practice Pointers

- Nephrology providers and trainees largely report that education in primary palliative and end-of-life care falls short of that required to feel competent in providing such care to their patients.
- Primary palliative care skills are effectively taught individually or as a multidisciplinary team.

Practice Improvement Opportunities

- All nephrology training programs should offer palliative care rotations or other structured palliative care experiences including observed trainee–patient interactions.
- Nephrology clinics and dialysis centers should identify team champions who are enthusiastic about primary palliative care education and willing to enact an education plan.

References

1. Parker MG, Ibrahim T, Shaffer R, Rosner MH, Molitoris BA. The future nephrology workforce: will there be one? *Clin J Am Soc Nephrol.* 2011;6(6):1501–1506.
2. Lupu D; American Academy of H, Palliative Medicine Workforce Task Force. Estimate of current hospice and palliative medicine physician workforce shortage. *J Pain Symptom Manage.* 2010;40(6):899–911.
3. Quill TE, Abernethy AP. Generalist plus specialist palliative care—creating a more sustainable model. *N Engl J Med.* 2013;368(13):1173–1175.
4. ACGME Program Requirements for Graduate Medical Education in Nephrology (Internal Medicine). www.acgme.org/Portals/0/PFAssets/ProgramRequirements/148_nephrology_2017-07-01.pdf?ver=2017-04-27-153225-583. Accessed February 28, 2019.
5. Combs SA, Culp S, Matlock DD, Kutner JS, Holley JL, Moss AH. Update on end-of-life care training during nephrology fellowship: a cross-sectional national survey of fellows. *Am J Kidney Dis.* 2015;65(2):233–239.
6. Holley JL, Carmody SS, Moss AH, et al. The need for end-of-life care training in nephrology: national survey results of nephrology fellows. *Am J Kidney Dis.* 2003;42(4):813–820.
7. Shah HH, Monga D, Caperna A, Jhaveri KD. Palliative care experience of US adult nephrology fellows: a national survey. *Ren Fail.* 2014;36(1):39–45.
8. Davison SN, Jhangri GS, Holley JL, Moss AH. Nephrologists' reported preparedness for end-of-life decision-making. *Clin J Am Soc Nephrol.* 2006;1(6):1256–1262.
9. Culp S, Lupu D, Arenella C, Armistead N, Moss AH. Unmet supportive care needs in U.S. Dialysis centers and lack of knowledge of available resources to address them. *J Pain Symptom Manage.* 2016;51(4):756–761 e752.
10. Beddhu S, Bruns FJ, Saul M, Seddon P, Zeidel ML. A simple comorbidity scale predicts clinical outcomes and costs in dialysis patients. *Am J Med.* 2000;108(8):609–613.
11. Cohen LM, Ruthazer R, Moss AH, Germain MJ. Predicting six-month mortality for patients who are on maintenance hemodialysis. *Clin J Am Soc Nephrol.* 2010;5(1):72–79.
12. Fadem SZ, Fadem J. HD mortality predictor. http://touchcalc.com/calculators/sq. Accessed February 28, 2019.

13. Moss AH. Revised dialysis clinical practice guideline promotes more informed decision-making. *Clin J Am Soc Nephrol.* 2010;5(12):2380–2383.
14. Ladin K, Pandya R, Perrone RD, et al. Characterizing approaches to dialysis decision making with older adults: a qualitative study of nephrologists. *Clin J Am Soc Nephrol.* 2018;13(8):1188–1196.
15. Latimer EJ, Kiehl K, Lennox S, Studd S. An interdisciplinary palliative care course for practicing health professionals: ten years' experience. *J Palliat Care.* 1998;14(4):27–33.
16. Koffman J. Multiprofessional palliative care education: past challenges, future issues. *J Palliat Care.* 2001;17(2):86–92.
17. Sanders JJ, Curtis JR, Tulsky JA. Achieving goal-concordant care: a conceptual model and approach to measuring serious illness communication and its impact. *J Palliat Med.* 2018;21(S2):S17–S27.
18. Schell JO, Cohen RA, Green JA, et al. NephroTalk: evaluation of a palliative care communication curriculum for nephrology fellows. *J Pain Symptom Manag.* 2018;56(5):767–773 e762.
19. The Pathways Project. http://go.gwu.edu/pathwaysprojectchangepackage. Accessed April 21, 2020.

Establishing Relationships With Specialty Palliative Care for More Complex Patient Needs

Kate Schueller and Joseph D. Rotella

Interdisciplinary palliative care teams can improve quality of life by addressing the needs and experience of the whole person with chronic kidney disease, including physical, psychological, social, spiritual, cultural, end-of-life, ethical, and practical concerns. Nephrology teams can develop the essential skills to provide primary palliative care for uncomplicated problems, but consultation with a specialty palliative care team is warranted for more severe, complex, or refractory problems. Although specialty palliative care can be delivered in any care setting, it may be a scarce resource outside of a hospital or hospice. Nephrology teams should identify all the specialty palliative care resources available in their community and consider engaging palliative care experts not only in patient care but also in advisory, educational, and quality improvement activities.

Case Study: A Difficult Decision

Mr. Thompson was a 78-year-old man with stage 4 chronic kidney disease (CKD) secondary to hypertension and polycystic kidney disease. He enjoyed drawing and discussing politics. He took daily walks with his wife and helped around the house. He had previously indicated to his nephrologist that he would not pursue dialysis if his renal function worsened. During a follow-up visit, he complained of mental cloudiness. His glomerular filtration rate had dropped to 9 mL/min. He was surprised because he had assumed any decline would be more physical than cognitive. He reconsidered his decision to forego dialysis. He remained conflicted after talking with his nephrologist, who referred him to specialty palliative care to help him sort out his options.

He and his wife met with the palliative care team, including a physician, a social worker, and a chaplain. They explored his priorities and preferences in more detail and outlined possible benefits and burdens of treatment options. The palliative care social worker documented the discussion and updated his advance directives. After deliberation, he decided on a trial of dialysis to improve his mental function so he could engage in the intellectual activities he enjoyed. If he didn't experience a meaningful improvement, he would stop dialysis. The team noticed his wife was unusually quiet.

With gentle probing, she expressed concern about the morality of stopping dialysis once it was initiated. This discordance strained their relationship and increased his ambivalence about dialysis.

The palliative care chaplain facilitated a discussion where the patient and wife considered their differing perspectives and religious beliefs. The chaplain helped his wife engage with her community pastor for further guidance. She learned that it was permitted in her faith to stop a life-prolonging treatment no longer thought to be beneficial. She was relieved that she could fully support her husband's decision for a dialysis trial.

In this chapter we'll review

1. Principles of palliative care as practiced at the primary and specialty level and when to refer to specialty palliative care.
2. Specialty palliative care service delivery in various settings of care.
3. How to find palliative care specialists.
4. How to manage communication and build relationships with palliative care consultants.

Primary and Specialty Palliative Care

Palliative care focuses on improving quality of life for people living with serious illness and their families. Serious illness has been described as "a health condition that carries a high risk of mortality AND either negatively impacts a person's daily function or quality of life, OR excessively strains their caregivers."[1p.S-8] It is estimated that up to 10% of the Medicare fee-for-service population meets this definition.[1] Even with solid growth in the specialty of hospice and palliative medicine over the past few decades, there are simply too few palliative care experts to meet the needs of this population using only a specialty care model. The wide gap between need and supply has led to calls for training all healthcare professionals who treat patients with serious illness in the essential skills of palliative care, such as management of uncomplicated symptoms and communication about prognosis and goals of care.[2] This essential knowledge and skillset for clinicians not specializing in palliative care has been called *primary palliative care* or *generalist palliative care*. Particularly when embedded in disease-specific care settings, such as oncology clinics or dialysis centers, whether at the primary or specialty level, it may be called *supportive care*.

The National Consensus Project Clinical Practice Guidelines for Quality Palliative Care (fourth edition) defines 8 domains of palliative care for patients with serious illness and their families:

1. Structure and processes of care
2. Physical aspects of care
3. Psychological and psychiatric aspects of care
4. Social aspects of care
5. Spiritual, religious, and existential aspects of care
6. Cultural aspects of care
7. Care of the patient nearing the end of life
8. Ethical and legal aspects of care[3]

The cornerstone of palliative care, whether at the primary or specialty level, is a comprehensive assessment by an interdisciplinary team to develop an individualized plan of care that addresses problems in all of these domains. Where primary and specialty palliative care differ is in the level of training of the interdisciplinary team members and their skills in addressing severe, refractory, or complex palliative care problems.

When to Consult Specialty Palliative Care

Many of the supportive care needs for CKD patients can and should be identified and managed by their interdisciplinary nephrology teams. However, when the actual or potential suffering associated with serious illness is more severe, refractory, or complex, consultation with a specialty-level palliative care service is warranted (see Table 7.1). Our case study illustrates some problems that are best addressed by a specialized interdisciplinary palliative care team, including complicated and shifting goals of care, nuanced treatment decisions, spiritual and family concerns, and refractory symptoms and emotional distress. Specialty palliative care

TABLE 7.1. Appropriate Involvement of Primary Palliative Care or Specialty Palliative Care in Nephrology

Primary Palliative Care		Specialty Palliative Care	
Appropriate Involvement	CKD-Specific Example	Appropriate Involvement	CKD-Specific example
Management of uncomplicated pain and symptoms	Initiating non-opioid (eg, gabapentin) or low-dose opioid analgesia (eg, oxycodone) for pain associated with dialysis treatments	Management of refractory pain or other symptoms	Opioid rotation d/t side effects. Methadone initiation/ titration for complex pain. Consideration of procedural options (lidocaine infusions) for symptom management
Management of uncomplicated depression and anxiety	Initiation of an SSRI Referral to mental health services/counseling	Management of more complex depression, anxiety, grief, and existential distress	Patient intolerance to SSRIs or need to consider additional non-SSRI treatments. Assistance with issues related to spiritual distress.
Discussions about Prognosis Goals of treatment Suffering Code status	Reviewing patient specific goals, priorities, and prognosis in the setting of known comorbidities. Using this knowledge to discuss options for treatment of ESKD: dialysis vs transplant vs medical management without dialysis	Assistance with conflict resolution regarding goals or methods of treatment: Within families Between staff and families Among treatment teams	Assisting with family meetings in the setting of prognostic uncertainty and patient/family/clinician disagreement about next steps. Ongoing support and goals of care discussions with patients/families in the setting of an additional concurrent serious illness (cardiac, oncology, respiratory)

Abbreviations: ESKD, end-stage kidney disease; SSRI, selective serotonin reuptake inhibitor.

consultation is appropriate at any point such needs arise in the course of serious illness, from diagnosis to end of life or survivorship. In its *Choosing Wisely* recommendations, the American Academy of Hospice and Palliative Medicine included the following, which is applicable to patients with advanced CKD who choose to pursue transplant or dialysis: "Don't delay palliative care for a patient with serious illness who has physical, psychological, social, or spiritual distress because they are pursuing disease-directed treatment."[4]

Making Difficult Decisions With Ambivalence and Conflicting Goals

Treatment decisions were challenging for this patient as his chronic kidney disease progressed. He was ambivalent about major interventions, and the balance for him between benefits and burdens was fragile and nuanced. There are tools available to nephrologists and patients to facilitate shared decision-making regarding initiation of dialysis.[5-7] However, even with these aids, it can be difficult to determine what trade-offs a patient will accept to meet multiple conflicting goals. In this case, the decision to initiate dialysis was complicated by his wife's religious beliefs regarding the permissibility of stopping it later. The nephrologist and other professionals managing his CKD did not have the training and special skills needed to facilitate making such a complex decision, particularly given his wife's spiritual concerns. They also were unlikely to have time available for multiple intensive family meetings, nor did they have a formal interdisciplinary team structure or process in place to integrate the kidney supportive care plan across all domains of potential suffering. Specialty palliative care teams may identify additional treatment options outside the typical all-or-none, take-it-or-leave-it paradigm; in this case, a time-limited trial of dialysis with a well-defined goal and end point was the best option.

Case Continued: Managing Symptoms and Comorbid Conditions

On follow up, Mr. Thompson reported the transition to home dialysis was initially overwhelming, but he was coping and his mentation had improved. He felt depressed but didn't want to bother his "busy" nephrologist about it. The palliative care team discussed medications and other treatments. He started journaling for mindfulness and was prescribed a selective serotonin reuptake inhibitor. After some medication adjustments, his mood improved, and he reported a good quality of life.

He managed well on home dialysis for the next 2 years, during which he continued to see his nephrology and palliative care teams. After he experienced new back pain, testing revealed metastatic prostate cancer. He explored treatment options with an oncologist, and his nephrology, primary care, and palliative care teams were looped into the discussion.

He decided against treatments he perceived as burdensome, including chemotherapy, but agreed to try hormonal therapy in hopes of lessening the pain. His oncologist and primary care doctor felt uncomfortable prescribing pain medication in the setting of end-stage kidney disease. His palliative care physician assumed responsibility for pain management, which worsened as his cancer progressed. He was initially treated with frequent doses of immediate-release hydromorphone, and then a fentanyl patch was added for long-acting control. Low-dose gabapentin was prescribed for the neuropathic component, and after he reported side effects, his long-acting opioid was rotated from fentanyl to methadone.

Managing Refractory Symptoms

As discussed in chapter 3, patients with kidney disease often experience a heavy burden of symptoms. Frequently, simply assessing symptoms with standardized and comprehensive tools and taking the first steps to treat them will bring a sufficient degree of relief. However, there are times when symptoms are more complex or refractory, and their medical management requires a more specialized approach. Moreover, suffering in the physical domain is usually accompanied by suffering in other domains, including psychological, social, and spiritual, as incorporated in Cicely Saunders's concept of *total pain*.[8] The specialty-level interdisciplinary palliative care team can take a deeper dive to develop an integrated approach to relieving suffering across the multiple domains of whole-person care. In the case outlined, the patient struggled with depression, which required ongoing adjustment of medications outside the comfort zone of the nephrologist. In addition, the nephrologist, primary care physician, and oncologist were uncomfortable prescribing and titrating opioids for treatment of his pain and appropriately asked the specialty palliative care team to take the lead.

Case Continued: Coordinating End-of-Life Care

Mr. Thompson continued home peritoneal dialysis, and his palliative care team supported him and his wife as they planned for the end of life. When his cancer progressed and his life expectancy was a few months, the palliative care team arranged a hospice referral.

He was admitted to hospice with a primary terminal diagnosis of metastatic prostate cancer. He continued to receive dialysis under his ESRD benefit as it was deemed unrelated to his terminal diagnosis, which allowed him the time and mental clarity to complete his end-of-life planning. When he became too weak to manage the peritoneal dialysis treatments safely at home, he stopped dialysis. He died comfortably at home a week later. The hospice team promptly notified his nephrology, oncology, palliative care, and primary care teams, who all expressed their condolences to his wife and other family members. Hospice provided bereavement services for the year following his death.

Ongoing Collaboration and Care Coordination

As time progressed, this patient again faced complex decisions around treatment of his cancer in the setting of end-stage kidney disease and ongoing dialysis. Palliative care teams collaborate with all other active healthcare teams to understand the medical situation and communicate the patient's goals and priorities. In this case, the specialty palliative care team helped the patient to navigate care in the different settings of outpatient primary care, other specialty care clinics, and home-based dialysis and hospice, assuring continuity wherever his illness took him. They made sure his decisions were in line with his evolving goals and priorities, his symptoms were managed to maintain a good quality of life despite the eventual clinical decline that was accelerated by his prostate cancer, his care was well coordinated, and his family and other healthcare teams were supported.

Specialty Palliative Care in Various Care Settings

Specialty palliative care can be delivered in any setting, and although overall access is increasing, it is currently more commonly available in the hospital and hospice than in outpatient or community-based settings. As of 2016, 75% of US hospitals with 50 or more beds reported having palliative care services.[9] Many inpatient palliative care teams, however, are not ideally staffed; in 2014, less than half the hospitals reporting palliative care consultation services met the Joint Commission standard of including on the team at least 1 physician, nurse, social worker, and chaplain.[10] In addition to consultation services, some hospitals have palliative care units where patients are managed primarily by the palliative care team. Specialty palliative care services may also be offered in an outpatient setting. These clinics can be independent or embedded within another specialty, most commonly oncology, or primary care. Increasingly, palliative care services are being offered in other specialty clinics, including cardiology, pulmonology, and neurology. There is ample opportunity to expand access to specialty palliative care within nephrology clinics and dialysis centers. In addition, specialty palliative care is increasingly being offered in community settings, including home-based palliative care services for patients wherever they reside.

The type of consultation offered by a palliative care service depends on the clinical situation. At times, there is a very specific concern to address, and the patient can be returned to the requesting service with recommendations and future follow-up as needed. At other times, a more ongoing collaborative co-management relationship with palliative care can be beneficial. For patients with CKD, palliative care consultants can assist with co-managing severe or complex symptoms or psychological, social, spiritual, or cultural concerns, whether they have opted for transplant, dialysis, or medical management without dialysis. Palliative care experts should work closely with the nephrology team to align their interventions with management of the underlying kidney disease.

How to Locate Specialty Palliative Care Resources

Specialty palliative care services operate within a broad range of practice structures and host organizations, and diligent investigation may be required to locate all the resources available within a particular community. Social workers and case managers are often the best team members to engage in identifying community resources. Palliative care services may be offered within broad health systems, academic medical centers, hospitals, Veteran's

Administration facilities, nursing facilities, community hospice or home health programs, primary care or specialty care clinics (particularly oncology), house call programs, and stand-alone palliative medicine practices. Some commercial payers offer palliative care as a benefit for special populations. Many states have set up palliative care advisory councils or enacted policies to foster increased access to palliative care.[11] The Center to Advance Palliative Care maintains a national Palliative Care Provider Directory, which can be searched by location and care setting.[8]

Managing Communication and Building Relationships With Specialty Palliative Care Teams

Consultation with a specialty palliative care team should be considered whenever there are severe or refractory symptoms, complex psychosocial, spiritual, cultural, or ethical concerns or difficult treatment decisions to make, at any stage in the course of a serious illness (see Box 7.1). In practice, however, palliative care consultations are often initiated very late in the disease process, when a hospice referral is appropriate. It is a disservice to both patients and colleagues to characterize palliative care—or, for that matter, hospice—as being focused on *death,* when, in fact, they are about *living* the best way possible under the circumstances. It is disappointing when patients or families ask for palliative care and are held off with a response like "It's not time for that."

When requesting a specialty palliative care consultation, it is helpful to specify what sort of assistance is desired. Is it support for exploring goals of care and making complex treatment decisions? Or, perhaps, there are difficult symptoms to manage. Often there is tension between the patient, family, and clinicians due to unresolved psychosocial, spiritual,

---

BOX 7.1. Which Patients with Stage 4 and 5 CKD to Consider for Palliative Care Consultation Referral

Complex symptoms (eg, pain, nausea, constipation) refractory to interventions
   Help with difficult decision making around treatments (initiation or cessation of)
   high levels of spiritual, emotional, and social stress
Poor functional status
Hesitance to engage in discussions around goals of care
Multiple hospitalizations
Diagnosis of an additional serious illness (ie, advanced CHF, advanced COPD, advanced dementia, advanced cancer)
Patient/family request for palliative care consultation

Abbreviations: CHF, congestive heart failure; CKD, chronic kidney disease; COPD, chronic obstructive pulmonary disease.

cultural, or ethical issues. The palliative care team will base its recommendations on a comprehensive assessment, but it is helpful to know upfront what needs the referring clinicians have already identified. It is also good consulting etiquette to specify whether one is asking for a 1-time consultation with recommendations, ongoing co-management of the patient, or transfer of primary responsibility to the palliative care service and to indicate the level of urgency.

Since palliative care experts are a scarce resource in many communities, it is helpful to build long-term relationships with them and look for ways to engage them in activities that add value beyond providing consultation on individual patients. Some organizations invite palliative care consultants to serve on their advisory boards or ethics committees. Many palliative care experts are happy to provide staff in-services to increase primary palliative care skills or to help design quality improvement projects, for example, to increase advance care planning in dialysis patients.[12] Palliative care experts can assist in developing policies and protocols for delivering primary palliative care with nonspecialized staff and defining how and when to escalate to specialty-level consultation.

Promising innovations to increase access to specialty palliative care for patients with kidney disease are emerging and are discussed in chapter 4.

Summary

Nephrology practices can develop the essential skills to provide primary palliative care, but, for complex problems, consultation with a specialty palliative care team is warranted. It may be challenging to locate palliative care specialists who can see patients in an outpatient setting. In addition to direct patient care, palliative care specialists can add value to development of clinical protocols and education and quality improvement initiatives.

Practice Pointers

1. When symptoms are severe, refractory, or complex, it is appropriate to consult with a specialty palliative care team.
2. Specialty palliative care is delivered by an interdisciplinary team including physicians, nurses, social workers, chaplains, pharmacists, and others. This approach helps address the different domains of suffering including physical, psychological, social, and spiritual aspects of care. The team may also assist with care coordination across settings and specialties.
3. There is a mismatch between the supply and need for specialty palliative care, and access varies by region and care setting. As a result, innovative models are currently in development. Nephrology teams should identify local resources and advocate for access to specialty palliative care.

Practice Improvement Opportunity

1. While it is frequently difficult to obtain outpatient palliative care consultation for seriously ill dialysis patients, nephrologists may want to make it a routine practice to obtain inpatient palliative care consultation for seriously ill patients with kidney disease to assist with goals of care clarification and symptom management.

References

1. Kelley AS, Bollens-Lund E. Identifying the population with serious illness: the "denominator" challenge. *J Palliat Med.* 2018;21(Suppl 2):S7–S16. doi:10.1089/jpm.2017.0548
2. Quill T, Abernethy AP. Generalist plus specialist palliative care—creating a more sustainable model. *N Engl J Med.* 2013;368(13):1173–1175. doi:10.1056/NEJMp1302093
3. National Consensus Project for Quality Palliative Care. *Clinical Practice Guidelines for Quality Palliative Care.* 4th ed. Richmond, VA: National Coalition for Hospice and Palliative Care; 2018. https://www.nationalcoalitionhpc.org/ncp
4. Fischberg D, Bull J, Casarett D, et al. Five things physicians and patients should question in hospice and palliative medicine. *J Pain Symptom Manag.* 2013;45(3):595–605. doi:10.1016/j.jpainsymman.2012.12.002
5. Davis JL, Davison SN. Hard choices, better outcomes: a review of shared decision-making and patient decision aids around dialysis initiation and conservative kidney management. *Curr Opin Nephrol Hypertens.* 2017;26(3):205–213. doi:10.1097/MNH.0000000000000321
6. Zimmermann C, Kanwar K, Campbell T, et al. Opportunities to improve patient engagement in dialysis decisions for older adults with life-limiting kidney disease (TH370B). *J Pain Symptom Manag.* 2018;55(2):589–590. doi:10.1016/j.jpainsymman.2017.12.062
7. Grubbs V. Time to recast our approach for older patients with ESRD: the best, the worst, and the most likely. *Am J Kidney Dis.* 2018;71(5):605–607. doi:10.1053/j.ajkd.2018.02.002
8. Richmond C. Dame Cicely Saunders. *BMJ.* 2005;331(7510):238–238. doi:10.1136/bmj.331.7510.238
9. Center for Advance Palliative Care. America's care of serious illness: 2015 state-by-state report card on access to palliative care in our nation's hospitals. https://reportcard.capc.org/wp-content/uploads/2015/08/CAPC-Report-Card-2015.pdf. Published 2015.
10. Spetz J, Dudley N, Trupin L, Rogers M, Meier DE, Dumanovsky T. Few hospital palliative care programs meet national staffing recommendations. *Health Aff (Millwood).* 2016;35(9):1690–1697. doi:10.1377/hlthaff.2016.0113
11. Donlon R, Purington K, Williams N. Advancing palliative care for adults with serious illness: a national review of state palliative care policies and programs. *National Academy for State Health Policy.* https://nashp.org/wp-content/uploads/2018/12/Palliative-Care-Brief-Final.pdf. Published December 2018. Accessed December 18, 2019.
12. Schmidt RJ, Weaner BB, Long D. The power of advance care planning in promoting hospice and out-of-hospital death in a dialysis unit. *J Palliat Med.* 2015;18(1):62–66. doi:10.1089/jpm.2014.0031

8

Physician Wellness in Nephrology and Palliative Care

Sarah Ramer and Holly Koncicki

Among many threats to physician wellness is burnout, which is associated with negative outcomes for patients and the healthcare system, in addition to the impact it has on physicians. Data on the prevalence, predictors, and consequences of burnout among nephrologists are very limited, but evidence from various sources suggests it might be a major issue. The prevalence of burnout among palliative care physicians is better-studied and appears to vary by country, with up to 60% of palliative care physicians in the United States suffering from burnout in a recent study. Various interventions for prevention and treatment of burnout have been tried, and some have been found to be effective. Controversy exists, however, over whether the individual or the system in which the individual works is more appropriately targeted for intervention. Learning palliative care skills, such as symptom management and advanced communication techniques, might lessen burnout and increase resilience in nephrologists.

Case

As she begins her second year with a nephrology group practice in the suburbs of a major US city, Lauren finds herself wondering how much longer she can tolerate her job. In a good week, she works 50 hours; in a bad week, 70 hours. Covering 16 weekends per year and taking overnight call 24 weeks per year, the bad weeks seem to far outnumber the good. In any given week she rounds at 3 hospitals and 4 dialysis units as well as sees patients in the office. As she drives from site to site, she often has to skip meals and even bathroom breaks. Most of her patients are pleasant and grateful for her care, but a few are demanding or even hostile.

Regardless of patient demeanor, it seems to her that too many encounters are consumed by patients and their family members venting about their frustration with the healthcare system, including her own practice. Lauren often agrees with them but feels powerless to change anything—in fact, she struggles to fill out all the forms and respond to all the messages that the office staff leave for her, and she gets a little angry that people think she has the time for this kind of thing.

At least once a week, Lauren learns that one of her dialysis or clinic patients has died, often after a long hospitalization that included several invasive procedures. With each death, she questions whether she failed the patient in some way. Seeing new patients in the hospital,

Lauren estimates that at least half of them will die within 6 months, but it seems like no one is talking about prognosis. Furthermore, as a consultant whose livelihood depends on the satisfaction of the physicians consulting her, she doesn't feel empowered to start conversations about goals of care or treatment preferences. She also has to admit that she doesn't have the training or time to engage in these conversations herself, even if she had license to. She's additionally aware that she lacks the training and time to treat most of her patients' symptoms, so she ends up paying more attention to her patients' numbers than to their quality of life. As a result, she frequently goes home at night feeling like she's accomplished nothing at work.

At home, Lauren only gets an hour or so with her 2 young children before they go to bed.

Afterwards, she usually fires up the electronic medical record on her laptop to finish her documentation from the day. Sometimes she nods off sitting up in bed with the computer still in her lap and wakes up to the piercing cry of her pager. At least once every few weeks, she needs to go into the hospital in the middle of the night for an emergent consult. She suffers from guilt that she's not available enough to her husband, children, or aging parents; she also regrets that she doesn't have enough time to exercise, finish knitting projects, or keep up with her friends.

Seeking a solution to her predicament, Lauren has noticed that the hospitalists who consult her work far fewer hours than she does for equivalent or even higher pay. She's started to investigate finding a job as a hospitalist. She'd miss her longitudinal relationships with patients and some aspects of nephrology, but for the sake of her family and herself, she knows she needs to make a major change.

The Physician Wellness Crisis

In recent years, the wellness of physicians and other healthcare workers has garnered a significant amount of attention from both researchers and the general public. A growing literature documents the high prevalence of depression,[1] suicidal ideation,[2] and especially burnout[3] among physicians. These wellness problems affect not just physicians and their families but also patients and the healthcare system as a whole. A recent systematic review and meta-analysis found that physician burnout, defined as a syndrome of emotional exhaustion, depersonalization, and a reduced sense of personal accomplishment,[4] is associated with an increased risk of patient safety incidents, lower quality of care due to less professionalism, and lower patient satisfaction.[5] Furthermore, physicians reporting burnout are more likely to plan on reducing their clinical hours, leaving their current practice, or retiring early (Box 8.1).[6,7]

BOX 8.1. Correlates of Physician Burnout

For the individual patient
- Increased risk of patient safety incidents
- Lower quality of care due to less professionalism Lower patient satisfaction

For the healthcare system
- Reduction in clinical hours
- Leaving current practice
- Early retirement

The search for solutions to physician wellness problems has encompassed interventions aimed at both the individual and at the system in which the individual works, with considerable controversy over which entity is more appropriately targeted.[8-10] This chapter will first review what is known about burnout and other wellness issues among nephrology and palliative care physicians and then focus on fixes that have been tried in various areas of medicine. Not surprisingly, palliative care leads nephrology in recognition and discussion of physician wellness issues. What's more, incorporation of palliative care into nephrology may enrich not only nephrology practice but also nephrologist wellness.

Burnout and Other Wellness Issues in Nephrology

Although there is some literature examining burnout in nephrology and dialysis nurses, no such literature examines the same in nephrologists. The only available data on the prevalence of burnout and other wellness problems in nephrologists come from Medscape surveys, which rely on a voluntary sample of Medscape member physicians who practice in the United States. In the survey released in 2019, completed by roughly 150 nephrologists, 32% reported burnout, which was the second-lowest prevalence among 29 surveyed specialties. It should be noted that this survey assessed burnout by asking participants if they felt burned out, not by having them fill out a validated burnout scale. This relatively low prevalence of burnout was despite the fact that 68% of nephrologists reported working more than 51 hours per week, ranking nephrology fifth among the 29 specialties for percentage working such long hours. Only 26% of nephrologists said they were happy at work, but only 19% said they would consider seeking professional help for burnout or depression, the fourth-lowest percentage among the 29 specialties.[11]

As the field of nephrology struggles to recruit trainees in the United States,[12] Canada,[13] and the United Kingdom,[14] leaders in the specialty have speculated as to why nephrology is not a more attractive career choice. One of the proffered reasons is nephrologist burnout, inferred from observations made by physicians both within and outside of the field.[15] Australian trainees who had been exposed to nephrology but chose other specialties noted that nephrologists work long, unpredictable hours caring for medically complex patients whose prognosis will often remain poor regardless of what their doctor does. In this particular study, "consultant 'burnout' . . . [was] described as negatively affecting the trainees' experiences in nephrology"; furthermore, "complicated medical issues were cited as making routine on-calls more demanding than in other specialties."[16] A recent analysis of all patients seen by any doctor in a single Canadian province confirmed this medical complexity of nephrology patients: Among 13 types of physicians, nephrologists saw the most medically complex patients, as determined by both an overall measure of complexity and several sub-measures.[17]

Perhaps the most detailed data on the conditions that foster burnout among US nephrologists are derived from surveys conducted by the American Society of Nephrology. In 2018, over 20% of US nephrology fellows responding to the annual fellows' survey said they would not recommend nephrology to current medical students and residents, citing "the heavy workload, low compensation, difficult schedule relative to hospital medicine and other specialties, [and] undervaluing of the specialty by other specialties."[18] A 2017 survey of US early-career nephrologists (defined as having completed training between 1 and 6 years prior) found that only 46% were satisfied or very satisfied with their work hours and only 39% were satisfied or very satisfied with their work–life balance. Over 60% were spending at least 40 hours per week on patient care, with 21% spending at least 60 hours per week on patient care. Forty-three percent were working more than 1 weekend per month, and nearly 30% were taking weeknight calls at least half the weeks of the year.[19]

Burnout and Other Wellness Issues in Palliative Care

In contrast to nephrology, palliative care as a field has paid much more attention to the wellness of its workforce, including physicians. It is somewhat intuitive that, in a specialty often consulted specifically to address extreme physical and emotional suffering, conflicts between patients, caregivers, and medical personnel, and death and dying, the practitioners might face a higher risk of burnout than most. On top of this, palliative care programs commonly deal with higher demand for services than they are able to provide. But along with the greater opportunities for burnout in palliative care comes the possibility of greater protective factors, namely, the meaning and personal satisfaction that palliative care clinicians derive from their work and the likelihood that those who selected the field did so with self-assurance that they could cope with the unique challenges.[20]

The most comprehensive study of the prevalence of burnout in US palliative care clinicians (including not just physicians but also nurse practitioners, physician assistants, nurses, social workers, and chaplains), a survey sent to members of the American Academy of Hospice and Palliative Medicine in 2013, found that 62% of the respondents were experiencing burnout. Interestingly, the rate was higher in nonphysicians (66%) than in physicians (60%), of whom at least 691 responded. Besides clinician type, being younger than 50, working more than 50 hours per week, working with 3 or fewer colleagues, and working weekends often or all of the time were all independently associated with burnout. Among all clinicians, work setting (hospice, nonhospice, or both) was not associated with burnout. Thirty-three percent of the clinicians felt that their work schedule did not leave enough time for personal and family life, and 11% felt "downhearted and blue" all, most, or a good bit of the time. For burnout management, the 3 activities that respondents said were most important were talking with family, friends, and significant others; engaging in exercise and hobbies; and taking vacations. The activities that were least used and judged to be least important were journaling or reflective writing and seeing a counselor or therapist.[20]

Solutions to Burnout and Other Wellness Issues

The increasing recognition of burnout in medicine has been accompanied by dozens of studies of interventions designed to reduce burnout. Two recent systematic reviews and meta-analyses concluded that various interventions tested in randomized trials and before-after cohort studies can reduce burnout in small but clinically significant ways.[21,22] The first systematic review and meta-analysis, from West and colleagues,[21] included 15 randomized controlled trials involving 716 physicians and 37 cohort studies involving 2914 physicians. One cohort study specifically looked at 17 palliative care physicians; no study specifically looked at nephrologists. The majority of the studies employed individual interventions, including facilitated and nonfacilitated small group curricula, stress management and self-care training, communication skills training, and mindfulness-based approaches. The rest of the studies employed structural interventions, including shortened attending rotations, shortened resident shifts, resident duty hour limitations, practice delivery changes, and modifications to clinical work processes. Overall there did not appear to be a significant difference in efficacy between individual and structural interventions, and the authors opined that both types are probably necessary, although recommendations will depend on much more research yet to be done.[21]

The second systematic review and meta-analysis, from Panagioti and colleagues,[22] included 19 studies involving 1550 physicians from 5 different continents. No study specifically examined physicians from either nephrology or palliative care. In contrast to West et al,[21] this systematic review and meta-analysis found greater reductions in burnout from structural interventions, which, in the authors' view, provided evidence for organizational problems being more to blame for burnout than personal physician problems. The authors also noted that the diversity of interventions, physicians, and healthcare settings and the overall low quality of evidence precluded firm recommendations on a best approach to burnout reduction.

As researchers and policymakers try to elucidate the factors that diminish physician wellness with the goal of finding ways to improve it, the concept of resilience has attracted increasing interest. Defined in many ways, including as "the ability of an individual to respond to stress in a healthy, adaptive way such that personal goals are achieved at minimal psychological and physical cost,"[24] (p. 301) resilience is thought to be an antidote to burnout and a key to physician wellness.[25] Resilience has become such a hot topic that a recent systematic review located 22 studies describing interventions to foster physician resilience, 16 of which were published between 2014 and 2016. The review ultimately concluded that "this research area is in its infancy and currently suffers from the lack of consideration or use of pertinent theory, a lack of consistency in outcome measurement, and substantive methodological weaknesses. In the absence of theoretically valid, evidence-based interventions, it is not possible to provide best practice guidance on how to improve resilience."[27] Furthermore, empirical evidence for a correlation between more resilience and less burnout in physicians is scant[26] (p. 168). In addition, many physicians bristle at the idea that a lack of resilience, inferred to be their own fault and therefore theirs alone to fix, is the source of their burnout, rather than the numerous systemic challenges they face at work.[23]

Perhaps the most practical approach to building resilience without inflating its relative importance in palliative care physician wellness comes from Back and colleagues.[28] (p. 286) Recognizing that both personal resources and work demands influence clinician wellness, the authors sketch out an intervention for hospital-based palliative care teams intended to build resilience skills and assess what they call "workplace engagement factors," noting that the responsibility for addressing the latter falls not only to clinicians but also to service leaders and administrators. With regards to resilience skills, the authors draw a parallel between these and communication skills, explaining that prior to the publication of research into communication skills training, there was a widespread belief that some people are good communicators and others are not, and one's communication skills could not improve with training. Back et al point out that palliative care training usually doesn't include resilience training. By extension, clinicians shouldn't feel that it's their fault if they find themselves lacking resilience skills when in fact they were never taught these skills. Fortunately, resilience skills, like communication skills, can be taught, according to the authors' hypothesis.

Summary

Physicians face many threats to their wellness; prominent among them is burnout. If burnout only impacted physicians, it would deserve serious attention; that it also impacts patients and the healthcare system as a whole only makes the imperative for research into reduction and prevention that much more pressing. Practitioners in both nephrology and palliative medicine care for some of the sickest, most medically complex patients—in fact, often the same patients. The respective responses of each field to that shared responsibility markedly diverge, however. Whereas palliative care physicians have sought to better characterize burnout among themselves and have begun to test interventions for lessening or avoiding it, nephrologists have so far undertaken few, if any, efforts in this area. The difficulty recruiting physicians into nephrology in several Western countries and the challenges of nephrologists' work suggest that such efforts are long overdue.

In thinking about what might underlie burnout in nephrology, one has to wonder if a major contributor is a mismatch between nephrologists' skills and the needs of their patients. As Back et al[28] state, "Put simply, burnout occurs when work demands outstrip personal resources. Conversely, resilience occurs when personal resources can rise to meet work demands"[28] (p. 286). One of nephrologists' most common "work demands" is the highly symptomatic kidney disease patient with multiple treatment options but a short life expectancy regardless of which option is chosen. If the nephrologist doesn't have the "personal resource" of primary palliative care training to assist the patient in choosing a treatment that reflects his values, might this demand without a resource to meet it fuel burnout? And will not the patient be worse off, dealing with untreated symptoms and undergoing a treatment unlikely to help him attain his goals? On the other hand, if the nephrologist knows how to address common symptoms and talk with her patient about prognosis and treatment options such that the patient picks a treatment in line with his priorities, might this demand met by a resource promote resilience? If nothing else, the nephrologist might feel fulfilled being able to get at what matters to the patient and not just the patient's numbers.

Nephrologists not only can learn from palliative care by studying burnout among themselves, but they can also learn from palliative care by actually learning some palliative care skills, which intensifies the importance of integrating palliative care into nephrology. The presumption has been that palliative care benefits nephrology patients. The possibility that it also benefits the nephrologists who learn to provide it merits consideration and future research.

Practice Pointers

- A high prevalence of physician burnout is associated with an increased risk of patient safety incidents, lower quality of care due to less professionalism, and lower patient satisfaction.
- Data on the prevalence and consequences of burnout among nephrologists are very limited, but evidence from various sources suggests it might be a major issue.
- A recent survey suggests up to 60% of palliative care physicians in the United States might be suffering from burnout. But controversy remains over whether the individual or the system in which the individual works is more appropriately targeted for burnout intervention and treatment.

Practice Improvement Opportunities

- Nephrologists and palliative care clinicians can probably learn resilience skills like they can learn communication skills. But to be effective and gain buy-in, interventions for burnout need to address the system in which the individual works as well as the individual's skills.
- Learning primary palliative care skills might lessen burnout and increase resilience in nephrologists. This possibility deserves future research.

References

1. Mata DA, Ramos MA, Bansal N, et al. Prevalence of depression and depressive symptoms among resident physicians: a systematic review and meta-analysis. *JAMA*. 2015;314(22):2373–2383.
2. Shanafelt TD, Hasan O, Dyrbye LN, et al. Changes in burnout and satisfaction with work-life balance in physicians and the general US working population between 2011 and 2014. *Mayo Clinic Proc*. 2015;90(12):1600–1613.
3. Rotenstein LS, Torre M, Ramos MA, et al. Prevalence of burnout among physicians: a systematic review. *JAMA*. 2018;320(11):1131–1150.
4. Maslach C, Jackson SE, Leiter MP. *Maslach Burnout Inventory Manual*. 4th ed. Menlo Park, CA: Mind Garden; 2017.
5. Panagioti M, Geraghty K, Johnson J, et al. Association between physician burnout and patient safety, professionalism, and patient satisfaction: a systematic review and meta- analysis. *JAMA Intern Med*. 2018;178(10):1317–1330.
6. Shanafelt TD, Raymond M, Kosty M, et al. Satisfaction with work–life balance and the career and retirement plans of US oncologists. *J Clin Oncol*. 2014;32(11):1127–1135.
7. Dewa CS, Loong D, Bonato S, Thanh NX, Jacobs P. How does burnout affect physician productivity? A systematic literature review. *BMC Health Serv Res*. 2014;14:325.
8. Oliver D. David Oliver: when "resilience" becomes a dirty word. *BMJ*. 2017;358:j3604.
9. Card AJ. Physician burnout: resilience training is only part of the solution. *Annal Fam Med*. 2018;16(3):267–270.
10. Shanafelt T, Trockel M, Ripp J, Murphy ML, Sandborg C, Bohman B. Building a program on well-being: key design considerations to meet the unique needs of each organization. *Acad Med*. 2019;94(2):156–161.
11. Kane L. Medscape National Physician Burnout, Depression and Suicide Report 2019. https://www.medscape.com/slideshow/2019-lifestyle-burnout-depression- 6011056#1. Published 2019. Accessed February 23, 2019.

12. Berns JS, Ellison DH, Linas SL, Rosner MH. Training the next generation's nephrology workforce. *Clin J Am Soc Nephrol*. 2014;9(9):1639–1644.
13. Ward DR, Manns B, Gil S, Au F, Kappel JE. Results of the 2014–2015 Canadian society of nephrology workforce survey. *Can J Kidney Health Dis*. 2016;3:25.
14. Barat A, Goldacre MJ, Lambert TW. Career choices for nephrology and factors influencing them: surveys of UK medical graduates. *JRSM Open*. 2018;9(8):2054270418793024.
15. Roberts JK. Burnout in nephrology: implications on recruitment and the workforce. *Clin J Am Soc Nephrol*. 2018;13(2):328–330.
16. Lane CA, Brown MA. Nephrology: a specialty in need of resuscitation? *Kidney Int*. 2009;76(6):594–596.
17. Tonelli M, Wiebe N, Manns BJ, et al. Comparison of the complexity of patients seen by different medical subspecialists in a universal health care system. *JAMA Netw Open*. 2018;1(7):e184852.
18. Quigley L, Salsberg E, Collins A. *Report on the Survey of 2018 Nephrology Fellows*. Washington, DC: American Society of Nephrology; 2018.
19. Quigley L, Salsberg E, Collins A. *Early Career Nephrologists: Results of a 2017 Survey* Washington, DC: American Society of Nephrology; 2018.
20. Kamal AH, Bull JH, Wolf SP, et al. Prevalence and predictors of burnout among hospice and palliative care clinicians in the U.S. *J Pain Symptom Manage*. 2016;51(4):690–696.
21. West CP, Dyrbye LN, Erwin PJ, Shanafelt TD. Interventions to prevent and reduce physician burnout: a systematic review and meta-analysis. *Lancet*. 2016;388(10057):2272–2281.
22. Panagioti M, Panagopoulou E, Bower P, et al. Controlled interventions to reduce burnout in physicians: a systematic review and meta-analysis. *JAMA Int Med*. 2017;177(2):195–205.
23. Podgurski L, Greco C, Croom A, Arnold R, Claxton R. A brief mindfulness-based self-care curriculum for an interprofessional group of palliative care providers. *J Palliat Med*. 2019;22(5):561–565.
24. Epstein RM, Krasner MS. Physician resilience: what it means, why it matters, and how to promote it. *Acad Med*. 2013;88(3):301–303.
25. Zwack J, Schweitzer J. If every fifth physician is affected by burnout, what about the other four? Resilience strategies of experienced physicians. *Acad Med*. 2013;88(3):382–389.
26. Fox S, Lydon S, Byrne D, Madden C, Connolly F, O'Connor P. A systematic review of interventions to foster physician resilience. *Postgrad Med J*. 2018;94(1109):162–170.
27. Reed S, Kemper KJ, Schwartz A, et al. Variability of burnout and stress measures in pediatric residents: an exploratory single-center study from the Pediatric Resident Burnout-Resilience Study Consortium. *J Evid Based Integr Med*. 2018;23:2515690X18804779.
28. Back AL, Steinhauser KE, Kamal AH, Jackson VA. Building resilience for palliative care clinicians: an approach to burnout prevention based on individual skills and workplace factors. *J Pain Symptom Manage*. Aug 2016;52(2):284–291.

SECTION III

Patient-Centered Care—Values Guide Care

The Shared Decision-Making Process as the Recommended Standard for Treatment Decisions in Kidney Disease and Requisite Communication Skills to Implement the Process

Ernest I. Mandel, Jane O. Schell, and Robert A. Cohen

Shared decision-making (SDM) is the accepted standard of care paradigm for medical decision making between patient or surrogate and clinician. In its Choosing Wisely campaign, the American Society of Nephrology (ASN) recommended SDM prior to the initiation of dialysis. Evidence suggests that SDM enhances patients' understanding of their illness and satisfaction with the decision-making process, but at present SDM is poorly integrated into dialysis decision-making. Dialysis patients often describe a passive role in the decision to start dialysis, reinforcing the need for implementation of SDM in decision-making with patients with kidney disease. The hallmark feature of SDM is collaboration between the clinician and the patient or surrogate whereby the patient's expertise in the realm of values and priorities is elicited while the clinician's medical expertise is shared. The ultimate treatment decision results from the integration of their respective expertise. The Agency for Healthcare Research and Quality SHARE Approach outlines the components of SDM, and frameworks such as the Serious Illness Conversation Guide, REMAP, and SPIRES are roadmaps for those components. Communication tools and mnemonics also facilitate SDM conversations. With knowledge and application of these frameworks and tools, the nephrology community will be better positioned to fulfill the mandate embodied in the ASN Choosing Wisely campaign to employ the SDM process in renal replacement therapy decisions.

Framing Case

Mr. Z is a 78-year-old man with coronary artery disease and hypertension seen in follow-up for chronic kidney disease (CKD) stage 4 with an estimated glomerular filtration rate now of 19 mL/min/1.73m^2. He recently moved into an assisted living facility having suffered 2 falls and a hip fracture in the past year and has had worsening mobility. His kidney function has slowly declined over the past 4 years, and although he has no trouble with volume control or uremic symptoms, you, his nephrologist, are concerned that a decision needs to be made soon regarding options for end-stage kidney disease (ESKD) treatment. You intend to broach the issue at this visit. How can we help this patient decide on the best treatment option for ESKD that matches the potential burdens and benefits of the different treatment options with the patient's priorities and preferences?

Introduction

Shared decision-making (SDM) involves eliciting values and preferences, sharing medical information, and then helping patients weigh both in making medical decisions.[1] It combines the ethical principle of respect for patient autonomy with the legal doctrine of patient self-determination through informed consent. Recently, as part of the ABIM Foundation Choosing Wisely campaign, the American Society of Nephrology recommended that decisions regarding renal replacement therapy (RRT) be made using the SDM process.[2] Despite this recommendation, decisions about ESKD management are often made without an informed discussion that takes into account the expected prognosis with patient priorities and preferences.[3,4] Patients on dialysis report the perception that they had no choice in decisions about dialysis or believed that choices had been made for them by a clinician.[5] This view of dialysis as the default option persists despite patient preferences supporting medical management without dialysis.[6] This chapter reviews the supportive evidence, timing, and context for SDM within the kidney disease trajectory; components of the process including frameworks to guide the approach; and specific communication tools that facilitate the process.

Evidence Favoring SDM

SDM has become the standard of care for medical decision making. The benefits of SDM span three realms: (i) affective-cognitive, which includes patient understanding, satisfaction, and trust in their provider; (ii) behavioral, which relates to patient adherence; and (iii) health outcomes, which includes quality of life measures as well as physiologic or other measures of disease control.[7] The majority of evidence supporting the effectiveness of SDM has focused on the affective-cognitive domain. Several studies have demonstrated that SDM improves patient understanding of their illness and treatment options and patient satisfaction in the decision process and, in some instances, enhances trust between patient and clinician.[7] Evidence for effectiveness in the behavioral and health outcomes domains, however, is lacking.

Timing and Setting of SDM in the Disease Course

The kidney disease trajectory is defined by multiple opportunities for SDM; SDM has a role in addressing treatment decisions with regard to (i) progressive CKD including treatment for

ESKD; (ii) goals of care in response to changing clinical status after ESKD treatments have been instituted; and (iii) acute kidney injury.

Chronic Kidney Disease

SDM is the appropriate approach for decisions throughout the course of CKD, ranging from dietary recommendations with moderate kidney impairment to deciding between RRT and medical management without dialysis as ESKD approaches. If RRT is selected, SDM is also suitable for decisions about specific dialysis modalities (hemodialysis or peritoneal dialysis), considerations of access type and timing, and pursuit of transplantation. Additionally, SDM is appropriate for discussions about a potential time-limited trial of chronic dialysis.

End-Stage Kidney Disease

For patients who are already undergoing treatment for ESKD, whether medical management without dialysis or RRT, additional SDM opportunities are prompted by changes in clinical status leading to a reconsideration of goals of care. Such conditions include the development of poorly controlled symptoms, newly diagnosed clinical issues that raise the possibility for additional interventions, recurring or prolonged hospital admissions, deterioration in overall quality of life with progression of comorbid illness, or challenges specific to dialysis, such as access complications or treatment intolerance. Potential decisions within this context are whether to pursue aggressive intervention, whether to undergo access salvage procedures, whether to prioritize symptom management and other kidney supportive care interventions, and whether to withdraw from dialysis.

Acute Kidney Injury

The development of acute kidney injury, especially if superimposed on pre-existing CKD, often necessitates consideration of RRT. SDM is suitable for decisions about whether to initiate RRT, the parameters of a possible time-limited trial of RRT, and when, in some instances, to discontinue RRT.

Shared Decision-Making Components

The Agency for Healthcare Research and Quality has defined a 5-step process for achieving SDM, SHARE.[8] The SHARE process consists of 5 components shown in Table 9.1. Done correctly, these components ensure that the SDM process combines evidence-based information and provider experience with the patient's elicited values and preferences to reach a treatment decision. The frameworks and decision aids discussed in the following text that are designed to guide the SDM process contain the components of the SHARE model.

TABLE 9.1. SHARE Approach in Context

SHARE Component	Explanation	Example	Skill
Seek	*Seek* the patient's participation	We are approaching a major decision about what to do as your kidney function worsens.	SICG and SPIRES Setup REMAP Reframe
		Who do you like to have present when you make such decisions?	
		What has been your experience making major decisions?	
		Is there an approach that has worked for you in the past?	
Help	*Help* the patient compare and explore treatment options	Is it all right if we discuss the next steps?	Ask (Ask–Tell–Ask)
		I'm worried that some of the treatments for worsening kidney function might not help as much as harm.	Tell (Ask–Tell–Ask)
		I can see how hard it is to think about these matters.	Respond to emotion
		Could we talk about the different options and consider some of the benefits and burdens of each?	Ask (Ask–Tell–Ask)
		Discuss treatment.	Tell (Ask–Tell–Ask)
		To make sure we are on the same page, could you share with me your understanding of these options?	Ask (Ask–Tell–Ask)
Assess	*Assess* the patient's values and preferences	Would it be all right with you if we talk about your priorities to help with this decision?	Ask (Ask–Tell–Ask)
		If you become sicker, what is most important to you?	Open-ended questions
		What else? What worries you as you think about your health? Tell me more about that.	Open-ended questions
		What I hear you saying is that you are concerned about spending too much time in the hospital and also about losing more independence.	Tell (Ask–Tell–Ask)
		Is that correct?	Ask (Ask–Tell–Ask)
Reach	*Reach* a decision with the patient	Would it be all right if I offer a recommendation based on what we have talked about?	Ask permission to make a recommendation
		Based on what you have said about not being hospitalized and maintaining independence, I think we should consider medical management without dialysis. With this approach we will focus on quality of life while not doing dialysis and other procedures that might send you back to the hospital or worsen your functional status.	SICG Close/Make a Recommendation REMAP Propose a Plan SPIRES Recommendation

TABLE 9.1. Continued

SHARE Component	Explanation	Example	Skill
Evaluate	*Evaluate* the patient's decision	Given the decision about conservative management, what seems to be working? Is there anything you think we might do differently? What questions do you have?	SPIRES Summarize and Strategize Ask (Ask-Tell-Ask)

Frameworks for SDM Conversations

Although eliciting patient values and preferences is a fundamental element of the SDM process, clinicians frequently find this activity challenging. Potential barriers to exploring values and preferences include a lack of training in how to engage in such conversations, fear of upsetting patients or removing hope, and insecurity in the ability to respond to the strong emotions arising in patients.[9-11] Using a guide for such conversations provides the clinician with direction and suggested language that helps to overcome these barriers. Several frameworks are appropriate for use in advanced kidney disease. These include the Serious Illness Conversation Guide (SICG),[12] REMAP,[13] and SPIRES.[14] Among their common elements are (i) requesting permission to have a conversation; (ii) ascertaining patient understanding about their health status; (iii) sharing relevant prognostic information; (iv) recognizing and responding to emotional cues; (v) eliciting patient values; and (vi) making a recommendation that incorporates patient values with what is clinically appropriate.

SICG is a structured tool designed to assist clinicians in navigating these challenging conversations. The SICG prescribes 9 communication steps for conducting serious illness conversations (Table 9.2).[12] The conversation opens with (i) *setup*, which includes asking permission to engage in the conversation and, in the context of SDM, framing the conversation as a necessary prerequisite to discussing and reaching a shared decision; (ii) *understanding*, which involves exploring the patient's understanding of their illness, and in the context of SDM, their understanding of the treatment options, including risks and benefits of treatments under consideration; (iii) *prognosis*, which includes sharing either a time-based prognosis expressed as a range (weeks to months), perhaps informed by an available prognosis calculator; a functional prognosis focused on likelihood of return of, or improvement in, function and expected trajectory in quality of life as it relates to anticipated future hospitalizations, procedures, or other medical setbacks; or an acknowledgement of the uncertainty of prognosis and the possibility of sudden unexpected decline; (iv) *goals* and (v) *fears*, both of which involve eliciting patients' health-related and personal goals and fears; (vi) *sources of strength*, which involves exploring patient sources of strength such as family, friends, faith, or any other sources; (vii) *acceptable or critical function*, which involves inquiring about what circumstances or possible outcomes might inform or alter the patient's desired course of action; exploring (viii) *trade-offs*, which involves discussing what medical interventions might be acceptable to the patient to achieve their previously stated goals and preferences; and (ix) *family*, which includes exploring the extent to which the patient desires their family to be involved in discussions or decision-making. The SICG ultimately prescribes summarizing the

TABLE 9.2. The Serious Illness Conversation Guide

Component	Explanation	Sample Language
Setup	Introduce the concept of the conversation and benefits and ask permission.	"I'm hoping we can talk about where things are with your kidney disease and where they are going. Is this OK?"
Understanding	Assess patient (surrogate) understanding of the illness and information preferences—how and what they wish to be told.	"What is your understanding now of where you are with your kidneys?" "How much information of what is likely to be ahead with your kidney disease would you like me to share?"
Prognosis	Share prognosis tailored to information preferences. This can include a time-based prognosis, a functional prognosis, or acknowledgement of the uncertainty of prognosis.	"I'm worried time might be short" "I'm worried this may be as good as you feel" "I'm worried things could change suddenly"
Goals	Explore goals—both health-related and personal.	"What are your most important goals for your future"
Fears	Explore fears and worries—both health-related and personal.	"What are your biggest fears and worries about the future"
Sources of strength	Explore sources of strength for coping with illness and challenges, which often include family, friends, or faith.	"What gives you strength as you think about the future with your health"
Acceptable or critical function	Explore what functions or abilities are critical to the patient even in declining health.	"What abilities are so critical to your life or sense of self that you cannot imagine living without them?" "What level of dependence or independence is critical to you?"
Trade-offs	Explore what trade-offs the patient would be willing to make for the promise of more time or improved quality of life.	"What would you be willing to go through for the promise of more time or better quality of life?"
Family	Explore to what extent the patient has discussed these preferences with family and to what extent they desire to in the future.	"How much does your family know about your priorities and wishes?"
Close	Summarize the conversation, make a recommendation, and affirm commitment to the patient.	"It sounds like _____ is very important to you." "Based on what we have discussed of your priorities and wishes, I would recommend _____." "I will be there with you to help navigate these challenges."

Adapted from Mandel EI, Bernacki RE, Block SD. Serious Illness Conversations in ESRD. *Clin J Am Soc Nephrol.* 2017;12:854–863.

TABLE 9.3. The REMAP Approach

Component	Explanation
Reframe	Alert the patient that the clinical situation has worsened and introduce the necessity to discuss the next potential treatments given this prognostic shift.
Expect emotion	Expect and respond to emotion to show empathy by employing strategies such as naming the emotion.
Map out patient values	Explore what matters most to patient, goals, fears, to help inform the recommendation.
Align with patient values	Reflect back what the patient shared to demonstrate understanding.
Propose a plan	Make a treatment recommendation that incorporates the values elicited in the conversation.

key points of what has been discussed and, when appropriate, making a recommendation that accounts for both medical realities and elicited values.

REMAP is a framework for a goals of care conversation later in the patient's course (Table 9.3).[13] As with the SICG, it acknowledges that conversations should begin with the clinician inquiring about the patient's understanding of his or her illness. Next, it suggests asking permission for the clinician to provide a summary of the patient's shifting health status. The *reframe* is defined as a concise prognostic "headline" that alerts the patient that the clinical situation has worsened and the necessity to discuss the next potential treatments given this prognostic shift. *Expect emotion* and respond empathically recognizes that providing prognostic information frequently triggers emotions. When strong emotions arise, it presents a temporary pause to allow time for the patient to process information. By acknowledging or validating these emotions, the clinician helps the patient cope with the prognostic information and other serious news raised in the conversation. When the patient is ready to move forward in the conversation, the clinician pivots away from discussing specific treatment instead to *map out patient values*, exploring what matters most to the patient by using open-ended questions that query a patient's hopes, goals, and worries. *Align with values* is the act of the clinician reflecting back the patient values voiced to let the patient know that he or she has been heard and to gain further clarification of elicited priorities. Once the exploration has yielded appropriate information, the clinician proceeds to requesting permission for offering a treatment recommendation. *Propose a plan* is a treatment recommendation that incorporates the values elicited in the conversation.

SPIRES is another stepwise communication framework for ESKD treatment decision-making in frail, older patients (Table 9.4).[14] Its steps are similar to those of SICG and REMAP.

Communication Tools for SDM

Effective collaboration is enhanced through use of specific communication tools (Table 9.5) during SDM conversations (Table 9.1).[15] "Ask–Tell–Ask" is a skill in which the first

TABLE 9.4. The SPIRES Framework

Component	Explanation
Setup	Advance preparation and information gathering, including prognostic information, key participants, and asking permission to engage in the conversation.
Perceptions and perspectives	Explore, with open-ended questions, the patient's understanding of their health, as well as their hopes and concerns regarding their quality of life and health.
Invitation	Ask permission to share a recommendation that integrates medical realities and prognostic information with the patient's stated hopes and concerns.
Recommendation	Make the recommendation.
Empathize	Expect emotion and respond accordingly with empathy.
Summarize and strategize	Assess the patient's response to the recommendation, outline next steps, and document the discussion.

"ask" assesses patient understanding and/or asks permission before giving information. The "tell" provides information in clear language and in small chunks. The second "ask" assesses the patient's understanding of the information provided. The following is an example: the clinician asks, "What is your understanding of how the kidneys are functioning?" The patient provides his or her perception, which may not capture the serious change. The clinician then asks permission to provide more information and proceeds to let the patient know that the kidney function has worsened to the point that decisions should be considered about what to do next. Ultimately, the clinician checks for patient understanding of the prognostic information provided. For example, "What will you take away from our conversation today?"

Open-ended questions promote exploration of patient values, preferences, and goals, encouraging the patient to articulate these with the depth required to inform the SDM process. Further, if the clinician is unsure about the meaning or implication of a patient's

TABLE 9.5. Communication Tools

Tool	Example
Open-ended questions	"What else" or "Tell me more" or "Help me understand."
Ask–Tell–Ask	Ask: "What is your understanding of the risks and benefits of preemptive access creation." Tell: Clinician shares risks/benefits, referencing known patient preferences and concerns. Ask: "So I can be sure we are on the same page, what will you tell your spouse about what we discussed today."
Wish–Worry–Wonder	"I wish things were different." "I worry that your health might decline." "I wonder what you would say if you became more dependent on others."
Employ Silence	After sharing prognosis or difficult news, resist the urge to fill the silence. Rather, allow the patient space to absorb what was shared, collect their thoughts, and reengage.

statement, expressing curiosity through open-ended exploratory questions or statements leads to clarification of emotions and values. Two examples of such statements are "Tell me more" or "Help me understand."

Aligning with the patient's wishes and hopes strengthens the patient–clinician bond and often moves the conversation toward a collaborative decision. Such support is demonstrated by using language embodied in the "hope for the best and plan for the worst" formulation. An example is "I hope that everything remains stable. At the same time, can we talk about what might happen if the situation worsens?" Other language formulations that align with the patient include "wish-worry-wonder" statements. A "wish statement" joins the patient in acknowledging that circumstances have changed for the worse, as in, "I wish things were different." A "worry" statement expresses concern about a shifting clinical or functional trajectory. For instance, "I worry that the disease will progress." "Wonder" statements ask the patient to consider less desirable possibilities. For example, "I wonder what you would hope for if that doesn't happen?"

Conversations about serious illness or goals of care frequently elicit strong emotions. When strong emotions arise, whether sadness, anger, or fear as examples, it is critical that the clinician recognize them and be prepared to respond empathically. Emotions, whether manifested verbally or nonverbally, are diagnostic, indicating that the patient or surrogate has absorbed the serious news. Since emotions serve as a barrier to further understanding, responding to emotion offers the possibility of helping the patient adapt to serious information to allow a more cognitive discussion to ensue. One approach for responding to emotion is to acknowledge or validate the patient's emotion, for example by saying "I can't imagine how difficult it is to hear this news." The NURSE mnemonic (Table 9.6) is a tool that assists clinicians in making empathic statements.[16] Another approach is allowing for some silence after serious news is given and following with an empathic statement. The former offers the patient space to become emotional, and the latter provides time for the patient to respond to the empathic statement. It also provides a moment for the clinician to determine if the patient is ready to move forward with other parts of the conversation or if more time is needed to acknowledge the emotion.

TABLE 9.6. The NURSE Approach

Component	Explanation	Example
Name	Name the emotion the patient is experiencing or exhibiting.	"You seem upset at this news."
Understand	Express understanding, but do not overstate and suggest you "know" how they feel.	"I understand that this is not what you wanted to hear."
Respect	Demonstrate empathy by expressing respect for what the patient is going through or experiencing or their coping skills.	"You have really been doing your best to take care of yourself."
Support	Offer support to the patient, possibly by expressing concern or willingness to help.	"We will continue to see each other regularly and I will help you to the best of my ability."
Explore	Explore some aspect of the emotion further to further demonstrate empathy.	"Could you tell me more about what you are feeling right now."

Decision Aids for SDM

Patient decision aids (PDAs) can also facilitate SDM. These are tools that explain the medical information and choices in clear, simple language. Some also help the patient weigh preferences for a given decision. Booklets and videos, such as the Yorkshire Dialysis Decision Aide (YoDDA), explain the options for management of ESKD, educating about dialysis modalities, transplantation, and medical management without dialysis.[17] Other available PDAs, which combine information with exercises that assist with eliciting preferences, include My Kidneys; My Choice; and My Life, My Dialysis Choice. Preference calculators that pose questions about health status and certain priorities (such as those available at the Alberta Health Services website Conservative Kidney Management: https://www.ckmcare.com/CKMPathway/PathwayIntroduction) use the patient's inserted data to tailor information about management options to the patient's health status and priorities. Prognosis calculators, both for survival/mortality as well as disease progression, also assist clinicians and patients in the SDM process.

Summary

SDM is the accepted standard of care paradigm for medical decision-making between patient or surrogate and clinician. Evidence suggests that SDM enhances patient understanding of their illness and satisfaction with their decision-making process. Dialysis patients often describe a passive role in the decision to start dialysis, reinforcing the need for implementation of SDM in decision-making with patients with kidney disease. The hallmark feature of SDM is collaboration between the clinician and the patient or surrogate. In the process, the patient's expertise in the realm of values and priorities is elicited while the clinician's medical expertise is shared. The ultimate treatment decision results from the integration of their respective expertise. Frameworks such as the SICG, REMAP, and SPIRES are guides for the SDM process. Communication tools and mnemonics facilitate SDM conversations. With knowledge and application of these frameworks and tools, the nephrology community will be better positioned to fulfill the mandate embodied in the ASN Choosing Wisely campaign recommendation to employ the SDM process in RRT decisions.

Practice Pointers

- SDM is standard of care for medical decision-making, involving eliciting patients' values and preferences, sharing medical information, and then helping patients weigh both in making medical decisions.
- Evidence for SDM is primarily in the affective-cognitive domain, with studies showing that SDM enhances patient understanding of their condition and satisfaction with their decision-making process.

Practice Improvement Opportunities

- Employ frameworks for eliciting goals and preferences and making recommendations, such as SICG, REMAP, and SPIRES and communication tools, such as open-ended questions, "Ask–Tell–Ask," "wish–worry–wonder" statements, and the NURSE mnemonic.
- Use of evidence-based PDAs enhances patient understanding by providing prognostic information (prognosis calculators) or explaining the medical choices and information clearly (booklets, videos, or other multimedia). Some PDAs combine information with exercises that elicit values and preferences applied to decision-making.

References

1. Charles C, Gafni A, Whelan T. Decision-making in the physician-patient encounter: revisiting the shared treatment decision-making model. *Soc Sci Med.* 1999;49:651–661.
2. American Society of Nephrology. Five things physicians and patients should question. https://www.choosingwisely.org/wp-content/uploads/2015/02/ASN-Choosing-Wisely-List.pdf. Published 2012. Accessed April 30, 2019.
3. O'Hare AM, Armistead N, Schrag WL, Diamond L, Moss AH. Patient-centered care: an opportunity to accomplish the "three aims" of the National Quality Strategy in the Medicare ESRD program. *Clin J Am Soc Nephrol.* 2014;9:2189–2194.
4. Wong SP, Hebert PL, Laundry RJ, et al. Decisions about renal replacement therapy in patients with advanced kidney disease in the US Department of Veterans Affairs, 2000–2011. *Clin J Am Soc Nephrol.* 2016;11:1825–1833.
5. Ladin K, Lin N, Hahn E, Zhang G, Koch-Weser S, Weiner DE. Engagement in decision-making and patient satisfaction: a qualitative study of older patients' perceptions of dialysis initiation and modality decisions. *Nephrol Dial Transplant.* 2017;32:1394–1401.
6. Wong SPY, McFarland LV, Liu CF, Laundry RJ, Hebert PL, O'Hare AM. Care practices for patients with advanced kidney disease who forgo maintenance dialysis. *JAMA Intern Med.* 2019;179(3):305–313.
7. Shay LA, Lafata JE. Where is the evidence? A systematic review of shared decision making and patient outcomes. *Med Decis Making.* 2015;35:114–131.
8. The SHARE approach: a model for shared decisionmaking—fact sheet. *Agency for Healthcare Research and Quality.* http://www.ahrq.gov/professionals/education/curriculum-tools/shareddecisionmaking/tools/sharefactsheet/index.html. Last reviewed September 2016.
9. O'Hare AM, Szarka J, McFarland LV, et al. Provider perspectives on advance care planning for patients with kidney disease: whose job is it anyway? *Clin J Am Soc Nephrol.* 2016;11:855–866.
10. Schell JO, Patel UD, Steinhauser KE, Ammarell N, Tulsky JA. Discussions of the kidney disease trajectory by elderly patients and nephrologists: a qualitative study. *Am J Kidney Dis.* 2012;59:495–503.
11. Davison SN, Jhangri GS, Holley JL, Moss AH. Nephrologists' reported preparedness for end-of-life decision-making. *Clin J Am Soc Nephrol.* 2006;1:1256–1262.
12. Mandel EI, Bernacki RE, Block SD. Serious illness conversations in ESRD. *Clin J Am Soc Nephrol.* 2017;12:854–863.
13. Childers JW, Back AL, Tulsky JA, Arnold RM. REMAP: A Framework for Goals of Care Conversations. *J Oncol Pract.* 2017;13:e844–e850.
14. Schell JO, Cohen RA. A communication framework for dialysis decision-making for frail elderly patients. *Clin J Am Soc Nephrol.* 2014;9:2014–2021.
15. Vital Talk. Three fundamental skills. https://www.vitaltalk.org/guides/responding-to-emotion-respecting/. Published 2018. Accessed April 30, 2019.
16. Vital Talk. Nurse statements for articulating empathy. https://www.vitaltalk.org/guides/responding-to-emotion-respecting/. Published 2018. Accessed April 30, 2019.
17. Davis JL, Davison SN. Hard choices, better outcomes: a review of shared decision-making and patient decision aids around dialysis initiation and conservative kidney management. *Curr Opin Nephrol Hypertens.* 2017;26:205–213.

10

Advance Care Planning to Elicit and Respect Patient Values and Preferences

Jean L. Holley and J. April Yasunaga

Advance care planning (ACP) is a patient-centered process to elicit patient and family goals and values that shape medical decision-making and form the basis for completing written advance directives. Advance directives such as healthcare power of attorney, surrogate decision-maker identification, and living wills are executed by the patient. These may be supplemented by provider orders such as resuscitation status (do not resuscitate/do not attempt resuscitation) and provider orders for life-sustaining treatment. Provider input into ACP is required as patients and families need information on prognosis and risks and benefits of interventions to make informed decisions. Because health states influence decisions for ongoing care, ACP is a process that requires revisiting wishes and goals via discussions at stages throughout a patient's life. All healthcare systems through which a patient passes will need to be involved and cognizant of advance directives to ensure a patient's wishes are honored. Dialysis units are an integral part of the healthcare system for end-stage kidney disease patients and need to be engaged in the ACP process. Consensus statements, guidelines, and tools exist to facilitate ACP in end-stage kidney disease and chronic kidney disease patients.

Case

EA is a 92-year-old woman with a history of hypertension, stage 3 chronic kidney disease (CKD), osteoporosis, and mild cognitive impairment who was transferred from an outside hospital after a fall with concerns for a cerebral vascular accident. Shortly after her admission, she required transfer to the intensive care unit and was treated for sepsis secondary to pneumonia. Her hospitalization was complicated by significant delirium, suspected aspiration, and acute kidney injury. After several days, she was transferred out of the intensive care unit. While her delirium improved, her cognitive function did not return to baseline, and she was not able to understand or process the complexity of her care. Her kidney function continued to decline, and discussions began regarding renal replacement therapy.

A family meeting with the patient, her healthcare surrogate (son), palliative care, and nephrology revealed that EA had been followed closely by her nephrologist and had been informed that with progressive kidney failure, dialysis would become an option at some future time. EA had decided that she would not pursue dialysis if it were offered. Further, about 5 years earlier, when she moved to an independent living facility, EA and her son met with her primary care provider, updated her living will, and completed a provider orders for life-sustaining treatment (POLST) form. At that time, she reiterated her decision not to pursue dialysis if it were offered. Several years later when EA transitioned to a facility with a higher level of support, she again confirmed her prior wishes to her provider and son.

During current discussions with her son about EA's overall goals of care, her son felt confident making decisions due to the advance care planning (ACP) process that had occurred over the years and EA's active engagement in that process. Her acute conditions stabilized without dialysis, and it was noted that medical management without dialysis was to be followed according to her previously expressed and confirmed wishes.

Advance Care Planning—Definitions

ACP is the process of discussing wishes for end-of-life care and situations in which a patient may not be able to make his or her own decisions, clarifying values and goals that inform those wishes, and documenting those care preferences by completing written documents and medical orders. ACP is a patient-centered process adapting over time and influenced by the patient's medical state, values, and family circumstances. Healthcare providers are vital to the ACP process because explanations of illness, consideration of prognosis, and discussion about the risks and benefits of interventions are required for informed decision-making by patients and families. The ACP process ideally engages the patient, their families/surrogates, and healthcare providers and is supported by all of the healthcare systems through which the patient moves.

A recent expert consensus definition stated:

> Advance care planning is a process that supports adults at any age or stage of health in understanding and sharing their personal values, life goals, and preferences regarding future medical care. The goal of advance care planning is to help ensure that people receive medical care that is consistent with their values, goals and preferences during serious and chronic illness."[1]

This definition identifies two parts to the ACP process: (i) discussion(s) to understand the patient's values, preferences and life goals and (ii) a system to document patients' values, preferences, and goals in a way that ensures that patients receive medical care that aligns with those preferences. This chapter concentrates on the first aspect while chapter 12 discusses the second.

Evidence of Effectiveness

Although ACP is recommended for all populations, there is limited information about the effects of ACP on the overall healthcare of individuals and families. ACP can improve end-of-life care and reduce inappropriate life-sustaining treatments while increasing the use of hospice and supportive care as well as ensure compliance with patient wishes.[2-4] Effective

ACP may also relieve burdens on loved ones, especially surrogate decision makers, reduce grief and uncertainty surrounding death, and create the appropriate circumstances and setting to avoid suffering and intensive, unsuccessful care at the end of life.

The Outputs of Advance Care Planning

ACP outputs include (i) documentation of the conversation itself, (ii) legally enforceable documents initiated by the patient, termed "advance directives," and (iii) medical orders to implement patient preferences. (Table 10.1). Advance directives are patient-initiated written documents such as living wills and forms naming a healthcare agent, proxy, or surrogate. Although completing advance directive documents is an aspect of ACP, contemporary ACP tends to focus more on conversations around goals and values with the understanding that ACP is a process that will occur over time, require revisions depending upon the health state and specific patient circumstances, and prepare patients and surrogate decision makers for "in the moment" decision-making.[5] The documentation of patients' wishes is an important step for having those wishes honored. All health systems through which the patient passes should be able to receive, record, and retrieve patients' previously completed advance directives.

TABLE 10.1. Advance Care Planning Outputs

Advanced directives refer to several types of patient-initiated documents. People can complete these forms at any time and in any state of health that allows them to do so.

Types	Description
Advance directive (living will)	A written (or video) statement about the kinds of medical care a person does or does not want under certain specific conditions if no longer able to express those wishes
	Resources: http://caring info.org; http://theconversation project.org
Durable power of attorney for healthcare	Identifies the person (the healthcare agent) who should make medical decisions in case of the patient's incapacity. Name of document is state-dependent (eg, healthcare proxy, healthcare surrogate, etc.)
	Resource: http//caringinfo.org

Medical orders are created with and signed by a health professional, usually a physician (in some states, a nurse practitioner or physician assistant), for someone who is seriously ill. Because they are actual doctor's orders, other health professionals, including emergency personnel, are required to follow them.

Types	Description
Physician/medical orders for life-sustaining treatment (POLST/MOLST)	Physician orders covering a range of topics likely to emerge in care of the patient near the end of life. The orders cross care settings and are honored in the community in an emergency
	Resource: http://POST.org
Do-not-resuscitate, do-not-intubate, do-not-hospitalize orders	Medical orders covering specific treatments that are written in a healthcare facility, but do not cross care settings and are not necessarily honored in the community.

Adapted from the Institute of Medicine. 2015. *Dying in America: improving quality and honoring individual preferences near the end of life.* Washington, DC: The National Academies Press; 119–123.

Provider orders are often used to supplement advance directive completion by patients. Do not resuscitate (DNR) orders, do not attempt resuscitation (DNAR) orders, and POLST are provider-generated and not usually classified as advance directives. These orders require a healthcare professional's signature to be effective and can be completed in conjunction with the patient's healthcare legal agent if the patient lacks decision-making capacity. Advance directive completion is limited to patients who have decision-making capacity (Table 10.1).

POLST forms (also called medical orders for life-sustaining medical orders for life-sustaining treatment [MOLST]) have been adopted by many states.[6] POLST forms are recommended for individuals with significant chronic medical conditions who have expected reduced survival. If a provider answers "no" to the surprise question ("Would you be surprised if this patient died within the next 6 months or year?"), it is appropriate to initiate a POLST or MOLST form as part of the ACP process.[6] POLST forms typically address resuscitation status, level of care desired, and choices about artificial nutrition. They may also include information about other potential medical interventions as well as an area for documenting a designated healthcare decision maker.

Like hospitals and nursing homes, dialysis units are tasked with providing written material on ACP to patients under the Patient Self-Determination Act. Effective ACP extends beyond merely providing materials and should encompass the ongoing discussions as previously described. The delivery of ACP will vary from unit to unit. In some units, the social worker may take the lead; in others, the nurse or the advanced care provider. For some patients, the primary care provider will need to be contacted to ensure that appropriate advance directives are available to all. A team effort is required; each unit should designate a responsible person for this task.[7]

Advance Care Planning in CKD and ESKD—Current Use

Despite widely held belief that conversations about end-of-life care wishes should occur,[8] only about a third of any group examined, including those with end-stage kidney disease (ESKD) or chronic kidney disease (CKD), complete written advance directives.[9,10] The elderly are more likely to complete advance directives and those of many ethnic groups less likely to complete them. Moreover, dialysis withdrawal is rarely considered in written documents, even by dialysis patients who complete advance directives.[10]

Many factors contribute to the low adoption of ACP, including patient factors (ethnicity, younger age), provider factors (failure to introduce ACP discussions for a variety of reasons such as prognostic uncertainty, lack of time, lack of competence), and uncertainty about illness trajectories.[7,10,11] Efforts to understand and address barriers to the adoption of ACP are ongoing within the nephrology community. Programs to improve nephrologists' comfort and confidence in communication skills with patients and families have been developed and are now available.[12] Nephrology societies have endorsed the need for ACP within the framework of kidney support care for the population[13,14] and promoted guidelines for this area of nephrology care (Table 10.2).[15] Widely available resources including toolkits and references are available for nephrologists (Table 10.2).[15-17]

TABLE 10.2. Guidelines Addressing Advance Care Planning in CKD, ESKD and Tools for Implementation

Resource	Summary
Guideline	
Choosing Wisely®, American Society of Nephrology[14]	Recommendation no. 4: Institute advance care planning
KDIGO controversies conference in supportive care in chronic kidney disease[12]	Treatment care team should engage in advance care planning. ACP discussions should start early in the illness trajectory and should include health states in which patients would want to withhold or withdraw dialysis
Toolkit	
The Conversation Project®	The Conversation Project® is a public engagement initiative with a goal to have every person's wishes for end-of-life care expressed and respected. It is not ESKD specific.
	http://theconversationproject.org
	Choosing or being a healthcare proxy:
	https://theconversationproject.org/wp-content/uploads/2017/03/ConversationProject-ProxyKit-English.pdf
Conversation Ready	Conversation Ready is a companion project by the Institute for HealthCare improvement provides provider focused resources to implement patient preferences. http://www.ihi.org/Engage/Initiatives/ConversationProject/Pages/ConversationReady.aspx
	http://ihi.org/resources/Pages/IHIWhitePapers/ConversationReadyEndofLifeCare.aspx
Prepare for Your Care	Website helps patients understand and fill out easy to read advance directives.
	www.prepareforyourcare.org/page
	The Prepare advance directive form is easy to read. Multiple languages legal in all states are downloadable
	https://prepareforyourcare.org/advance-directive-library
Caring Info	State-specific legal forms in all states
	www.caringinfo.org/i4a/pages/
My Way	Make Your Wishes About You (My Way) From the Coalition for Supportive Care of Kidney Patients
	Staff curriculum guide for advance care planning with CKD patients
	https://cpb-us-w2.wpmucdn.com/blogs.nursing.gwu.edu/dist/a/4/files/2019/05/CurriculumGuideAdvanceCarePlan4302018bWeb.pdf
	Patient education brochure
	https://cpb-us-w2.wpmucdn.com/blogs.nursing.gwu.edu/dist/a/4/files/2019/05/ACPforCKDbrochure4302018Web.pdf
Medicare billing for ACP	Frequently Asked Questions about Billing the Physician Fee Schedule for Advance Care
	Planning services
	https://www.cms.gov/Medicare/Medicare-Fee-for-Service-Payment/PhysicianFeeSched/Downloads/FAQ-Advance-Care-Planning.pdf

Abbreviation: ACP, advance care planning.

ACP Guidelines and Consensus Statements in CKD and ESKD

Table 10.2 lists some of the available guidelines and consensus statements addressing ACP in CKD and ESKD. These can be used as resources for nephrologists and dialysis units interested in adopting policies and procedures to address ACP in their patients. There is widespread congruence among the guidelines in terms of recommendations for ACP in the ESKD and CKD populations.

Although guidelines may be helpful in identifying and addressing care needs, they have not resulted in more advance directive completion. There is a need for continued education for patients, families, and providers about the benefits of ACP within the context of CKD, emphasizing discussions about values and goals as a means of addressing care needs and desires. In addition, changes to incorporate ACP within existing workflows—as discussed in chapter 12—can create the expectation and support for making this a normative part of care.

Steps in the Process of ACP in ESKD and CKD Patients

As suggested in the Renal Physicians Association's Clinical Practice Guideline,[15] ACP is often an iterative process, repeated as changes in life circumstances and health states necessitate revisiting goals and values. Figure 10.1 illustrates an ACP process that can be followed with a CKD or ESKD patient, and Box 10.1 suggests questions that can be posed by providers to initiate and direct the conversation. The patient's values and goals provide the foundation of

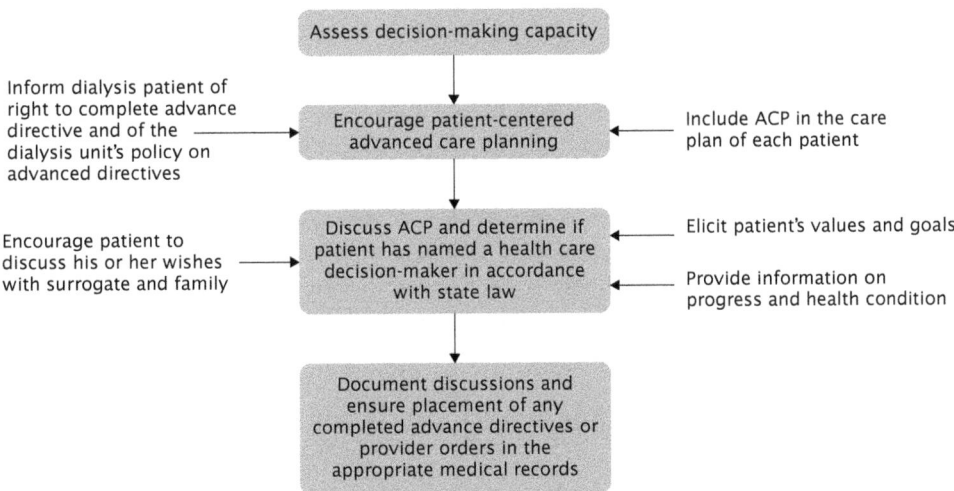

FIGURE 10.1. Steps to implement ACP in chronic kidney disease and end-stage kidney disease patients. Adapted from Renal Physicians Association. *Shared decision-making in the appropriate initiation of and withdrawal from dialysis, clinical practice guideline.* 2nd ed. Rockville, MD: RPA; 2010.

Abbreviation: ACP, advance care planning.

> **BOX 10.1. Questions to Facilitate Advance Care Planning and Elicit Patients' Values and Goals**
>
> Would you be open to talking about how we should care for you if you became very ill?
> What is most important to you?
> What makes life worth living for you?
> Are there things you want to accomplish before you die?
> If your time was limited, how would you want to spend that time?
> Is it more important to you to live as long as possible, despite some suffering or discomfort, or would you choose to live a shorter period of time without suffering or discomfort?
> If something were to happen to you so that you could not communicate your wishes for care, is there someone you would want to make those decisions for you? If so, have you discussed your wishes, what's most important to you living a good or acceptable life with that person?
> Do you have a healthcare proxy or surrogate?
> Do you have a living will?
> Are there circumstances in which life would not be worth living for you?
> Where do you prefer to die and who do you wish to be with you when that happens?
> Under what circumstances, if any, would you choose to stop dialysis?

their end-of-life choices and guide their advance directives. It is the clinician's role to provide information vital to the patient's and family's understanding of medical conditions, including prognosis and course of disease as well as the risks and benefits of possible interventions.

As shown in Figure 10.1, it is important to ensure the patient is capable of understanding the situation and making his or her own decisions. This is assured by assessing decision-making capacity. Tools are available to assist in this process[15,16] If the patient lacks decision-making capacity and a healthcare surrogate was previously identified and named, discussions about ACP will occur with that healthcare surrogate or proxy. If there is no formally identified healthcare surrogate, family members will be asked to fill that role following state and local policies. Families should be encouraged to designate one person to be the primary decision maker and communicator with the healthcare providers.

Dialysis Decision-Making as Part of ACP in CKD and ESKD

In CKD and ESKD patients, additional topics for ACP may include decisions and wishes around renal replacement therapies. ACP around dialysis may include decisions about starting or stopping dialysis. The RPA guideline[15] has specific recommendations about these issues and the National Kidney Foundation (www.kidney.org) and Coalition for the Supportive Care of Kidney Patients[16] have patient, family, and professional provider resources addressing these issues. If a patient does articulate conditions regarding starting or stopping dialysis, these should be noted in documentation of the discussion in the advance directives and in the POLST or other medical orders.

Eliciting Patient Values and Goals—The Cornerstone of ACP

Since ACP is a patient-centered process supporting patients and families in understanding and documenting preferences for future medical care, it is important to realize that personal values, life goals, and health states and circumstances will inform and influence preferences for care. The goal of ACP is to help ensure that people receive medical care that is consistent with their values, goals, and preferences, recognizing that goals and preferences may change over time and in different circumstances and health states. Thus, eliciting values and goals (Box 10.1) is the central tenet to be followed in ACP discussions, ensuring that each discussion is unique because it is patient-centered.

Initiating a conversation about goals and values can be approached by inviting the patient to discuss these issues (eg, "Would you be open to talking about how we should care for you if you became very ill and couldn't speak for yourself?"). Often, the initial topic of conversation can be centered around identifying a healthcare power of attorney or surrogate decision maker. For many people, this is the least threatening aspect of ACP discussions. Subsequent open-ended questions can be used to elicit values and goals that will influence patients' decisions about end-of-life care (Box 10.1).[18] A discussion about goals of care may not always result in completion of an advance directive and sometimes may not be viewed by patients and families as an ACP discussion. Opening the conversation by specifically asking to discuss wishes for care in the event of serious illness may help produce shared understanding.

Summary

ACP is an important aspect of kidney supportive care and is an ongoing process framed by the patient's and family's values, goals, and desires. Most CKD and ESKD patients welcome ACP discussions but rely on providers to initiate the process. Provider involvement is required to achieve informed decision-making because information on risks and benefits of interventions and expected prognosis is integral to making informed choices. Although societies and the government all promote ACP and completion of advance directives, only about a third of individuals complete written advance directives. Reasons for the lack of widespread adoption of written advance directives are complex and both patient/family- and provider-based. Efforts to improve the communication skills of nephrologists and other providers playing a role in the ACP process among CKD and ESKD patients may facilitate ACP in this population in a way that societal and governmental recommendations have not. Physician orders for end-of-life care such as DNAR, POLST, or MOLST forms are recommended for patients for whom the answer to the surprise question ("Would you be surprised if this patient died within the next 6 months to a year?") is no.

Practice Pointers

- ACP is a patient-centered process that begins with a discussion about the patient's values and goals as well as consideration of their health state and prognosis. It is an ongoing process that should be revisited as health status changes.
- Advance directives are written patient-generated documents outlining wishes for end-of-life care and/or designating a healthcare decision maker.
- DNR or DNAR and POLST or MOLST forms are provider-generated orders addressing choices the patient or family makes for end-of-life care.

Practice Improvement Opportunities

- It is incumbent upon nephrologists and dialysis unit–associated healthcare providers to introduce ACP as part of the overall care plan for each CKD or ESKD patient and to revisit such discussions throughout the course of the patient's life as his or her circumstances, health state, and goals change.
- Clearly designate who within the practice or unit is responsible for holding conversations, updating on regular basis, and including documentation in chart.

References

1. Sudore RL, Lum HD, You JJ, et al. Defining advance care planning for adults: a consensus definition from a multidisciplinary Delphi panel. *J Pain Symptom Manage*. 2017;53 (5):821–832.
2. Brinkman-Stoppelenburg A, Rietjens JA, van der Heidea. The effects of advance care planning on end-of-life care: a systematic review. *Palliat Med*. 2014;28:1000–1025.
3. Houben CHM, Spruit MA, Groenen MTJ, et al. Efficacy of advance care planning: a systematic review and meta-analysis. *JAMA*. 2014;15 (7):477–489.
4. Kirchoff KT, Hammes BJ, Kehl KA, Briggs LA, Brown RL. Effect of a disease-specific advance care planning intervention on end-of-life care. *J Am Geriatr Soc*. 2012;60 (5):946–950.
5. Sudore RL, Fried TR. Redefining the "planning" in advance care planning: preparing for end-of-life decision making. *Ann Intern Med*. 2010;153 (4):256–261.
6. National POLST. [Home page]. http://polst.org. Accessed January 30, 2019.
7. O'Hare AM, Szarka J, McFarland L V, et al. Provider perspectives on advance care planning for patients with kidney disease: whose job is it anyway? *Clin J Am Soc Nephrol*. 2016;11(5):855–866.
8. The Conversation Project. [Home page]. https://theconversation project.org. Accessed January 15, 2019.
9. Ra JR, Anderson LA, Lin FC, Laux JP. Completion of advance directives among US consumers. *Am J Prev Med*. 2004; 46(1):65–70.
10. Feely MA, Hildebrandt D, Eadkkanambeth VJ, Mueller PS. Prevalence and contents of advance directives of patients with end-stage renal disease receiving dialysis. *Clin J Am Soc Nephrol*. 2016;11(12):2204–2209.

11. Davison SN. End-of-life care preferences and needs: perceptions of patients with chronic kidney disease. *Clin J Am Soc Nephrol*. 201; 5 (2):195–204.
12. Schell JO, Cohen RA, Green JA, et al. Nephrotalk: evaluation of a palliative care communication curricula for nephrology fellows. *J Pain Symptom Manage*. 2018;56 (5):767–773.
13. Davison SN, Levin A, Moss AH, et al. Executive summary of the KDIGO controversies conference in supportive care in chronic kidney disease: developing a roadmap to improving quality care. *Kidney Int*. 2015;88 (3): 447–459.
14. American Society of Nephrology. Don't initiate chronic dialysis without ensuring a shared decision-making process between patients, their families, and their physicians. April 4, 2012 https://www.choosingwisely.org/clinician-lists/american-society-nephrology-chronic-dialysis-without-shared-decision-making/. Accessed April 13, 2020.
15. Renal Physicians Association. *Shared decision-making in the appropriate initiation of and withdrawal from dialysis: clinical practice guideline*. 2nd ed. Rockville, MD: RPA; 2010.
16. Coalition for Supportive Care of Kidney Patients. [Home page]. http://kidneysupportivecare.org. Accessed January 30, 2019
17. Anderson E, Aldous A, Lupu D. Make your wishes about you (MY WAY): using motivational interviewing to foster advance care planning for patients with chronic kidney disease *Nephrol Nurs J*. 2018;45 (5):411–421.
18. Mandel EI, Bernacki RE, Block SD. Serious illness conversations in end-stage renal disease. *Clin J Am Soc Nephrol*. 2016;12(5):854–863.

Involving Family and Friends in Palliative Care for Persons With Kidney Disease

Elizabeth Anderson and David M. White

Family-centered palliative care for patients with kidney disease shows great promise in alleviating the suffering of patients with collateral benefits to family members. Engaging family caregivers is particularly valuable for those with kidney disease, given often multiple comorbidities, impact of dialysis on quality of life, and often conflicting end-of-life decisions. Family caregivers are at high risk for burnout, increasing the likelihood that patients themselves will not receive end-of-life care or support. Important components of family-centered palliative care include assessment, emotional support, education, assertive communication skills, referrals, and grief and bereavement support. It is crucial that the care team recognize the role of cultural norms, family beliefs, and communication patterns, tailoring family-centered care to meet the needs of each individual patient.

Case

Sondra is a 73-year old African-American widow living in the Washington, DC, with her daughter and son-in-law Angela and Raymond and their children, Aurora (aged 16) and Ray Jr. (aged 10). Sondra retired from her job as a secretary in 2008 and was an active member of her block association and church.

Sondra began in-center dialysis in 2013 after many years of struggling with the management of diabetes and high blood pressure. She took it with her well-known grace and enthusiasm, putting herself in charge of keeping up the other patients' spirits while also continuing her existing outside activities.

Sondra's health has taken a turn for the worse, and she now uses a walker, limiting her ability to get to church and block association meetings. She now needs assistance from Angel and Aurora with getting dressed, taking a bath, and cooking meals for the family.

Sondra reports a loss of appetite and uncomfortable muscle cramps. She misses being able to get around on her own and being active, and she is not always as upbeat at the clinic as she used to be. She worries about being a burden on family members, who are busy with full-time jobs, school, and activities. Sondra often comments, "I don't like just sitting around all day. I feel like I'm not contributing."

Current Evidence

Family care often occupies a central role in end-stage kidney disease (ESKD), dialysis, and palliative care. Family is not used here in the strict sense as "blood relatives" but is relative to the individual's circumstances and culture and is ultimately defined by the individual. Hepworth, Rooney, Rooney, and Gottfried state that family's purpose is to attend to the "health, well-being and mutual care of its members that are unlike those of any other social system"[1] (p. 253). Families are a natural and underutilized resource in providing such care.

Family systems theory suggests that families function as a system in which each individual members impact other members and the family system as a whole.[2] Families create patterns, belief and value systems, boundaries, structures, roles, rules and communication patterns.[2] A change in the health status of one family member often causes significant stress and emotional imbalance on the entire family system, requiring members to readjust boundaries, roles, rules, and communication.[3] Families have the capacity not only to survive crisis, but to thrive above and beyond prior functioning. Work with the family can be complex because it requires a provider to consider the perspectives of multiple people who may have different priorities and values.

Case vignette: Angela and Raymond juggle their work schedules so that someone is home to provide care. Since Angela and Raymond take turns, the care team get different messages depending on who is providing information.

Family Involvement

Family involvement is important to patients with kidney disease, who rely heavily on family caregivers and readily recognize the importance of that reliance.[4,5] Family caregivers are often responsible for managing a patient's multiple conditions and activities of daily living.[4] Studies indicate that most patients discuss end of life care with their family[6] but some hemodialysis family members have expressed regret that conversations about withdrawing dialysis occurred without the family members being present[7] underscoring how underutilized family members often felt in the care of persons with kidney disease.

Case vignette: Sondra is losing energy to go to dialysis daily and wants more time to travel to see her grandchildren. She says, "I know my time is near," and family quickly respond with "Don't say that; you are doing great!" Family members are worried about Sondra's deteriorating health, but the increased caregiving demands have made for more busy schedules, putting off any discussion about the future with "We'll have time for that later."

Positive Outcomes

For patients on hemodialysis, family members have been a key factor in weighing dialysis options[8] while improving patient understanding of dialysis.[9] More broadly, family involvement has had a positive correlation with behavioral changes including decreased smoking, drinking, increased cancer screenings, better nutrition, decreased heart rate, and blood pressure.[10] When a companion accompanies a patient to a doctor visit, patients are more likely to ask questions and have more focused discussions.[11] Extensive family counseling with the chronically ill has been shown to decrease the length of stay in intensive care units by a day.[12] It is not surprising, then, that family involvement is correlated with patient quality of life,[13] decreased depression, and care more congruent with patient values.[14]

Case vignette: Sondra tells her family that the doctor says that she might be able to get palliative care services to help her with the chronic pain. Angela gets upset that the physician mentioned palliative care, feeling concerned that she is going to die soon. Angela asks Sondra questions about palliative care, and Sondra states "I get things mixed up sometimes and I forget to ask questions when I go to the doctor alone. I feel better when someone is with me." When Angela accompanies Sondra on her next doctor visit, Angela is relieved to learn that there are other support options to help care for her mom.

Family and Patient Stress

Patients worry about being a burden on their relatives and often feel that dependence on family members is a violation of privacy.[4] Adding to the complexity, caregivers may blame the patient for years of poor health decisions leading to dialysis.[4] Considering how important family members are to patients, it is not surprising that family caregivers of patients with kidney disease are at high risk of burnout, with as many as one-third of ESKD unpaid caregivers reporting moderate to severe caregiver burden.[15]

Hemodialysis family members report that as their loved one's health deteriorate, they worry about when to call an ambulance and when to allow resuscitation or withdrawal from dialysis and feel responsible for ensuring that the patient has a peaceful death.[7] End-of-life family caregivers in general report that they often experience emotional distress thinking about the impending loss of their loved one or watching their loved one suffer, often with more limited social support than earlier years.[16] When providers engage in conversations concerning supportive care for patients, caregiver burden decreases.[17] Including family caregivers in conversations with patients not only may relieve caregiver burden but should also help the patient receive care consistent with their own values.

Case vignette: Sondra moved in with Angela as her health declined. Angela managed her mother's healthcare, diet, appointments, and activities of daily living. Sondra began missing dialysis sporadically and became ill. Angela had also gotten sick and was in the hospital dealing with chronic back pain and struggling to cover the cost of transportation to dialysis and healthy food at the grocery store. Angela reported feeling overwhelmed with providing increased care for her mother, and for herself, and she often felt alone in her decision-making. Sondra was tearful in the conversation with the team but expressed appreciation at having the opportunity to discuss the barriers to care.

Challenges

Palliative care providers, often skilled in family-centered end-of-life conversations, are often underutilized within the nephrology community.[18] Ideally, such family conversations would occur before dialysis is initiated, but dialysis is often initiated in emergent situations where such conversations are difficult.[9] On the whole, family members are just becoming aware of how important their role can be to the well-being of the person receiving care and how they can fit into the relationships appropriately.

Case vignette: Example conversation from the care team is as follows:

> Angela, thank you so much for coming in today. We have found that family members play such a vital part of the healthcare of our patients. Right now your Mom is doing

so well. However, if things ever change, as they probably will, it is important to me that I have a relationship with you so we can work together to give your Mom the best care possible.

Cultural Humility in Family Meetings

Some would argue that the very lens through which we view family theory is overly focused on Western individualism and largely ignores the more collective approaches other cultures enjoy.[2] Family functioning is often dictated by cultural norms, and each family will have unique views, belief systems, and values.[3] While it is important that the care team recognize cultural differences, providers must also avoid overgeneralizing or making assumptions about differences as well. Providers should recognize their own beliefs about family functioning to avoid imposing their own biases. Likewise, it is important to recognize the roles racism and oppression have played in creating trust issues with health providers. It requires the providers to practice cultural humility, a willingness to be present, listen, and learn from patients, with a genuine desire to create therapeutic rapport. Cultural humility, unlike cultural competence, recognizes that no person can never know all that there is to know about another person's culture, respecting the roles of diversity, difference, and power in relationships.

Case vignette: A white male care team member working with Sondra and her family, he notes, "One thing that I have learned is not to make any assumptions related to my patients because we all have different perspectives." He then asks, "What would be important for me to know about your family in terms of providing support to you throughout this process?"

Guidelines for Providing Family-Centered Care

The Pathways Project seeks to provide patient-centered care to people with kidney disease.[19] The project has created evidence-based recommendations to improve supportive care for patients with kidney disease, including family engagement. Recommendations include annual caregiver assessments, respite and support resources lists, family meeting rooms, educational material, and bereavement support.

Practice Pointers

To date, there are no formal guidelines or consensus statements directly related to family centered palliative care for nephrology; however the following practice pointers follow the existing literature from other professions.

At the most basic level, the care team is encouraged to *invite and include family caregivers to all meetings*.[9] Working with families offers a unique opportunity for the care team to empower family members to help each other, rather than having the provider as the sole individual giving advice and support.[3] Meetings should include assessment, (Box 11.1), emotional support (Box 11.2), and support resources (Box 11.3), including supportive care for patients with kidney disease. Conversations regarding such supportive care often eases family caregiver anxiety about the future[17] and has been recommended for providers of patients

> **BOX 11.1. Family Caregiver Assessment Questions**
>
> - How is caregiving going for you?
> - How is the family doing?
> - Sometimes when a family member gets sick it raises concerns for us. What are some of your own concerns?
> - What are your hopes for your family member?

with ESKD.[18] Conversations regarding supportive care can help prepare the family and patient for the coming losses and emotional roller coaster.[18]

The Caregiving Stress Appraisal Tool is often used by providers during the first visit to capture baseline caregiver burden.[15] The *assessment tool* serves to direct caregiver conversations and education on resources and problem solving. Example questions include "How is caregiving going for you?" or "How is the family doing?"[20] Specific guidance can be found in chapter 9 on serious illness conversations for patients with ESKD.

Emotional Support

On average, hospital patients are interrupted every 11 seconds by a physician (Box 11.2).[21] Offering emotional support requires the care team to focus on listening to the patient and family member's concerns and responding to their emotional needs. Hemodialysis family caregivers have expressed that they would like the healthcare team to acknowledge them, especially during some of the most challenging emotional times.[7] Research suggests that family caregivers of patients on hemodialysis often suppress their feelings for fear that they will upset the patient,[7] which can lead to depression. The care team should offer the opportunity for reflection, emotional support, and empathy by recognizing and validating common feelings regarding caregiving and fears of life-limiting illness.[23]

Family caregivers who have a positive view of caregiving are less likely to experience caregiver burden and are therefore more emotionally available to help in the care of the patient.[15] Affinito and Louie suggest cognitive reframing skills and identifying positive impacts of caregiving.[15] In a cognitive behavioral theoretical framework, conflict may arise from *miscommunication with unrealistic expectations*.[3] The care team can help avoid

> **BOX 11.2. Emotional Support Steps**
>
> - Identify patient or family member emotion and reflect it back to the patient. "It sounds like this is a painful area to consider."
> - Reflect back patient and family concerns.
> - Validate common feelings related to caregiving and fears of life-limiting illness.
> - Resist the urge to "fix it" when patients or family members share something emotional. Instead, stay present, listen, and reflect.

> **BOX 11.3. Referral Suggestions**
> - Palliative care
> - Hospice
> - Bereavement services
> - Adult day care
> - Respite
> - Home care
> - Social worker, therapist, or counselor
> - Support groups

conflict by providing education and information on what to expect as a patient declines. Other strategies may include coping techniques such as teaching family caregivers deep breathing exercises to help them through during difficult periods and identifying necessary communication skills and anger management strategies when family caregivers report feeling stress.[15]

Referrals to Support

Family caregivers often have reduced support systems because of the demands of providing care, thus taking time away from other natural support systems in the community such as work, spiritual care, and hobbies (Box 11.3). Doneath found that when a general practitioner provider referred an informal caregiver to counseling or a support group, the utilization rate of the support increased 4-fold and 5-fold, respectively, indicating that informal caregivers take providers suggestions seriously.[22] Examples of resources to provide include local palliative care organization, hospice organization, counselors or therapists, adult day care, respite, home care, and social workers,[21] as well as local support groups.[22] Many hospices offer free bereavement services to the community as well.

Education for Family Members About End of Life

Family caregivers of patients with ESKD emphasize that as their responsibility for the patient increases, so does their uncertainty and fear of the future.[7] Family caregivers have expressed a desire that someone share more with them about the dying process, including written information about what to expect, how to be supportive, and how to cope with the changes in health.[7]

Bereavement services have been reported as the least met supportive need.[19] Family caregivers of patients on dialysis at the end of life report on the strain of knowing death was near, often feeling alone when dialysis staff did not contact them following the death of a loved one.[7] Sending bereavement notes from staff and referrals to bereavement programs can help family members of patients who have died.

Summary

The inclusion of family is essential to the provision of quality patient centered palliative care to patients with advanced kidney disease. Engaging families in meetings and patient visits provides a firm layer of support, increases positive outcomes, and allows patients to receive care that is more congruent with their values. Assessing and addressing caregiver burden in family members of patients can further facilitate higher quality of life for the patient as well as the family member, can reduce burnout, and can reduce complicated grief. Counseling patients one on one in palliative care requires a complex skill set, which is compounded when family members are included. The care team must recognize that family engagement requires additional skills, including assessment of the family caregiver, eliciting family member feedback, listening attentively to caregiver concerns, emotional caregiver support, and the use of referrals, education, and bereavement services. Those skilled in caregiver/family communication are in a much better position to assist patients and family caregivers through difficult end-of-life care and decisions.

Concerns about the time challenges of providing such emotional support should be evaluated in light of ethical principles to provide holistic care and in consideration of the significant unmet palliative care needs of patients with kidney disease. Development and evaluation of a family-centered best-practice tool for the care team could serve to address this need and ultimately provide patients with holistic palliative care.

Practice Pointers

- Involving family in conversations has numerous positive outcomes including an increase quality of life, a decrease in depression, and care that is congruent with patient values.
- Family caregivers experience increased stress and burden, making family caregivers more vulnerable to burnout. Assessing and addressing family caregivers can serve to alleviate burnout.
- Patients and family members would prefer to have more conversations about preferences at the end of life.

Practice Improvement Opportunities

- Assess and engage family members and provide education about disease progression and supportive care options.
- Provide emotional support to family caregivers of patients with kidney disease.
- Create referral resources for family members, including access to grief and bereavement services.

References

1. Hepworth DH, Rooney RH, Rooney GD, Strom-Gottfried K. *Direct Social Work Practice: Theory and Skills.* 10th ed. Boston, MA: Cengage Learning; 2017.

2. Hutchinson ED. *Dimensions of Human Behavior: Person and Environment.* 5th ed. Thousand Oaks, CA: SAGE; 2016.
3. Shulman L. *The Skill of Helping Individuals, Families, Groups and Communities.* 8th ed. Boston, MA. Cengage; 2016.
4. da Silva Jacobi C, Beuter M, Girardon-Perlini NMO, Timm AMB, Bruinsma JL, Mistura C. The care of elderly patients receiving pre-dialysis treatment: a descriptive study. *Online Braz J Nurs.* 2016;15(4):713–723.
5. Silva-Gane D, Farrington K. Supportive care in advanced kidney disease: patient attitudes and expectations. *J Renal Care.* 2014:40(S1):30–35.
6. Weiner S. End-of-life care discussions: a survey of patients on dialysis and professionals. *J Pain Symptom Manage.* 2010;39(2):395–396.
7. Axelsson L, Klang B, Lundh Hagelin C, Jacobson SH, Gleissman SA. Meanings of being a close relative of a family member treated with haemodialysis approaching end of life. *J Clin Nurs.* 2015:24(3–4):447–456.
8. Morton RL, Tong A, Howard K, Snelling P, Webster AC. The views of patients and carers in treatment decision making for chronic kidney disease: systematic review and thematic synthesis of qualitative studies. *BMJ.* 2010;340(7742):350. doi:10.1136/bmj.c112.
9. Sheu J, Ephraim PL, Powe NR, et al. African American and non-African American Patients' and families' decision making about renal replacement therapies. *Qual Health Res.* 2012;22(7):997–1006. doi:10.1177/1049732312443427.
10. Seeman TE. Social health promoting effects of friends and family on health outcomes in older adults. *Am J Heal Promot.* 2000;14(6):362–371. doi:10.4278/0890-1171-14.6.362.
11. Wolff JL. Family matters in health care delivery. *JAMA.* 2012;308(15):1529–1530. doi:10.1001/jama.2012.13366.
12. Shier G, Ginsburg M, Howell J, Volland P, Golden R. Strong social support services, such as transportation and help for caregivers, can lead to lower health care use and costs. *Health Aff (Millwood).* 2013;32(3):544–551. doi:10.1377/hlthaff.2012.0170.
13. Braveman P, Egerter S, Barclay C. *Issue Brief Series: Exploring the Social Determinants of Health: Income, Wealth, and Health.* Princeton, NJ: Robert Wood Johnson Foundation; 2011.
14. Symister P. Beyond social support: using family expectations to predict psychological adjustment in end-stage renal disease patients. *J Health Psychol.* 2011;16(7):1015–1026. doi:10.1177/1359105311398680.
15. Affinito J, Louie K. Positive coping and self-assessed levels of health and burden in unpaid caregivers of patients with end stage renal disease receiving hemodialysis therapy. *Nephrol Nurs J.* 2018;45(4):373–379.
16. De Korte-Verhoef MC, Pasman HRW, Schweitzer BP, Francke AL, Onwuteaka-Philipsen BD, Deliens L. Burden for family carers at the end of life: a mixed-method study of the perspectives of family carers and GPs. BMC Pall Care. 2014;13(1):16.
17. Hoffman A, Tranter S, Josland E, Brennan F, Brown M. Renal supportive care in conservatively managed patients with advanced chronic kidney disease: a qualitative study of the experiences of patients and their carers/families. *Ren Soc Australas J.* 2017;13(3):100–106.
18. Mandel EI, Bernacki RE, Block SD. Serious illness conversations in ESRD. *Clin J Am Soc Nephrol.* 2016;12(5): 854–863. doi:10.2215/CJN.05760516
19. Culp S, Lupu D, Arenella C, Armistead N, Moss AH. Unmet supportive care needs in US dialysis centers and lack of knowledge of available resources to address them. *J Pain Symptom Manage.*2016;51(4):756–761.
20. Rabow MW, Hauser JM, Adams J. Perspectives on care at the close of life: supporting family caregivers at the end of life: "they don't know what they don't know." *JAMA.* 2004;291(4):483–491.
21. Ospina NS, Phillips KA, RodriguezGutierrez R, et al. Eliciting the patient's agenda: secondary analysis of recorded clinical encounters. *J Gen Intern Med.* 2019;34(1):36–40.
22. Donath, C., Gräßel, E., Großfeld-Schmitz, et al. Effects of general practitioner training and family support services on the care of home-dwelling dementia patients-results of a controlled cluster-randomized study. *BMC Health Serv Res.* 2010;10(1):314.

12

The System to Implement Advance Care Planning and Make Proxies, Advance Directives, and Portable Medical Orders Available and Actionable Across Care Settings

Valerie Satkoske and Alvin H. Moss

> Few would debate that thoughtful advance care planning conversations between providers, patients, and patients' loved ones reflect a respect for the right to direct one's end-of-life care based upon personal values, preferences, and goals. Previous research suggests that advance directives and medical orders are the vehicles to enable patient wishes to be known. However, without ensuring clinician access to those documents, the chances that a patient will receive the desired level of treatment at the end of life diminish significantly. This chapter explores the impediments to accessing and acting upon advance directives and medical orders and suggests a comprehensive system that improves access to completed advance care planning documents for providers and patients. It reviews the successes with such a system in a state—West Virginia—and the positive outcomes with employing components of the proposed system with chronic kidney disease and dialysis patients.

Case

Mrs. Johnson, a 67-year old woman with end-stage kidney disease (ESKD) from polycystic kidney disease, was recently transported to the hospital from an outpatient dialysis clinic after she had become unresponsive. The patient had multiple hospitalizations over the previous 6 months and frequently required admission to the intensive care unit (ICU). During her most recent admission she spent 10 days in the ICU, requiring ventilator support for 7 days. When Mrs. Johnson arrived at the emergency department (ED) this time, she was too sick to discuss her wishes. The accompanying paperwork from the dialysis clinic included a note from the clinic social worker that said the patient had advance directives and a physician orders for life-sustaining treatment (POLST) form, but they were not in her transfer packet from the dialysis clinic, the patient's chart in the hospital's electronic medical record system, or in the state's end-of-life advance directive and medical order registry. The ED nurse and unit clerk were unable to contact the patient's son, who the dialysis social worker said was the patient's medical power of attorney representative. The ED physician was hesitant to limit treatment since she did not know what the patient's advance directives and POLST form said. As Mrs. Johnson was in respiratory failure, she was transferred to the ICU where she was once again intubated.

The Process of Advance Care Planning

Mrs. Johnson had engaged in advance care planning (ACP) and expressed her wishes in writing for medical care in the event she lost decision-making capacity at some time in the future, but sadly her advance directive and POLST form were not available when needed in the time of a medical emergency. Her case illustrates why when a multidisciplinary international panel of ACP experts developed a consensus definition of ACP, they included 2 parts to the ACP process: (i) discussion(s) to understand the patient's values, preferences, and life goals and (ii) a *system* to document patients' values, preferences, and goals in a way that ensures that patients receive medical care that aligns with their wishes.[1] They included the second component because they understood that even when providers do engage in those discussions, the systems for documenting patient wishes, storing documents so they are retrievable across settings, and honoring those wishes are not reliable. For example, if ACP is discussed and forms completed, but the clinician does not document the conversation or enter (scan) the documents into the electronic medical record, then it is up to patients and families to remember to bring those documents every time they have a clinical encounter. When such clinical encounters are emergent, stressed family members may not remember to bring such documents and may not find, retrieve, or provide them to the treating facility during the course of a patient's admission. The lack of systemic processes for documenting, storing, retrieving, and acting on patient wishes is ethically problematic in that it undermines both patient autonomy and a clinician's ability to respect patients' end-of-life treatment preferences.

This chapter will provide an overview of implementing the second part of the ACP definition so that advance directives and portable medical orders of patients with kidney disease are reliably available and actionable across care settings. See chapter 10 for a discussion of the first part of ACP.

The Failure of Dialysis Patients' Advance Directives to Address Dialysis

Because of the ethical principle of respect for patient autonomy, physicians and other health professionals involved in the care of patients with advanced chronic kidney disease and ESKD are obligated to document patients' values, preferences, and goals in a manner that enables them to be known and respected at the time of a medical crisis. Because dialysis patients are dependent on a life-sustaining treatment for survival, it is especially important for them to document their preferences to continue or stop dialysis so they can be respected in the future when they may be unable to participate in decision-making. Even dialysis patients who complete advance directives rarely indicate their preference for whether to stop dialysis at the end of life or discuss this particular circumstance with their proxy decisionmaker.[2,3] The failure of ACP with dialysis patients to include their preferences with regard to stopping dialysis underscores the challenge for a system that is attempting to know and respect dialysis patients' wishes with regard to management of dialysis at the end of life.

Nonetheless, dialysis patients have strong preferences about health states in which they would want to stop dialysis. In a study of 95 Canadian hemodialysis patients who were asked their preferences for life-sustaining treatments in a variety of health states, only 25% wanted to continue dialysis in the event of a severe stroke, 19% if they had severe dementia, and 14% if they were in a permanent coma.[4] A successful system of ACP for dialysis patients will need to more intentionally address patients' preferences for dialysis at the end of life. This chapter will use West Virginia's nationally recognized system for ACP as a model for successful implementation of a system to promote ACP best practices for patients with chronic kidney disease and ESKD.[5]

The Components of a Comprehensive Advance Care Planning System: West Virginia's Example

As the definition for ACP indicates, effective ACP requires a system to guide and support end-of-life discussions and decision-making and consistent, reliable methods of documenting, storing, and accessing ACP documents—advance directives and medical orders (do not resuscitate [DNR] and POLST). West Virginia has such a system (Figure 12.1) with a mature POLST program (http://polst.org) and Internet-based registry.[5] The system includes the 7 components listed in Box 12.1.[6]

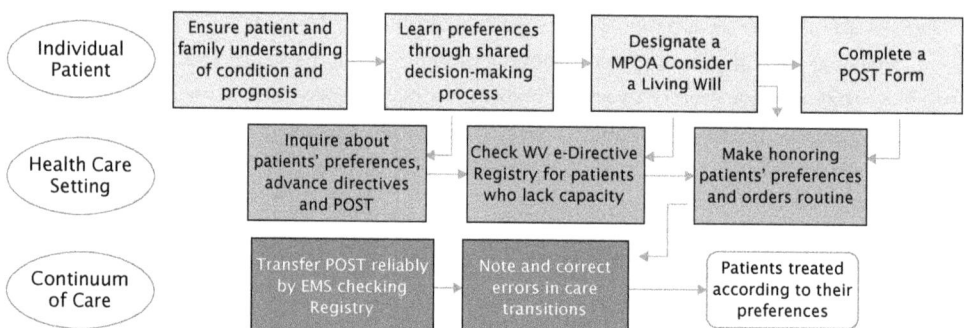

FIGURE 12.1. West Virginia's system to provide patient-centered, high-quality care for patients with advanced illness. Clinician asks oneself the surprise question, "Would I be surprised if this patient died in the next year?" A "No, I would not be surprised" response serves as a trigger to the clinician to initiate an advance care planning discussion. Figure used with the permission of the West Virginia Center for End-of-Life Care.

Abbreviations: EMS, Emergency Medical Services; LW, living will; MPOA, medial power of attorney; POST, Physician Orders for Scope of Treatment; WV, West Virginia.

> **BOX 12.1. Deliverables of the West Virginia System to Respect Patients' End-of-Life Wishes**
>
> - Standardized practices, policies (regulations/laws), and forms
> - Trained advance care planning facilitators
> - Timely discussions prompted by prognosis
> - Surprise question, "Would I be surprised if . . . ?"
> - Specific language on an actionable brightly colored, easily found POLST form
> - Orders honored throughout the system
> - QI activities for continual refinement
> - Online secure electronic registry for 24/7 access to patients' directives/orders
>
> Abbreviations: POLST, physician orders for life-sustaining treatment; QI, quality improvement.

In its 2014 report, *Dying in America: Improving Quality and Honoring Individual Preferences near the End-of-Life*, the Institute of Medicine (IOM) identified the POLST program as one of several promising innovations to improve end-of-life care in the United States. The IOM encouraged all states to adopt a POLST or similar type program and Internet-based registries as preferred practices to improve the care of the dying by honoring individuals' preferences near the end of life.[7]

West Virginia is 1 of only 3 states in the country considered to have a mature POLST program. To qualify to be considered mature, more than 50% of all healthcare setting (hospitals, nursing homes, and hospices) in all regions of the state had to be demonstrated to be using the POLST form. West Virginia has also garnered national attention because of its online West Virginia e-Directive Registry. This registry receives advance directives, DNR cards, POLST forms, surrogate selection forms, and guardianship papers from treating healthcare providers and the public and, with the consent of patients or their legal agents, releases them to treating healthcare providers at the time of a medical crisis. In a March 13, 2015, *New York Times* article, West Virginia was noted as a pioneer in end-of-life planning because of its POLST program and online registry.[8]

If a patient is seriously ill (including those with advanced kidney disease) and the physician would not be surprised if the patient died in the next year, as part of ACP, the IOM recommends completion of a POLST form (called physician orders for scope of treatment [POST] form in West Virginia and by other names in other states such as medical orders for life-sustaining treatment [MOLST] or medical orders for scope of treatment [MOST] form).[7] The value of the POLST form is that it translates the patients' wishes expressed in an advance directive into immediately actionable medical orders that do not require interpretation or further activation and that, by state law, are to be honored. POLST aims to provide continuity of care for patients according to their preferences across all care settings (eg, hospitals, hospice, long-term care and home) and is transferred with the patient throughout the healthcare system. In each state that has adopted a POLST program, leaders have conducted statewide education to support the use of POLST across the spectrum of healthcare settings.[9]

The power of the POLST form depends on the strength of the underlying patient–physician communication, the accurate translation of patients' wishes in a medical order form, and on the establishment of a statewide system for communicating and honoring those orders at the time of a medical crisis[9]. Ideally, in each statewide system POLST orders are identified by emergency medical services as they are transporting patients to EDs, and patients with a POLST form with limited treatment or comfort measures orders are spared unwanted intubation in the ED and mechanical ventilation in an ICU. West Virginia created the statewide Internet-based registry, the West Virginia e-Directive Registry (http://wvendoflife.org/for-providers/e-directive-registry/), to fulfill this.

Nephrology researchers have documented the value of conversations and POLST form completion with dialysis patients. They found that a system of care for dialysis patients including timely goals of care discussions and completion of POLST forms according to patients' wishes alters their care in the direction of an increased focus on comfort and a decreased emphasis on aggressive life support at the end of life. Nephrologist-led ACP discussions for 50 patients at 2 dialysis centers in Boston resulted in patients' preference for a DNR order increasing from 18% to 42% ($p = .0001$), and the completion of MOLST forms increasing from 10% to 90%.[10] In another dialysis center-based study, a nephrologist and nephrology nurse practitioner led an intervention in which 65 seriously ill patients were systematically engaged in an ACP discussion.[9] Of these patients, all completed a POLST form, 71% died out of the hospital, 51% decided to withdraw from dialysis, and of those who withdrew, the majority (58%) died with hospice care, which are much higher percentages than those reported in other studies of dialysis patients' end-of-life care.[11]

The West Virginia Center for End-of-Life Care has documented the following advantages of an Internet-based registry to store and provide access to patients' advance directives and medical orders (DNR and POLST):

- Accurate, relevant information available in a medical crisis
- 24/7 online access by healthcare providers
- Consumer able to confirm online accuracy of their advance directives and medical orders
- Patients' wishes accessible and respected throughout the continuum of care settings
- Password-protected and HIPAA compliant[12]

Based on market research surveys conducted by the West Virginia Center for End-of-Life Care, West Virginia is among the top states in advance directive completion with 49% of West Virginians reporting that they have executed a medical power of attorney, living will, or both. Research has shown, however, that advance directives are not as effective as initially thought. Research has demonstrated that advance directives alone do not impact a patient's site of death.[12] Although 92% of West Virginians state a preference to die outside of the hospital, only 57% of deceased West Virginians who have submitted advance directives to the West Virginia e-Directive Registry do, and there is no significant difference between this 57% and the 59% of all West Virginians who die outside of the hospital.[12]

In contrast to advance directives, the POLST form has been shown to have much more of an impact on where patients die. Eighty-eight percent of West Virginians who submitted a POLST form with comfort measure orders to the Registry died outside of the hospital.[12] This is as would be expected since the POLST comfort measure orders read, "Do not transfer to hospital for life-sustaining treatment. Transfer only if comfort needs cannot be met in current location."

In surveys conducted over the past decade, 75% of West Virginians (as do dialysis patients[13]) repeatedly say that at the end of life they would prefer to live a shorter period of time to avoid pain, suffering, and being kept alive on machines. The POLST form with medical orders that are followed throughout the continuum of healthcare (without the need for interpretation or the patient being declared incapacitated) more than advance directives allows patients with kidney disease with such preferences to be treated according to their wishes. The POLST form with comfort measures orders directs all treating healthcare providers to make patient comfort the first priority.[9]

Inpatient hospital palliative care consultation teams complete a large percentage of the POLST forms in West Virginia. However, dialysis patients, even when seriously ill, are rarely seen by inpatient palliative care consultation teams. One study found that inpatient palliative care occurred in less than 1% of hospitalizations of ESKD patients lasting more than 2 days nationally.[14] The researchers suggest that expanded access to inpatient palliative care with the resultant goals of care conversations may meaningfully shorten inpatient length of stay and alter the intensity of care delivered after discharge, reducing readmissions and perhaps smoothing transitions to hospice among patients with ESKD who are nearing the end of life.[14]

In addition to utilization of inpatient palliative care consultation, all clinicians who provide care to critically and chronically ill patients with advanced kidney disease should seek training in primary palliative care. Provider communication skills for shared decision-making and ACP are discussed in other chapters. However, as noted previously, the conversation itself is not sufficient. A system for converting patients' values identified from these conversations into advance directives and POLST forms and then storing them in a location from which they are reliably retrieved and honoring them is needed.[15]

Back to Mrs. Johnson

Mrs. Johnson and her dialysis team did many things right with regard to ACP. She took the steps necessary to ensure that her end-of-life wishes were recorded in a living will, and she appointed a loved one, her son, to be her medical power of attorney representative. Additionally, Mrs. Johnson and her physician completed a POLST form to make sure that her medical treatment wishes were immediately actionable. However, as is too often the case, a chart note signaling the existence of advance directives and/or medical orders, in the absence of *access* to those documents, does little to protect the patient's control over decisions made in her care. In reality, Mrs. Johnson and her care providers only accomplished the first part of ACP. Her case underscores why a comprehensive ACP system as outlined in this chapter is needed so that patients with kidney disease have their wishes known and respected at the end of life.

Summary

Dialysis patients and their families report that they welcome the opportunity to engage in ACP with their nephrologists, but only the minority has done so. Multiple national organizations have recommended a system to conduct ACP conversations and to document them in advance directives and medical orders stored in registries so that the documents are readily accessible at the end of life. This chapter presents the elements of a comprehensive ACP system using the system in West Virginia as a model. Use of the system including POLST forms has been shown to result in improved quality metrics for end-of-life care according to patients' wishes compared to advance directives alone. More frequent inpatient palliative care consultation for seriously ill patients with kidney disease is likely to lead to better identification of patients' values and completion of advance directives and POLST forms. The challenge for the nephrology community is to integrate these effective ACP components into the routine care of patients with kidney disease.

Practice Pointers

- Only 10% or less of dialysis patients report end-of-life care conversations with their nephrologists even though the vast majority of patients report they want to have them.
- Conversations with dialysis patients and documentation of their end-of-life treatment preferences in POLST forms has resulted in less aggressive care at the end of life. Seriously ill patients with POLST forms in the West Virginia registry were more than twice as likely to die outside the hospital and with hospice care.

Practice Improvement Opportunities

- Each nephrology practice should include in its performance improvement process regular audits and quality improvement projects to assure that updated ACP documents and/or POLST orders are readily retrievable for most patients, that these address patient's preferences for continuing or stopping dialysis, and that they are sent with patients when transferring settings.
- The nephrology community should collaborate with hospitals and nursing homes to increase participation in multisite ACP and POLST registries.
- Large dialysis organizations need to develop systematic ACP practices that utilize advance directives and medical orders and store them in accessible registries so that their patients' end-of-life treatment preferences are known and respected.

References

1. Sudore RL, Lum HD, You JJ, et al. Defining advance care planning for adults: a consensus definition from a multidisciplinary Delphi panel. *J Pain Symptom Manage*. 2017;53(5):821–832.
2. Feely MA, Hildebrandt D, Varayil JE, Mueller PS. Prevalence and contents of advance directives of patients with ESRD receiving dialysis. *Clin J Am Soc Nephrol*. 2016;11:2204–2209. doi:10.2215/CJN.12131115
3. Holley JL, Hines SC, Glover JJ, Babrow AS, Badzek LA, Moss AH. Failure of advance care planning to elicit patients' preferences for withdrawal from dialysis. *Am J Kidney Dis*. 1999;33(4):688–693.
4. Singer PA, Thiel EC, Naylor CD, et al. Life-sustaining treatment preferences of hemodialysis patients: implications for advance directives. *JASN*. 1995;6 (5):1410–1417.
5. US Government Accountability Office. Advance care planning: selected states' efforts to educate and address access challenges. GAO-19-231. https://www.gao.gov/products/GAO-19-231?utm_source=email&utm_medium=hc&utm_campaign=acp_i. Published February 21, 2019.
6. Moss AH. It takes a system to respect patients' wishes. *WV Medical J*. 2016;112:54–58.
7. Institute of Medicine. *Dying in America: Improving Quality and Honoring Individual Preferences near the End-of-Life*. Washington, D.C.: National Academies Press, 2014.
8. Span P. The trouble with advance directives. *New York Times*. http://www.nytimes.com/2015/03/17/health/the-trouble-with-advance-directives.html?_r=0. Published March 13, 2015.
9. Citko J, Moss AH, Carley M, Tolle SW. The National POLST Paradigm Initiative. 2nd ed. *Fast Facts and Concepts*. https://www.mypcnow.org/blank-k2dh9. Published 2010.
10. Amro OW, Ramasamy M, Strom JA, Weiner DE, Jaber BL. Nephrologist-facilitated advance care planning for hemodialysis patients: a quality improvement project. *Am J Kidney Dis*. 2016;68(1):103–109.
11. Schmidt RJ, Weaner BB, Long D. The power of advance care planning in promoting hospice and out-of-hospital death in a dialysis unit. *J Palliat Med*. 2015;18(1):62–66.
12. Pedraza SL, Culp S, Falkenstine E, Moss AH. POST forms more than advance directives associated with out-of-hospital death: insights from a state registry. *J Pain Symptom Manage*. 2016;51:240–246.
13. Hines SC, Glover JJ, Babrow AS, Holley JL, Badzek LA, Moss AH. Improving advance care planning by accommodating family preferences. *J Palliat Med*. 2001;4(4):481–489.
14. Chettiar A, Montez-Rath M, Liu S, Hall YN, O'Hare AM, Kurella Tamura M. Association of inpatient palliative care with health care utilization and postdischarge outcomes among medicare beneficiaries with end stage kidney disease. *Clin J Am Soc Nephrol*. 2018;13(8):1180–1187.
15. Sokol-Hessner L, Zambeaux A, Little K, Macy L, Lally K, McCutcheon Adams K. "Conversation ready": a framework for improving end-of-life care. 2nd ed. IHI White Paper. *Institute for Healthcare Improvement*. http://www.ihi.org/resources/Pages/IHIWhitePapers/ConversationReadyEndofLifeCare.aspx. Published 2019.

SECTION IV

Just Right Care—The Right Care to the Right Person at the Right Time

13

The Role of Estimating and Communicating Prognosis in Kidney Supportive Care

Bjorg Thorsteinsdottir and Michael J. Germain

> Most patients with advanced chronic kidney disease and end-stage kidney disease want to know their prognosis. Nephrologists report discomfort in communicating prognostic information to their patients and tend to avoid these discussions. This contributes to prognostic misperceptions among patients and overtreatment for patients for whom treatment benefit is questionable. Decisional regret and withdrawal rates are very high, especially among elderly dialysis patients. Prognosis lies at the center of good discussions about treatment goals that, in turn, facilitate shared decision-making. Good prognostic discussions thus have the potential to promote patient autonomy and facilitate goal concordant care. Several validated tools and frameworks are available to guide clinicians in these important conversations.

Case

Mrs. Jameson is an 85-year-old woman with end-stage kidney disease (ESKD), hypertension, advanced peripheral arterial disease, and early dementia. She is accompanied by her 87-year-old husband and their daughter. Mrs. Jameson has had slowly progressive chronic kidney disease (CKD) for a long time, but the past couple of months her glomerular filtration rate has been in the 14 to 15 range, and her blood urea nitrogen has been increasing. Mrs. Jameson says she is doing fine; she is still making urine, and she denies excessive swelling, shortness of breath, or nausea. Her caregivers report she seems close to her baseline cognitive functional status. She is sleeping a bit more, and her appetite has decreased. Mrs. Jameson has indicated to you in the past that she does not want dialysis because of going through it with her close friend who was on dialysis for many years. You have respected that wish but now you feel that a more formal discussion about treatment decisions needs to happen with her and her family.

There Is Equipoise Regarding the Benefits of Dialysis for Certain Patient Groups

Shared decision-making is the pinnacle of patient centered care,[1] and estimating and communicating prognosis are a central part of shared decision-making.[2] This is particularly important in decision-making regarding the appropriate initiation and withdrawal of dialysis.[3,4] Dialysis should be considered a preference-sensitive condition with patients' goals and preferences center stage.[5] For certain subgroups of patients, especially the frail elderly with multiple comorbidities, there is equipoise regarding the ability of dialysis to extend life when compared to medical management without dialysis.[6,7] In addition, elderly patients on dialysis experience rapid physical functional decline,[8] and dialysis patients as a whole suffer high symptom burden.[9] These facts raise important questions about the balance of benefit and burdens of dialysis treatment for these patient groups.[5] A substantial number of patients choose to discontinue dialysis when faced with superimposed acute illness or excessive treatment burden even if it means death in the short term.[10] Patients who overestimate their prognosis are more likely to delay advance care planning and pursue aggressive treatments near the end of life.[11,12] This has been shown to be particularly common in the dialysis population, where aggressive end-of-life care is the norm, and hospice and palliative care are underutilized.[10,13] Prognostic information may help many, if not most, patients make better decisions about both initiation and discontinuation of dialysis, ones that are consistent with their values, preferences, and goals.[4,14]

Without Prognostic Information, Patients Lack Autonomy When Making Decisions About Dialysis Initiation and Withdrawal

Unfortunately shared decision-making is poorly integrated into current nephrology practice[15,16] Discussions about prognosis have the potential to improve these conversations and are recommended by practice guidelines.[2,3] Many patients are unaware of their poor prognosis with ESKD and often overestimate both their survival and ability to qualify for transplantation.[17] There is also a significant discordance between the prognostic estimate of patients and their treating physicians.[17]

Case vignette: Mrs. Jameson has poor prognosis because of her age and comorbid burden, particularly dementia and peripheral vascular disease. Therefore, you decide to have a family conference to guide further treatment, emphasizing the value of kidney supportive care as an alternative to dialysis.

Patients Desire Information About Prognosis and Disease Progression

Several studies have shown that patients care about prognosis.[17,18] A qualitative study of elderly patients highlighted the uncertainty about disease progression, which, in turn, adversely affects their ability to prepare for living with dialysis.[19] Instead, patients coped with this uncertainty through avoidance and false hope. When surveyed, patients indicate that they would like information about prognosis. In a large Canadian survey of 584 patients with advanced kidney disease or ESKD (41% predialysis, 59% on kidney replacement therapy), 91% of patients felt that it was important to be informed about prognosis, and 83% indicated

TABLE 13.1. Prognostic Calculators for CKD and ESKD Patients Available Online

Name of Index	Purpose of Index	Website
Kidney Failure Risk Equation or Tangri	Gives estimates for 2- and 5-year risk of progression to ESKD	http://kidneyfailurerisk.com https://qxmd.com/calculate/calculator_308/kidney-failure-risk-equation-4-variable
Charlson Comorbidity Index	Overall comorbidity estimate has been used to predict mortality for dialysis patients in multiple studies	https://www.mdcalc.com/charlson-comorbidity-index-cci http://touchcalc.com/calculators/cci_js
REIN Index	Predicts 3-month mortality for incident elderly ESKD patients	https://qxmd.com/calculate/calculator_286/3-month-mortality-in-incident-elderly-esrd-patients
Cohen calculator	Predicts 6-month mortality for patients on hemodialysis has also been used to predict mortality for CKD patients	https://qxmd.com/calculate/calculator_135/6-month-mortality-on-hd http://touchcalc.com/calculators/sq
Thamer calculator	Predicts 6-month mortality at the start of dialysis.	http://www.pmidcalc.org/?sid=26123861&newtest=Y.
Obi calculator	Predicts 6-month mortality at the start of dialysis.	www.DialysisScore.com[53]

Abbreviations: CKD, chronic kidney disease; ESKD, end-stage kidney disease.

that it was important to be prepared and plan ahead in the case of death. Almost half (48%) of the patients indicated that they preferred to have those discussions with their nephrologist. Similarly, in a survey of 100 patients during their first visit to a nephrologist, an overwhelming majority of patients (97%) preferred to receive detailed information about survival during their first visit to a nephrologist, before making a decision about dialysis.[18] They expected nephrologists to volunteer this information without being prompted and indicated that they would desire as much information as possible, both good and bad. The patients agreed that this information would better prepare them (95%), affect their decision to start dialysis (78%), and alter their future lifestyle (83%).

Case vignette: You look up Mrs. Jameson life expectancy using online risk calculators (Table 13.1) and see that she is more likely than not to die within 6 months of starting dialysis. You decide to share this information with the family.

Nephrologists Feel Unprepared for Discussions About Prognosis and End of Life

Several studies have shown that nephrologists feel unprepared for these discussions and are hesitant to share this information with patients,[20,21] even when asked.[17] In a recent paired interview study of 62 patients with less than 20% 1-year life expectancy and their treating nephrologists, no patient reported that they had had a discussion about life expectancy with their nephrologist, and nephrologists reported having this discussion with only 2 patients. In the same study, the nephrologist gave the investigators estimates of life expectancy for 55 (89%) of the patients but indicated that for 33 (60%) of these patients they would refuse to provide these estimates to the patients even if they insisted on knowing.[17]

This reluctance is likely multifactorial. In a qualitative study of nephrologists and patients, nephrologists voiced concerns about upsetting patients and uncertainty of predictions as the major barriers of discussions about disease trajectories and prognosis.[19] A 2005 survey of 360 US and Canadian nephrologists showed that only 39% of respondents perceived themselves as very well prepared to make end-of-life decisions for patients.[21] Lack of emphasis on kidney supportive care and end-of-life care in nephrology fellowship training is a likely cause for this discomfort. In a survey of nephrology fellows, only two-thirds correctly estimated the annual gross mortality of patients on dialysis.[20]

The concern of taking away hope is a common reason physicians shy away from discussing prognosis with patients who have terminal diseases. A qualitative study of ESKD patients suggested the opposite—that timely and appropriate information to facilitate advance care planning can positively enhance patients' hope.[22] Other barriers include fear of litigation, the belief that patients have the right to demand treatment even if not indicated, time constraints, and economic pressures to keep dialysis units full.[23]

When Prognosis Is Poor, Quality of life Becomes More Important

Prognosis can help center treatment decisions regarding patient's goals and preferences especially when dealing with high-risk cases that are unlikely to benefit from dialysis or recover their physical functional status.[2,3] Many have argued that when prognosis is poor and dialysis is a destination treatment, aggressive treatment goals driven by quality metrics should give way to a focus on minimizing treatment burden and intrusiveness.[16,24,25] Finally, for patients with more than 50% predicted risk of death in 6 months, prognosis can be used to qualify the US patient for the Medicare hospice benefit, which is severely underutilized for dialysis patients.[16]

Case vignette: When presented with individualized information on her prognosis Mrs. Jameson and her family initially express shock at her prognosis. You are able to help them process this information and answer important questions about dialysis and other life extending treatment. At the end, Mrs. Jameson is able to express her relief that she does not have to adjust to a life on dialysis and a determination to fully enjoy the life she has left.

Existing Indices to Predict Life Expectancy

There are many validated indices available to help clinicians obtain prognostic estimates both for incident and prevalent dialysis patients.[2,26,27]

Our recent systematic review found that the most commonly used indices at dialysis start included Charlson Comorbidity Index (CCI), which has been modified by several research teams to better fit the dialysis population[28–32]; Khan Wright Index; and the REIN index.[33] Several other indices, including the Cohen, integrated prognostic model have been used in prevalent dialysis patients.[34] Finally the surprise question "Would you be surprised if this patient died in the next year?" has been successfully used as a predictor and at times outperforms indices using objective measures.[35,36]

The CCI assigns weights to various medical conditions for calculating a numerical score. Developed by Charlson et al (and then first applied to dialysis patients by Beddhu et al[30])as a general measure of disease burden, it has subsequently been widely used across health conditions. The length of prognosticated survival ranged from 1 to 5 years, and discrimination (C statistic) ranged from 0.631 to 0.90, where 0.7 is considered good prognostic ability. Only 1 study reported calibration for predicting 1- and 5-year mortality (positive predictive value, 78.7% and 79.4%; negative predictive value, 40.8% and 70.4%; and likelihood ratio, 1.1 and 7.0, respectively).[37]

The REIN score was developed by Couchoud et al[38] for a French cohort. It uses the following risk factors: body mass index less than 18.5, comorbidities, severe behavioral disorder, dependence for transfers, and the distinction of planned or unplanned dialysis initiation. In the development study, discrimination was good (C statistic, 0.70), and calibration was reported (Hosmer-Lemeshow $p = .93$). In 4 subsequent validations, discrimination was moderate to good (C statistic, 0.63–0.75).[39-41] In elderly dialysis patients, a score of 9 or more had a specificity of 80% to 92% for predicting death.[39] The length of prognostication was 6 months, but the index was also validated to predict 3-, 6-, and 12-month mortality, and it showed good discrimination (C statistic, 0.74).[40] Couchoud et al[42] subsequently updated and revalidated the score to predict 3-month mortality by reweighting the prognostic factors showing good discrimination (C statistic, 0.749).

Another commonly used index was the K–W Index ($n = 7$) developed by Wright[43] and modified by Khan et al.[44] It applies the following risk factors: age, diabetes mellitus, significant cardiovascular disease, and noncutaneous malignancy.[44] Discrimination measures were not reported in the development study. In subsequent validation studies, prognosticated survival ranged from 3 months to 10 years, and discrimination ranged from 0.54 to 0.908.[45-47]

Clinician intuition should not be underestimated. The surprise question has been shown to be a simple way for clinicians to stratify patients into high and low risk of imminent death. In a systematic review of the surprise question across different diseases, it was shown to have a pooled accuracy level of 74.8% with a C statistic of 0.735 for physicians, comparable to that of the best prognostic indices.[36] That being said, some studies note poor prognostic ability and that the accuracy of clinician's prognosis is inversely associated with how well they know the patient.[48] Several studies have looked at this in CKD and dialysis patients. In a study of 388 nondialysis patients with CKD stage 4 or 5, a "no" answer had a sensitivity of 66% and a specificity of 68%. When the researchers allowed for a neutral category, sensitivity for the answer "no" was 55% but specificity was better at 76%.[49] In another study of 367 peritoneal dialysis patients, a "no" answer was associated with a 3.6 hazard ratio of death and a specificity of 70%. Unfortunately, the positive predictive value was low at 24.8%.[50] Finally, in a prospective cohort study of 147 patients in 3 hemodialysis dialysis units, the surprise question was found to be effective in identifying dialysis patients with a high risk for early mortality for targeted kidney supportive care interventions.[51]

The Cohen prognostic model builds on the surprise question and was developed in 512 dialysis patients and includes age, albumin, dementia, and peripheral vascular disease as well as a yes or no answer to the surprise question "Would you be surprised if this patient died in the next year?"[34] This index had excellent performance in the derivation and validation cohort (another 514 patients) with a C statistic of 0.87 and 0.80, respectively, for predicting 6-month mortality.

In a recent validation study in patients with advanced CKD the c-statistic for predicting 12-month mortality in the validation cohort was 0.74.[52]

Newer indices continue to be developed and show promise in this patient population.[27,53-55]

Indices Available Electronically

Some of these indices are available as online calculators to help with patient-specific estimates of prognosis to inform shared decision-making as recommended by the Renal Physicians Association clinical practice guideline (see Table 13.1).[3] To give predialysis patients an idea of their risk of disease progression to ESKD, the internationally validated Kidney Failure Risk Equation is available.[56]

Summary

Communication of prognosis is an essential element of patient-centered care, because it is necessary for meaningful shared decision-making around both initiating and withdrawing dialysis. Prognostic tools are becoming increasingly available to help clinicians estimate patients' prognosis. More research is needed on the feasibility and acceptability of presenting estimates from prognostic tools at the bedside and their effect on treatment choice, measures of shared decision-making, and other outcomes important to patients.

Guidelines increasingly call for shared decision-making around the initiation and termination of renal replacement therapy. Prognosis is key to these discussions. Most patients with advanced CKD desire prognostic information. In the absence of being provided it, they tend to overestimate their prognosis. Misaligned prognostic expectations may decrease patients' interest in advance care planning and, in turn, contribute to high-intensity treatment at the end of life. There are many prognostic indices available to estimate life expectancy for patients with CKD and ESKD. Fellowship programs need to offer training for nephrologists in conducting prognostic discussions. More research is needed on how discussions of prognosis influence patient preferences, decision making and outcomes.

Practice Pointers

- Patients with ESKD have poor prognosis, yet many patients have overly optimistic prognostic expectations, which delays advance care planning and may drive overtreatment near the end of life.[12,17] Most patients desire prognostic information to help them plan and prioritize life goals.[18,19]
- Nephrologists feel compelled to offer, or even convince, patients to accept dialysis and shy away from discussions of prognosis for fear of taking away hope.[17,19]

- Several prognostic indices and discussion frameworks are available to help nephrologists and other clinicians navigate these discussions and facilitate advance care planning.[3,4]

Practice Improvement Opportunities

- Answer patients' questions about prognosis but start by asking about their prognostic expectations, goals, and values.
- Use one of the many available prognostic indices to provide patients with individualized prognostic estimate (Table 13.1).[27]
- Quality improvement and research projects focused on how to integrate prognostic discussions into routine clinical care and how to leverage the multidisciplinary team deserve more attention and have the potential to diminish treatment burden and improve quality of life.

References

1. Barry MJ, Edgman-Levitan S. Shared decision making—pinnacle of patient-centered care. *N Engl J Med.* 2012;366(9):780–781.
2. Germain MJ. How to integrate predictions in outcomes in planning clinical care. *Blood Purif.* 2015;39(1-3):65–69.
3. Renal Physicians Association. *Shared Decision-Making in the Appropriate Initiation of and Withdrawal from Dialysis. Clinical Practice Guideline.* Rockville, MD: Renal Physicians Association; 2010.
4. Michel DM, Moss AH. Communicating prognosis in the dialysis consent process: a patient-centered, guideline-supported approach. *Adv Chronic Kidney Dis.* 2005;12(2):196–201.
5. Thorsteinsdottir B, Swetz KM, Albright RC. The ethics of chronic dialysis for the older patient: time to reevaluate the norms. *Clin J Am Soc Nephrol.* 2015;10(11):2094–2099.
6. Verberne WR, Geers AB, Jellema WT, Vincent HH, van Delden JJ, Bos WJ. Comparative survival among older adults with advanced kidney disease managed conservatively versus with dialysis. *Clin J Am Soc Nephrol.* 2016;11(4):633–640.
7. Chandna SM, Da Silva-Gane M, Marshall C, Warwicker P, Greenwood RN, Farrington K. Survival of elderly patients with stage 5 CKD: comparison of conservative management and renal replacement therapy. *Nephrol, Dialy, Transpl.* 2011;26(5):1608–1614.
8. Kurella Tamura M, Covinsky KE, Chertow GM, Yaffe K, Landefeld CS, McCulloch CE. Functional status of elderly adults before and after initiation of dialysis. *N Engl J Med.* 2009;361(16):1539–1547.
9. Murtagh FEM, Addington-Hall J, Higginson IJ. The prevalence of symptoms in end-stage renal disease: a systematic review. *Adv Chronic Kidney Dis.* 2007;14(1):82–99.
10. United States Renal Data System. *USRDS 2016 Annual Data Report: Atlas of End-Stage Renal Disease in the United States.* Bethesda MD: National Institutes of Health, National Institute of Diabetes and Digestive and Kidney Diseases;2016.
11. Ghandourh WA. Palliative care in cancer: managing patients' expectations. *J Med Radiat Sci.* 2016;63(4):242–257.
12. O'Hare AM, Kurella Tamura M, Lavallee DC, et al. Assessment of self-reported prognostic expectations of people undergoing dialysis: United States Renal Data System Study of Treatment Preferences (USTATE). *JAMA Intern Med.* 2019. doi:10.1001/jamainternmed.2019.2879. [Epub ahead of print]
13. Wong SP, Kreuter W, O'Hare AM. Treatment intensity at the end of life in older adults receiving long-term dialysis. *Arch Intern Med.* 2012;172(8):661–663.

14. Couchoud C, Hemmelgarn B, Kotanko P, Germain MJ, Moranne O, Davison SN. Supportive care: time to change our prognostic tools and their use in CKD. *Clin J Am Soc Nephrol.* 2016;11(10): 1892–1901.
15. Wong SPY, Hebert PL, Laundry RJ, et al. Decisions about renal replacement therapy in patients with advanced kidney disease in the US Department of Veterans Affairs, 2000–2011. *Clin J Am Soc Nephrol.* 2016;11(10):1825–1833.
16. O'Hare AM, Armistead N, Schrag WL, Diamond L, Moss AH. Patient-centered care: an opportunity to accomplish the "three aims" of the national quality strategy in the Medicare ESRD program. *Clin J Am Soc Nephrol.* 2014;9(12):2189–2194.
17. Wachterman MW, Marcantonio ER, Davis RB, et al. Relationship between the prognostic expectations of seriously ill patients undergoing hemodialysis and their nephrologists. *JAMA Intern Med.* 2013;173(13):1206–1214.
18. Fine A, Fontaine B, Kraushar MM, Rich BR. Nephrologists should voluntarily divulge survival data to potential dialysis patients: a questionnaire study. *Perit Dial Int.* 2005;25(3):269–273.
19. Schell JO, Patel UD, Steinhauser KE, Ammarell N, Tulsky JA. Discussions of the kidney disease trajectory by elderly patients and nephrologists: a qualitative study. *American Journal of Kidney Diseases.* 2012;59(4):495–503.
20. Combs SA, Culp S, Matlock DD, Kutner JS, Holley JL, Moss AH. Update on end-of-life care training during nephrology fellowship: a cross-sectional national survey of fellows. *Am J Kidney Dis.* 2015;65(2):233–239.
21. Davison SN, Jhangri GS, Holley JL, Moss AH. Nephrologists' reported preparedness for end-of-life decision-making. *Clin J Am Soc Nephrol.* 2006;1(6):1256–1262.
22. Davison SN, Simpson C. Hope and advance care planning in patients with end stage renal disease: qualitative interview study. *BMJ.* 2006;333(7574):886.
23. Ladin K, Pandya R, Kannam A, et al. Discussing conservative management with older patients with CKD: an interview study of nephrologists. *Am J Kidney Dis.* 2018;71(5):627–635.
24. Vandecasteele SJ, Kurella Tamura M. A patient-centered vision of care for ESRD: dialysis as a bridging treatment or as a final destination? *J Am Soc Nephrol.* 2014;25(8):1647–1651.
25. Jassal SV. Four plus forty-four: hours to modify, theirs to enjoy. *Clin J Am Soc Nephrol.* 2015;10(2):169–171.
26. Davison SN, Levin A, Moss AH, et al. Executive summary of the KDIGO Controversies Conference on Supportive Care in Chronic Kidney Disease: developing a roadmap to improving quality care. *Kidney Int.* 2015;88(3):447–459.
27. Anderson RT, Cleek H, Pajouhi AS, et al. Prediction of risk of death for patients starting dialysis: a systematic review and meta-analysis. *Clin J Am Soc Nephrol.* 2019;14(8):1213–1227.
28. Charlson ME, Pompei P, Ales KL, MacKenzie CR. A new method of classifying prognostic comorbidity in longitudinal studies: development and validation. *J Chronic Dis.* 1987;40(5):373–383.
29. Liu J, Huang Z, Gilbertson DT, Foley RN, Collins AJ. An improved comorbidity index for outcome analyses among dialysis patients. *Kidney Int.* 2010;77(2):141–151.
30. Beddhu S, Bruns FJ, Saul M, Seddon P, Zeidel ML. A simple comorbidity scale predicts clinical outcomes and costs in dialysis patients. *Am J Med.* 2000;108(8):609–613.
31. Di Iorio B, Cillo N, Cirillo M, De Santo NG. Charlson Comorbidity Index is a predictor of outcomes in incident hemodialysis patients and correlates with phase angle and hospitalization. *Int J Artif Organs.* 2004;27(4):330–336.
32. Hemmelgarn BR, Manns BJ, Quan H, Ghali WA. Adapting the Charlson Comorbidity Index for use in patients with ESRD. *Am J Kidney Dis.* 2003;42(1):125–132.
33. Couchoud C, Labeeuw M, Moranne O, et al. A clinical score to predict 6-month prognosis in elderly patients starting dialysis for end-stage renal disease. *Nephrol Dial Transplant.* 2009;24(5):1553–1561.
34. Cohen LM, Ruthazer R, Moss AH, Germain MJ. Predicting six-month mortality for patients who are on maintenance hemodialysis. *Clin J Am Soc Nephrol.* 2010;5(1):72–79.
35. Barrett BJ, Parfrey PS, Morgan J, et al. Prediction of early death in end-stage renal disease patients starting dialysis. *Am J Kidney Dis.* 1997;29(2):214–222.
36. White N, Kupeli N, Vickerstaff V, Stone P. How accurate is the 'Surprise Question' at identifying patients at the end of life? A systematic review and meta-analysis. *BMC Medicine.* 2017;15:139.

37. Geddes CC, van Dijk PC, McArthur S, et al. The ERA–EDTA cohort study: comparison of methods to predict survival on renal replacement therapy. *Nephrol Dial Transplant.* 2006;21(4):945–956.
38. Couchoud C, Labeeuw M, Moranne O, et al. French Renal Epidemiology and Information Network (REIN) registry: a clinical score to predict 6-month prognosis in elderly patients starting dialysis for end-stage renal disease. *Nephrol Dial Transplant.* 2009;24(5):1553–1561.
39. Cheung KL, Montez-Rath ME, Chertow GM, Winkelmayer WC, Periyakoil VS, Kurella Tamura M. Prognostic stratification in older adults commencing dialysis. *J Gerontol A Biol Sci Med Sci.* 2014;69(8):1033–1039.
40. Otero-Lopez MS, Martinez-Ocana JC, Betancourt-Castellanos L, Rodriguez-Salazar E, Garcia-Garcia M. Two prognostic scores for early mortality and their clinical applicability in elderly patients on haemodialysis: poor predictive success in individual patients. *Nefrologia.* 2012;32(2):213–220.
41. Peeters P, Van Biesen W, Veys N, Lemahieu W, De Moor B, De Meester J. External Validation of a risk stratification model to assist shared decision making for patients starting renal replacement therapy. *BMC Nephrol.* 2016;17:41.
42. Couchoud CG, Beuscart JB, Aldigier JC, Brunet PJ, Moranne OP. REIN registry: development of a risk stratification algorithm to improve patient-centered care and decision making for incident elderly patients with end-stage renal disease. *Kidney Int.* 2015;88(5):1178–1186.
43. Wright LF. Survival in patients with end-stage renal disease. *Am J Kidney Dis.* 1991;17(1):25–28.
44. Khan IH, Catto GR, Edward N, Fleming LW, Henderson IS, MacLeod AM. Influence of coexisting disease on survival on renal-replacement therapy. *Lancet.* 1993;341(8842):415–418.
45. Marinovich S, Lavorato C, Morinigo C, et al. A new prognostic index for one-year survival in incident hemodialysis patients. *Int J Artif Organs.* 2010;33(10):689–699.
46. Postorino M, Marino C, Tripepi G, Zoccali C. Calabrian Registry of Dialysis and Transplantation: prognostic value of the New York Heart Association classification in end-stage renal disease. *Nephrol Dial Transplant.* 2007;22(5):1377–1382.
47. van Manen JG, Korevaar JC, Dekker FW, Boeschoten EW, Bossuyt PM, Krediet RT; NECOSAD Study Group; Netherlands Co-operative Study on the Adequacy of Dialysis. How to adjust for comorbidity in survival studies in ESRD patients: a comparison of different indices. *Am J Kidney Dis.* 2002;40(1):82–89.
48. Christakis NA, Lamont EB. Extent and determinants of error in doctors' prognoses in terminally ill patients: prospective cohort study. *BMJ.* 2000;320(7233):469–472.
49. Javier AD, Figueroa R, Siew ED, et al. Reliability and utility of the surprise question in CKD stages 4 to 5. *Am J Kidney Dis.* 2017;70(1):93–101.
50. Pang W-F, Kwan BC-H, Chow K-M, Leung C-B, Li PK-T, Szeto C-C. Predicting 12-month mortality for peritoneal dialysis patients using the "surprise" question. *Perit Dial Int.* 2013;33(1):60–66.
51. Moss AH, Ganjoo J, Sharma S, et al. Utility of the "surprise" question to identify dialysis patients with high mortality. *Clin J Am Soc Nephrol.* 2008;3(5):1379–1384.
52. Schmidt RJ, Landry DL, Cohen L, Moss AH, Dalton C, Nathanson BH, Germain MJ. Derivation and Validation of a Prognostic Model to Predict Mortality in Patients with Advanced Chronic Kidney Disease. *Nephrol Dial Transplant.* 2019;34(9):1517–1525.
53. Obi Y, Nguyen DV, Zhou H, et al. Development and validation of prediction scores for early mortality at transition to dialysis. *Mayo Clinic Proc.* 2018;93(9):1224–1235.
54. Floege J, Gillespie IA, Kronenberg F, et al. Development and validation of a predictive mortality risk score from a European hemodialysis cohort. *Kidney Int.* 2015;87(5):996–1008.
55. Wick JP, Turin TC, Faris PD, et al. A clinical risk prediction tool for 6-month mortality after dialysis initiation among older adults. *Am J Kidney Dis.* 2017;69(5):568–575.
56. Tangri N, Grams ME, Levey AS, et al. Multinational assessment of accuracy of equations for predicting risk of kidney failure: a meta-analysis. *JAMA.* 2016;315(2):164–174.

14

Active Medical Management Without Dialysis for Patients With Advanced Chronic Kidney Disease

Kelly Li and Mark Brown

This chapter outlines the management of patients with advanced chronic kidney disease for whom dialysis may not be beneficial or desired. Active medical management without dialysis should be offered to patients through a shared-decision making process as a viable alternative to dialysis. This is important as patients and families wish to consider not only survival, but also symptom control and QoL in their decision to pursue a dialysis or nondialysis pathway. A multidisciplinary team delivering good quality, active, and patient-centered care that combines chronic kidney disease management with the principles of palliative care can help patients achieve good symptom management and quality of life. Active and early planning for the end-of-life phase facilitates appropriate care for patients in acute and/or unexpected deterioration and helps achieve patient and family goals.

Case

George is an 82-year-old man with chronic kidney disease (CKD) secondary to ischemic nephrosclerosis, who has regular follow-up in the CKD clinic. His renal function has been declining over years, with estimated glomerular filtration rate (eGFR) now 15 mL/min/1.73m^2. His comorbidities include hypertension, moderate aortic stenosis, gout, and osteoarthritis. He has good cognition, lives independently with his wife, and uses a 4-wheel walker only for longer distances due to arthritic pain. The CKD nurse has flagged him for discussion regarding dialysis planning.

It is increasingly recognized that not all patients with advanced CKD derive benefit from commencing dialysis, with benefit broadly referring to an expectation of longer survival with an acceptable quality of life (QoL). It is therefore pertinent that CKD patients and their families understand the benefits and burdens of dialysis and are offered a viable alternative. Active medical management without dialysis, also termed comprehensive conservative care,[1] combines optimal nephrology practice with the principles of palliative care to provide a holistic, patient-centered management plan tailored to individualized goals and values, with emphasis on QoL. This requires an evidence-based approach tempered with flexible, practical, and personalized priorities to provide the right care to the right person at the right time.

The Right Person

It is important for nephrologists to recognize patients who are more likely to benefit from medical management without dialysis of advanced CKD or who might suffer harm from dialysis. This includes patients for whom dialysis is technically difficult such as those with severe hypotension from left ventricular dysfunction and patients with a terminal illness from nonrenal causes such as metastatic cancer or advanced dementia. Observational studies in recent years have identified patient groups for whom dialysis has been offered, but who subsequently have not derived a survival advantage despite commencing dialysis. This includes patients over age 75 with a high number of extra-renal comorbidities, particularly diabetes[2] and ischemic heart disease,[3] patients over age 80 regardless of comorbidities,[4,5] and patients over age 70 with poor performance status (World Health Organization Performance Score of 3 or more).[5] Nephrologists can refer to local and international guidelines, such as the Renal Physicians Association clinical practice guideline.[6] These and more recent evidence are summarized in Box 14.1.

Ideally, all decisions to commence or not commence dialysis should arise from the process of shared decision-making between the patient (and family) and nephrologist. (see chapter 9 of this volume). In everyday clinical practice, it is important for the nephrologist to make a recommendation as the technical expert in the shared decision-making process with detailed knowledge of available evidence. Patients and their families seek this guidance to facilitate good discussions. In more complex clinical scenarios, a second opinion from a nephrology colleague can provide more clarity. An experienced nephrologist knows the importance of living with uncertainty, inherent in any clinical decision despite available data and predictive tools. In regard to a decision to commence dialysis, it is pertinent to acknowledge this uncertainty and work with patients and their family in a shared decision-making process

---

BOX 14.1. Active Medical Management Without Dialysis May Be More Beneficial Than Dialysis for the Certain Patients

1. Patients for whom dialysis is technically difficult[6]
2. Patients with a terminal illness from nonrenal causes[6]
3. Patients over age 75 with 2 or more of the following poor prognostic criteria[6]:
   - Clinician's response of "No, I would not be surprised" to the surprise question (Would you be surprised if this patient died within the next 12 months?)
   - High comorbidities score
   - Significantly impaired functional status
   - Severe chronic malnutrition
4. Patients over age 80, regardless of comorbidities[4,5]

to negotiate a course of action consistent with their goals and values, rather than having dialysis being the default option just because there is uncertainty.

A trial of dialysis has been suggested as a middle ground when decisions regarding the benefits and harms of dialysis are difficult. While this can be an option for clinicians and patients, it has several problems and is not a pathway we follow. First, the decision to withdraw from dialysis is confronting, fraught with emotions, and adds stress to patients and families, generally more so than an initial decision not to commence dialysis. Second, patients who undergo a trial of dialysis followed by withdrawal are exposed to all the harms and burdens of dialysis including access creation, happening in the framework where the actual benefits in terms of survival and QoL are unclear. Finally, having commenced a patient on hemodialysis also means likely loss of residual glomerular filtration rate (GFR) and acceleration of time to death should dialysis turn out to be unacceptable.

It is more preferable to work with patients and their family in reaching a decision to pursue dialysis or active medical management without dialysis, rather than deferring this decision by offering a trial. Moreover, any patient commenced on dialysis should be informed that withdrawal is a choice they can make at any time when they feel it is no longer in their best interest and that the nephrology team will support them in their decisions.

The Right Time

It is well established that survival is poor for elderly patients on dialysis and can be worse than most cancers. Table 14.1 shows survival for incident dialysis patients in Australia, a country with good dialysis outcomes, compared to newly diagnosed cancers. Furthermore, dialysis withdrawal is common among elderly patients (Table 14.2), suggesting that for some, dialysis initiation may not have been the best option and that others may have reached a time point where the burdens of dialysis have superseded its benefits.

Active medical management without dialysis should be a viable option for patients either as CKD approaches stage 5, or at any time for those on dialysis who may have acquired

TABLE 14.1. Five-Year Survival of Australian Incident Dialysis Patients and Australian Cancer Patients

Patients	5-year survival (%)
Australian incident dialysis patients 2008–2017[32]	
Aged 65–74	50
Aged 75–84	33
Aged 85+	19
Australian cancer patients 2009–2013[33]	
Breast cancer (all)	90
Breast cancer (aged 75+ at diagnosis)	70
Colorectal cancer (all)	69
Colorectal cancer (aged 75+ at diagnosis)	61
Lung cancer (all)	16
Lung cancer (aged 75+ at diagnosis)	10

TABLE 14.2. Dialysis Withdrawal Rates

United States: all dialysis[a]		Australia: HD[b]		New Zealand: HD[b]	
All ages	Aged 85+	HD all ages	HD 75+	HD all ages	HD 75+
23%	34%	32%	41%	26%	43%

Abbreviation: HD, hemodialysis.
[a]United States—dialysis discontinuation before death.[34]
[b]ANZDATA: percentage of death listed as due to dialysis withdrawal.[32]

extra-renal comorbidities or are struggling to cope with dialysis due to progressive functional decline. At these appropriate time points, nephrologists should initiate and lead discussions around the option of nondialysis management. Patients for whom prognosis is particularly poor should be informed that dialysis might not confer a survival advantage or improve QoL or functional status over active medical management.[1] Provision of prognostic information to patients does not annihilate hope, and in fact, discussions earlier in the course of illness with focus on the impact of treatment to daily life can empower patients, sustain hope, and facilitate future planning and the setting of realistic goals.[7] In addition to survival, patients and families often value other aspects such as QoL and the anticipated effects of interventions—dialysis or nondialysis—on physical function, symptoms, and family and social circumstances. In an Australian study, patients were willing to forego 7 months of life expectancy to reduce the number of visits to hospital and 15 months to increase their ability to travel.[8] Available evidence suggest that QoL is similar in patients managed without dialysis compared with their age-matched dialysis patients,[3] and for those with progressive CKD, dialysis initiation is associated with significant decline in QoL, whereas those managed medically without dialysis maintained QoL.[9,10]

Overcoming Challenges

Despite its growing need and evidence base, active medical management without dialysis faces multiple challenges. First, nephrologists and fellows often feel inadequately prepared for discussions of prognosis and the challenges of managing end of life care,[11,12] and many feel uncomfortable not offering dialysis even if patients clearly have poor prognosis.[13] Skilled communications around difficult decisions and end-of-life care can be taught and improved with formalized training[14,15] and should be a core competency in nephrology practice (see chapter 6 of this volume). Second, lack of a structured program to support active medical management for end-stage kidney disease (ESKD) means that patients who opt for nondialysis management may lose their connection with the nephrology unit and be discharged into primary care. Having an active nondialysis pathway embedded within the existing nephrology service emphasizes the importance of ongoing medical management and reinforces the important principle of nonabandonment. Third, there can be misconception that a nondialysis pathway, or delivery of a kidney supportive care service, equates to end-of-life care, suggesting that patients who do not elect to have dialysis face an imminent death. Patients with poor prognosis may have similar survival on a dialysis or nondialysis pathway (particularly groups noted in Box 14.1). Functional decline in the nondialysis group generally occurs in the last 1 to 2 months of life,[16] meaning that these patients can expect to maintain their quality life for most of their median survival of 6 to 30 months.[17] Lastly, routine incorporation of active medical management without dialysis within a nephrology unit is a practice change that requires leadership by clinical champions, multidisciplinary team building, and support at a government or organizational level.[18]

The Right Care

Active medical management without dialysis should not be perceived as a substandard, second-rate alternative to dialysis. In the right patients, it is the optimal management option.

Patients managed without dialysis should follow up regularly with their primary nephrologist, usually at 2- to 3-months' interval, to optimize CKD management, until the terminal phase where focus shifts to end-of-life care. Continued care by a trusted provider adopts the principle of nonabandonment, defined as a longitudinal commitment from the physician to jointly seek solutions to problems with patients throughout their illness, as an open-minded, caring, and knowledgeable partner.[19]

A multidisciplinary team with a kidney supportive care focus and expertise, including (where resources permit) a palliative care physician, specialist nurse practitioners or consultants, social worker, psychologist, pharmacist, and dietician will provide additional care, ideally separate from the nephrology review so that emphasis can be redirected to symptom management and psychosocial assessment. This allows more frequent review and management for patients with high symptom burden, anxiety and depression, or difficult social circumstances, without overloading existing CKD clinics. Supportive care clinics offering more structured programs have been set up to address the increased demand for active medical management without dialysis, in an era of an aging population with increased number of elderly comorbid patients with ESKD. In recent years, many such programs have been established and continue to expand in developed countries including Australia,[10] United Kingdom,[20] and Canada[21] and are emerging in the United States.[22]

For nephrology units where resources are limited, active medical management can initially be provided by the existing team of nephrologist, specialist renal nurses, social worker, and dietician. Longer or separate appointments should be scheduled for these patients with specific focus on symptom assessment and management. It is important to establish a collaborative working relationship with the local specialist palliative care service to co-manage patients with more difficult symptoms and for end-of-life care (see chapter 7 of this volume).

Management needs to be active and at the same time flexible and patient-centered, reflecting the philosophy of kidney supportive care. Central components of medical management include interventions to delay CKD progression and managing CKD complications, symptom management, psychosocial and spiritual support, open and sensitive communication, and shared-decision-making including advance care planning (ACP; Box 14.2).[1] Online resources are also available (Box 14.3).

Hypertension Management

Blood pressure management should not be discontinued when patients enter a nondialysis pathway, provided treatment does not induce side effects. Optimizing blood pressure is

> **BOX 14.2. Components of Active Medical Management Without Dialysis**
>
> - Shared decision-making
> - Advance care planning
> - CKD management including but not limited to
>   - Hypertension management
>   - Anemia management
>   - Nutritional management
> - Meticulous symptom assessment and management
> - Psychosocial and family support

important in delaying CKD progression and preventing further cardiovascular comorbidities. General targets of 140 mmHg systolic or 90 mmHg diastolic for CKD patients[23] can be relaxed, although moderate to severe hypertension should be treated,[24,25] with slow dose titration and altering of treatment based on tolerability and side effects. Angiotensin-converting enzymes inhibitors or angiotensin receptor blockers are not contraindicated but should be used with caution due to the risk of hyperkalemia at low GFR.

Anemia Management

Anemia is a potentially treatable complication of advanced CKD and contributes significantly to patients' symptom burden. Basic anemia assessment should include any history of bleeding, full blood count and red cell indices, iron studies, and vitamin B12 and folate. Any easily reversible nonrenal cause of anemia should be identified and treated.

For anemia attributable to CKD, general recommendations applicable to the CKD population[26] can be adapted. This includes intravenous iron supplementation for symptomatic iron deficiency and erythropoietin-stimulating agents in iron-replete patients with symptomatic

> **BOX 14.3. Online Resources**
>
> Conservative kidney management: Alberta Health Services, Canada
> www.ckmcare.com
> British Columbia Renal Agency
> www.bcrenalagency.ca/health-professionals/clinical-resources/palliative-care
> www.bcrenalagency.ca/health-professionals/clinical-resources/symptom-assessment-and-management
> Renal and hypertension service: St George and Sutherland Hospitals, Australia
> www.stgrenal.org.au/renal-supportive-care
> Supportive care: Kidney Health Australia
> www.kidney.org.au/your-kidneys/support/kidney-disease/supportive-care

anemia. Once initiated, hemoglobin targets should be individualized to symptoms, although a target of 90 to 100g/L is reasonable for most. Red cell transfusions may be used for symptomatic anemia not responsive to iron and erythropoietin-stimulating agents. Ongoing transfusions should be based on severity of symptoms and the magnitude of benefit achieved.

Nutritional Management

In elderly patients with advanced CKD, nutritional management plays an important part in reducing symptom burden, supporting physical function and independence, and improving QoL.[27] Traditional CKD diet prescription is generally shifted to a more flexible and permissive style of eating, and an individualized dietary plan tailored to the patient.[27] Like other aspects of CKD management, dietary management needs to align with patient goals and empower patients to make informed dietary choices relevant to cultural, social, and personal circumstances.

Key themes in providing nutritional support include:

- Education regarding dietary goals, for example, biochemistry that can be acutely unsafe (hyperkalemia) compared with long-term complications (hyperphosphatemia) that are less relevant in this population.[27]
- Personal, religious, and cultural values need to be considered, and social aspects of eating such as participating in family gatherings may be more important than the food consumed.[28]
- Specific dietary interventions are important in managing several common symptoms in advanced CKD, such as xerostomia, dysgeusia, nausea, dyspnea from fluid overload, and constipation.[27]

Symptom Management

Patients with stage 5 CKD managed without dialysis experience a considerable symptom burden that is comparable to populations with advanced cancer.[29,30] The prevalence and severity of symptoms may be underappreciated, and regular and structured symptom assessments using validated tools (see chapter 5 of this volume) are necessary to fully elicit symptoms that are of most concern to patients and help direct consultation toward patient-centered goals.

For patients managed on a nondialysis pathway, it is possible to maintain and improve symptom control. In a prospective observational study of 122 stage 5 CKD patients managed without dialysis, over two-thirds of patients achieved improvement in symptom burden by 6 and 12 months despite declining GFR. In this study, symptoms were routinely assessed at each clinic visit with the Palliative care Outcomes Scale—Symptoms (renal) POS-S (renal), and a multidisciplinary team including a palliative care physician was involved in patient care.[10] This is important as patients and families wish to consider not only survival, but also symptom control and QoL in their decision to pursue a dialysis or nondialysis pathway.

Advance Care Planning and End-of-Life Care

In patients actively managed without dialysis, ACP should be discussed early in the course of CKD and documentation of the choice of medical management without dialysis pathway made clear to all relevant persons particularly nominated surrogate decision makers, all members of the nephrology team, and primary care physicians (see chapter 10 of this volume). Other end-of-life care preferences, such as dying at home or hospice, unwanted aggressive treatments, and psychosocial and spiritual needs, should also form part of ACP. Where possible, ACP documents should be placed in the electronic medical records of the local hospital so that they can be easily accessible in an emergency setting.

Quality Assurance

The quality of a medical management program should be assessed both by the clinical outcomes of patients within the service and its overall impact on the relevant patient population within the nephrology unit. The New South Wales, Australia, model, for example, has predetermined outcome and performance measures to ensure ongoing quality assurance of its effectiveness.[31] Patient outcomes are measured using validate clinical tools (see Box 14.4) and patient and family satisfaction surveys. Appropriate utilization of the service and its impact within the nephrology unit and local healthcare providers can be ascertained by determining the percentage of ESKD patients medically managed without dialysis and dialysis withdrawals accessing the service until death. Economic impact of the service such as hospital utilization and emergency presentations may also be relevant from a funding and service planning perspective.

Case Revisited

For George, dialysis is technically possible, and his family was willing to support him in practical ways should he choose to commence dialysis. George was also offered active medical management without dialysis, and the following points discussed:

- As George is over 80, current evidence suggest that he may not live longer with dialysis compared with no dialysis. At his age he was estimated to have about 16 months survival.[10]
- QoL may decrease with the commencement of dialysis.
- If he chooses a nondialysis pathway, it does not mean all his treatments will cease. He will have ongoing CKD management by his nephrologist, including appropriate medications and nutritional counseling.
- He will have additional support (depending on local resources) from a multidisciplinary team with kidney supportive care expertise to focus on symptom management and psychosocial and family support.

BOX 14.4. Clinical Tools Used in Active Medical Management Without Dialysis to Assess Patient Outcomes

- iPOS Ren.al (symptom burden)
- EuroQol 5 dimensions EQ-5D-5L (QoL)
- Australian Karnofsky Performance Scale (functional status)
- Subjective Global Assessment (nutritional status)

From ACI Renal Network NSW Renal Supportive Care Service Model.[31]

- With appropriate assessment and management, it is possible to improve symptoms for the majority of patients on nondialysis pathway despite progressive decline in renal function.

George chose to have active medical management without dialysis and continued to be followed up in both the CKD and renal supportive care clinics. He and his family received support from a team consisting of a palliative care physician, specialist nurses, dietician, social worker, and pharmacist. He made an advance care plan with the team, outlining his wishes regarding future medical treatment. He lived a further 16 months and remained at home until the final month, when his function declined and home was too difficult. He died in the local palliative care (hospice) unit.

Summary

Active medical management without dialysis that is delivered by a multidisciplinary team, integrating palliative care principles with CKD management, is a viable and preferred option for CKD patients with poor prognosis for whom dialysis is unlikely to provide benefit. Effective communication of prognosis and shared understanding of treatment goals and individualized priorities allow the nephrologist to make appropriate treatment recommendations and to continue to be actively involved in patient care (see Box 14.5).

> **BOX 14.5. Active Medical Management Without Dialysis: A Quick Guide**
>
> - Decisions about nondialysis management *should be made early* in the course of CKD (we recommend at eGFR around 15 ml/min/1.73m^2) and not be left until late stage 5 ESKD.
> - Nondialysis management must be *active* and high-quality, underpinned by evidence and research. Nephrologists treating these patients should remain aware of the available literature on this topic.
> - *Nonabandonment*: nephrologists should continue to care for patients regardless of their treatment pathway, even if the patient also sees the palliative care team.
> - Focus on *patient-centered goals* such as QoL alongside disease-centered goals such as life prolongation.
> - Discussions about *prognosis* based on evidence is possible and important. Nephrologists need to instigate these discussions even though they can be difficult.
> - Adopt *shared decision-making* and acknowledge prognostic uncertainty; discussions should occur early in the course of CKD.
> - Nephrologists should initiate ACP discussions.
> - At all times, consider family, culture, and spirituality.
> - *Communication skills* are essential for nephrologists and others in this field.
> - If the palliative care team is not embedded within the renal team for these patients, then engage the local specialist palliative care service for difficult cases.

Practice Pointers

- Older patients with many comorbidities or frailty are likely to experience a decline in QoL but unlikely to derive a survival advantage from dialysis. Furthermore, some patients value QoL over survival, and these values should be elicited and used in care planning.
- Nondialysis management must be *active* and high quality, underpinned by evidence and research. Nephrologists treating these patients should remain aware of the available literature on this topic.
- For patients managed on a nondialysis pathway, it is possible to maintain and improve symptom control.

Practice Improvement Opportunities

- Focus on patient-centered goals such as QoL alongside disease-centered goals such as life prolongation.
- Initiate discussions about prognosis based on evidence, even though such discussions can be difficult. If the palliative care team is not embedded within the renal team for these patients, then engage the local specialist palliative care service for difficult cases.
- Active and early planning for the end-of-life phase is critical. This includes close liaison with emergency physicians and intensivists to ensure ACPs are accessible to them when a patient presents to hospital can facilitate appropriate care for patients in acute and/or unexpected deterioration.

References

1. Davison SN, Levin A, Moss AH, et al. Executive summary of the KDIGO Controversies Conference on Supportive Care in Chronic Kidney Disease: developing a roadmap to improving quality care. *Kidney Int.* 2015;88(3):447–459.
2. Chandna SM, Da Silva-Gane M, Marshall C, Warwicker P, Greenwood RN, Farrington K. Survival of elderly patients with stage 5 CKD: comparison of conservative management and renal replacement therapy. *Nephrol Dialy Transpl.* 2010;26(5):1608–1614.
3. O'Connor NR, Kumar P. Conservative management of end-stage renal disease without dialysis: a systematic review. *J Palliat Med.* 2012;15(2):228–235.
4. Verberne WR, Geers AT, Jellema WT, Vincent HH, van Delden JJ, Bos WJW. Comparative survival among older adults with advanced kidney disease managed conservatively versus with dialysis. *Clin J Am Soc Nephrol.* 2016;7;11(4):633–640.
5. Hussain JA, Mooney A, Russon L. Comparison of survival analysis and palliative care involvement in patients aged over 70 years choosing conservative management or renal replacement therapy in advanced chronic kidney disease. *Palliat Med.* 2013;27(9):829–839.
6. Renal Physicians Association. *Shared Decision-Making in the Appropriate Initiation of and Withdrawal From Dialysis: Clinical Practice Guideline.* 2nd ed. Rockville, Maryland, 2010.
7. Davison SN, Simpson C. Hope and advance care planning in patients with end stage renal disease: qualitative interview study. *BMJ.* 2006;333(7574):886.
8. Morton RL, Snelling P, Webster AC, et al. Factors influencing patient choice of dialysis versus conservative care to treat end-stage kidney disease. *CMAJ.* 2012;184(5):E277–E283.

9. Da Silva-Gane M, Wellsted D, Greenshields H, Norton S, Chandna SM, Farrington K. Quality of life and survival in patients with advanced kidney failure managed conservatively or by dialysis. *Clin J Am Soc Nephrol.* 2012;7(12):2002–2009.
10. Brown MA, Collett GK, Josland EA, Foote C, Li Q, Brennan FP. CKD in elderly patients managed without dialysis: survival, symptoms, and quality of life. *Clin J Am Soc Nephrol.* 2015;10(2):260–268.
11. Davison SN, Jhangri GS, Holley JL, Moss AH. Nephrologists' reported preparedness for end-of-life decision-making. *Clin J Am Soc Nephrol.* 2006;1(6):1256–1262.
12. Combs SA, Culp S, Matlock DD, Kutner JS, Holley JL, Moss AH. Update on end-of-life care training during nephrology fellowship: a cross-sectional national survey of fellows. *Am J Kidney Dis.* 2015;65(2):233–239.
13. Shah HH, Monga D, Caperna A, Jhaveri KD. Palliative care experience of US adult nephrology fellows: a national survey. *Ren Fail.* 2014;36(1):39–45.
14. Schell JO, Cohen RA, Green JA, et al. NephroTalk: evaluation of a palliative care communication curriculum for nephrology fellows. *J Pain Symptom Manage.* 2018;56(5):767–773.
15. Cohen RA, Jackson VA, Norwich D, et al. A nephrology fellows' communication skills course: an educational quality improvement report. *Am J Kidney Dis.* 2016;68(2):203–211.
16. Murtagh FE, Addington-Hall JM, Higginson IJ. End-stage renal disease: a new trajectory of functional decline in the last year of life. *J Am Geriatr Soc.* 2011;59(2):304–308.
17. Wongrakpanich S, Susantitaphong P, Isaranuwatchai S, Chenbhanich J, Eiam-Ong S, Jaber BL. Dialysis therapy and conservative management of advanced chronic kidney disease in the elderly: a systematic review. *Nephron.* 2017;137(3):178–189.
18. Lam DY, Scherer JS, Brown M, Grubbs V, Schell JO. A conceptual framework of palliative care across the continuum of advanced kidney disease. *Clin J Am Soc Nephrol.* 2019;14(4):635–641.
19. Quill TE, Cassel CK. Nonabandonment: a central obligation for physicians. *Ann Intern Med.* 1995;122(5):368–374.
20. Roderick P, Rayner H, Tonkin-Crine S, et al. A national study of practice patterns in UK renal units in the use of dialysis and conservative kidney management to treat people aged 75 years and over with chronic kidney failure. *Health Services and Delivery Research.* 2015;3(12). https://www.ncbi.nlm.nih.gov/books/NBK284925/.
21. Alberta Health Services CKM. Conservative kidney management. http://www.ckmcare.com. Published 2016.
22. Scherer JS, Wright R, Blaum CS, Wall SP. Building an outpatient kidney palliative care clinical program. *J Pain Symptom Manage.* 2018;55(1):108–116.
23. James PA, Oparil S, Carter BL, et al. 2014 evidence-based guideline for the management of high blood pressure in adults: report from the panel members appointed to the Eighth Joint National Committee (JNC 8). *JAMA.* 2014;311(5):507–520.
24. Davison SN, Tupala B, Wasylynuk BA, Siu V, Sinnarajah A, Triscott J. Recommendations for the care of patients receiving conservative kidney management: focus on management of chronic kidney disease and symptoms. *Clin J Am Soc Nephrol.* 2019;14(4):626–634.
25. Musini VM, Tejani AM, Bassett K, Wright JM. Pharmacotherapy for hypertension in the elderly. *Cochrane Database Syst Rev.* 2009(4):CD000028.
26. Outcomes KDIG, Group AW. KDIGO clinical practice guideline for anemia in chronic kidney disease. *Kidney Int Suppl.* 2012;2:279–335.
27. Stevenson J, Meade A, Randall AM, et al. Nutrition in renal supportive care: patient-driven and flexible. *Nephrology.* 2017;22(10):739–747.
28. Holmes S. Importance of nutrition in palliative care of patients with chronic disease. *Nurs Stand.* 2010;25(1):48–56; quiz 58.
29. Murtagh FE, Addington-Hall JM, Edmonds PM, et al. Symptoms in advanced renal disease: a cross-sectional survey of symptom prevalence in stage 5 chronic kidney disease managed without dialysis. *J Palliat Med.* 2007;10(6):1266–1276.
30. Brennan F, Collett G, Josland EA, Brown MA. The symptoms of patients with CKD stage 5 managed without dialysis. *Progr Palliat Care.* 2015;23(5):267–273.

31. ACIRenalNetwork. NSW renal supportive care service model. *Agency for Clinical Innovation*. www.aci.health.nsw.gov.au/_data/assets/pdf_file/0020/443072/Renal-Supportive-Care-Service-Model.pdf. Published 2018.
32. ANZDATA Registry. 41st report, chapter 3: mortality in end stage kidney disease. Australia and New Zealand Dialysis and Transplant Registry, Adelaide, Australia. http://www.anzdata.org.au. Published 2018.
33. Australian Institute of Health and Welfare. Cancer in Australia 2017. AIHW, Canberra. 2017. https://www.aihw.gov.au/reports/cancer/cancer-in-australia-2017/data. Accessed April 27, 2018.
34. United States Renal Data System. Chapter 12: end-of-life care for patients with end-stage renal disease: 2000–2014. In *2016 USRDS Annual Data Report: Epidemiology of Kidney Disease in the United States*: Bethesda, MD: National Institutes of Health, National Institute of Diabetes and Digestive and Kidney Diseases; 2016. https://www.usrds.org/2016/view/

15

Systematic Pain Assessment and Management

Sara N. Davison

Patients with chronic kidney disease suffer from high rates of pain. Pain is a highly complex, multi-dimensional, and personal phenomenon with far reaching physical and psychosocial consequences if the pain progresses to become a chronic disorder. Systematic integration of global symptom screening needs to be incorporated into routine kidney care, followed by a comprehensive pain assessment for those with clinically significant pain, keeping in mind the overall goal is to promote functionality and quality of life and not to necessarily completely resolve the pain. There is tremendous variability within and between countries in the management of pain, including the prescribing patterns of analgesics. This chapter outlines a systematic approach to the assessment and management of acute and chronic pain with both nonpharmacologic and pharmacologic interventions.

Introduction

Pain is a common, distressing, and inadequately treated symptom experienced by many patients with chronic kidney disease (CKD) throughout their illness.[1,2] A large body of literature shows that almost 70% of patients with end-stage kidney disease (ESKD) on dialysis experience recurrent acute or chronic pain, approximately 30% report moderate or severe bone/joint pain, and approximately 30% report moderate or severe muscle pain.[1] There is also evidence that patients at earlier stages of CKD also suffer from high rates of pain.[1] People living with chronic pain experience a lower quality of life (QOL) that is associated with disability, depressive thoughts, conflicts in close relationships, and reduced participation in many social aspects of everyday life.[3,4]

Patients with advanced CKD have highlighted improving the burden of symptoms, including better management of pain, as a top priority.[5] Pain assessment and management need to be integrated into routine care early in CKD treatment with regular reassessment throughout the patient's illness. There is tremendous variability within and between countries in the management of pain, including the prescribing patterns of analgesics.[6] This chapter outlines a systematic approach to the assessment and management of acute and chronic pain with both non-pharmacologic and pharmacologic interventions.

Categorizing Pain

The International Association for the Study of Pain defines pain as "an unpleasant sensory and emotional experience associated with actual or potential tissue damage or described in terms of such damage."[7p210] This definition reflects pain as a complex and multidimensional phenomenon with physical, psychosocial, and spiritual components and reinforces the need for a broad perspective when assessing and treating pain.

Pain should be described in terms of chronicity (Table 15.1). Acute pain is generally due to tissue injury. It is important to treat underlying causes of acute pain to ensure long-term resolution. As pain persists and becomes more chronic, the original injury becomes less important than the psychological factors that contribute to pain. As a result, patients with chronic pain often do not have a clear and treatable underlying cause. Patients with chronic pain require nonpharmacologic assessment and support as pharmacologic therapy alone

TABLE 15.1. Categories of Pain

Chronicity of Pain		
	Acute Pain	**Chronic Pain**
Pain characteristics	• Typically persists for less than 3 months. • Associated with tissue damage. • Usually episodic with periods without pain.	• Often defined as any painful condition that persists for greater than 3 months. • Usually initiated by tissue injury but is perpetuated by neurophysiological changes, which take place within the peripheral and central nervous system, leading to continuation of pain once healing has occurred. • Severity is often out of proportion with the extent of the originating injury.
Clinical implications	• Tends to last a predictable period, have no progressive pattern, and subside as healing occurs. • Tends to respond well to pharmacologic therapy: titrating analgesics against pain intensity is usually effective.	• More likely to result in functional impairment and disability, psychological distress, sleep deprivation, and poor QOL compared with acute pain. • The pain experience may be impacted substantially by mood, stress, and social circumstances. • May not respond well to analgesics, including opioids, except early in the course of treatment.
Type of pain		
	Nociceptive Pain	**Neuropathic**
Pain characteristics	• Results from tissue damage in the skin, muscle, or other tissues, causing stimulation of sensory receptors. • May be described as sharp or knife-like and is often felt at the site of damage. • With stimulation of visceral nociceptors, may be experienced as dull, aching, and poorly localized.	• Results from damage to the nervous system resulting in either dysfunction or pathological change. • May be felt at a site distant from its cause (eg, in the distribution of a nerve). • Common descriptors include burning, shooting, and electrical. • May be associated with episodes of spontaneous pain, hyperalgesia, and allodynia. • The presence of allodynia is pathognomonic.
Clinical implications	• Tends to respond to analgesics.	• Responds poorly to analgesics and typically requires adjuvant therapy.

Abbreviations: QOL, quality of life.

is unlikely to be sufficient. Recurrent pain results from recurrent tissue injury, which may occur over long periods of time (eg, pain from needling fistulas, intradialytic steal syndrome, and intradialytic headaches and cramps. It should be distinguished from chronic pain as management is more in keeping with acute pain. Management for recurrent pain focuses on strategies to minimize tissue injury and, if the cause cannot be avoided, the addition of concurrent short-term pharmacologic management.

Pain should also be classified as either neuropathic or nociceptive in nature (Table 15.1). Nociceptive pain is caused by tissue damage and, in the short term, typically responds well to nonopioid and opioid analgesics. In contrast, neuropathic pain results from the abnormal stimulation of sensory receptors due to nerve damage and is poorly responsive to nonsteroidal anti-inflammatory drugs (NSAIDs) and opioid analgesics or requires doses for response that are associated with unacceptable toxicity. The pain experienced by patients with CKD is frequently a mix of different types of pain including neuropathic pain, pain due to ischemia, and pain due to calciphylaxis.

A Systematic Approach to Pain Assessment

Patients often do not readily communicate with healthcare providers that they are experiencing pain. To address this, Kidney Disease: Improving Global Outcomes (KDIGO) recommends incorporating regular symptom screening using validated tools into routine clinical practice throughout the illness trajectory starting in the earlier stages of the disease.[8] Routine screening for symptoms helps to focus care on a more patient-centered model. The assessment of pain requires a comprehensive evaluation and physical examination of the patient that is best facilitated using a multidisciplinary approach. Four key aspects of the patient's assessment essential to determining a comprehensive approach to pain management include determining (i) pain intensity; (ii) chronicity and possible reversible causes for the pain; (iii) the type of pain (nociceptive, neuropathic, or combined); and (iv) treatment goals.

Determine Pain Intensity

Pain is subjective and unique to each individual and, as such, can only be measured by that individual. Culture, ethnicity, mood, and the patient's perceived meaning of pain may influence how pain is experienced and reported. The concept of "total pain" refers to the physical, psychological, social, and spiritual influence on a patient's perception of pain. Pain that is perceived by the patient as mild (ie, reported as a score of 1 to 3 out of 10) does not usually require initiation of or a change in pain management. Pain perceived as moderate (ie, reported as a score of 4 to 6 out of 10) generally means therapy should be initiated or changed as pain management is inadequate. Pain described as severe (ie, rated as a 7 to 10 out of 10(typically requires immediate attention. Regular follow-up to evaluate changes in the severity of pain is also critical in the process of pain management.

Determine the Chronicity of Pain

Although we still do not fully understand the development of chronic pain, lessons learned from patients undergoing surgery have taught us that good acute pain control reduces the likelihood of experiencing chronic pain. This means a comprehensive assessment and

TABLE 15.2. The PQRST Approach to Evaluating Pain

Components of the Assessment	Example Questions to Explore
P = Provokes and Palliates	What causes the pain or makes it worse? What makes the pain better?
Q = Quality	What does the pain feel like? Is it sharp? Dull? Stabbing? Burning? Crushing?
R = Region and Radiation	Where is the pain located? Does the pain radiate? If so, where to?
S = Severity	How severe is the pain?
T = Time (or Temporal)	When did the pain start? Is it present all the time? Are you pain-free at night or during the day?

physical exam should be undertaken to determine possible reversible causes for the pain along with careful attention to effective acute pain management strategies. For patients with chronic pain, treatment will most likely focus on nonpharmacologic therapies.

Determine the Nature of the Pain

The choice of initial analgesic treatment is dependent upon whether the pain is neuropathic or nociceptive in nature. The PQRST approach (provokes and palliates, quality, region and radiation, severity, and time; see Table 15.2) can help elucidate the chronicity and nature of the pain (see Table 15.1).

Establish Treatment Goals

Developing a treatment plan includes explaining the nature of the pain condition and setting appropriate treatment goals. Since complete relief of pain is generally not possible, particularly with chronic pain, the goal of therapy is to relieve the pain to a tolerable level to allow for acceptable function and QOL. For most patients this is a target of ≤3 out of 10. Clinicians should assess the impact of the pain on patient's physical and psychosocial function and QOL. The functional goals that a patient sets such as the ability to ambulate, sleep, or interact socially will need to be incorporated into the management plan and follow-up assessments.

Pain Assessment Tools for Patients With CKD

Screening for the presence of pain is best done as part of a global assessment of symptoms. This facilitates a better understanding of the patient's overall physical and psychological symptom burden and the multidimensional context within which the pain is being experienced. Listening to the patient validates the significance of their symptoms and their suffering and is an important part of the therapeutic intervention. Screening tools should be short and simple to minimize patient and staff burden. These tools must also be appropriate for use in high-risk patients such as those who are frail and those with cognitive impairment.

The most widely used screening tools with evidence for validity in patients with CKD are the Edmonton System Assessment System–Revised: Renal (Figure 15.1) and the

Edmonton Symptom Assessment System Revised: Renal (ESAS-r:Renal)

Please circle the number that best describes now you feel Now:

No Pain	0	1	2	3	4	5	6	7	8	9	10	Worst Possible Pain
No Tiredness *(Tiredness = lack of energy)*	0	1	2	3	4	5	6	7	8	9	10	Worst Possible Tiredness
No Drowsiness *(Drowsiness = feeling sleepy)*	0	1	2	3	4	5	6	7	8	9	10	Worst possible Drowsiness
No Nausea	0	1	2	3	4	5	6	7	8	9	10	Worst possible Nausea
No Lack of Appetite	0	1	2	3	4	5	6	7	8	9	10	Worst possible Lack of Appetite
No Shortness of Breath	0	1	2	3	4	5	6	7	8	9	10	Worst possible Shortness of Breath
No Depression *(Depression = feeling sad)*	0	1	2	3	4	5	6	7	8	9	10	Worst possible Depression
No Anxiety *(Anxiety = feeling nervous)*	0	1	2	3	4	5	6	7	8	9	10	Worst possible Anxiety
Best Wellbeing *(Wellbeing = how you feel overall)*	0	1	2	3	4	5	6	7	8	9	10	Worst possible Wellbeing
No itching	0	1	2	3	4	5	6	7	8	9	10	Worst possible Itching
No Problem Sleeping	0	1	2	3	4	5	6	7	8	9	10	Worst possible Problem Sleeping
No Restless Legs	0	1	2	3	4	5	6	7	8	9	10	Worst possible Restless Legs
No Other Problem *(for example constipation)*	0	1	2	3	4	5	6	7	8	9	10	Worst possible

Patient's Name _____

Date _____ Time _____

Completed by (check one):
☐ Patient
☐ Family caregiver
☐ Health care professional caregiver
☐ Caregiver-assisted
Body Diagram on Reverse

Developed by the Edmonton Zone Palliative Care Program and the kidney Supportive Care Research Group, Northern Alberta Renal Program Revised 2018-04

You hurt:

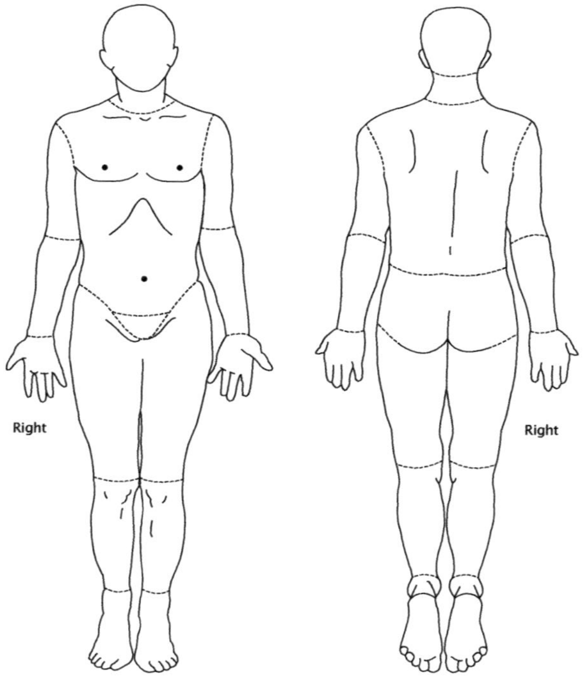

Right

Right

FIGURE 15.1. The Edmonton Symptom Assessment System–Revised: Renal.

Integrated Palliative Care Outcome Scale–Renal. See chapter 5 of this volume for additional information on tools to assess pain and other symptoms.

Once pain is recognized, its impact on function and QOL should be assessed. This requires careful communication with the patient that can be facilitated by a multidimensional pain assessment tool. The Brief Pain Inventory is one of the most commonly used multidimensional assessment tools. It assesses location, type (nociceptive vs neuropathic) and severity of pain; the pain's impact on function, mood, and QOL; pain medications being used and their perceived effectiveness; and the patient's treatment goals.

Nonpharmacological Approaches to Pain Management

A vital component of the management of pain, especially chronic nonmalignant pain, is the use of nonpharmacological therapies.[9] Unfortunately, there is a significant lack of nonpharmacological intervention studies in patients with CKD. The available evidence is synthesized in Table 15.3.

TABLE 15.3. Nonpharmacological Approaches to Pain

Treatment	Evidence
Physical therapies	
Exercise	• Osteoarthritis: guidelines found the level of evidence ranged from low to high, but the overall recommendation was strong.[9-11] • Chronic low back pain: a 2018 meta-analysis found that both aerobic training and progressive resistance training reduced the severity of pain about equally.[12]
Yoga	• An RCT found that a 12-week yoga-based rehabilitation program reduced pain by 37% (along with fatigue and insomnia) in 19 hemodialysis patients compared to 18 control patients.[13] • Chronic low back pain: the American College of Physicians Guideline recommends yoga, albeit based on low-quality evidence.[14]
Weight reduction	• Osteoarthritis pain of the knees: strongly recommended across all guidelines although the effects of weight reduction varied.[15]
Acupuncture	• Chronic musculoskeletal pain: good evidence for efficacy.[16] • Osteoarthritis: a systematic review of guidelines recommended acupuncture.[11] • Neuropathic pain: insufficient evidence to support or refute its use.[17] However, a meta-analysis of pain management in diabetic peripheral neuropathy and carpal tunnel syndrome showed benefit, although caution was expressed regarding the methodology in the RCTs examined.[18]
Behavioral therapies	
Education	• Education and self-management are core recommendations in all major guidelines for chronic noncancer pain generally and for specific pain syndromes such as osteoarthritis, although reviews of their role show a spectrum of results from positive to no effects.
Psychological	• Chronic nonmalignant pain: reviews of CBT, mindfulness-based interventions, and stress-management training are generally positive, although studies are of low to moderate quality.[15] • Chronic nonmalignant pain (excluding headache): a 2012 systematic review of 42 RCTs found CBT to have a small to moderate effect on pain.[19]

Abbreviations: cognitive-behavioral therapy; RCT, randomized controlled trial.

A Systematic Pharmacological Approach to Pain Management

The pharmacologic management of pain has recently been reviewed in detail.[20] While medication should not be the sole focus of treatment for chronic nonmalignant pain, it may be required in conjunction with nonpharmacologic treatment modalities to meet treatment goals. There are 5 essential principles for the pharmacologic management of pain, which are described in Table 15.4.

Pharmacologic Approach to Neuropathic Pain

The stepwise selection of analgesics using the World Health Organization analgesic ladder is outlined in Figure 15.2. The pharmacologic treatment of neuropathic pain starts with an adjuvant drug, which is a drug that is not primarily indicated to control pain but can be used for this purpose. The pain experienced by patients with CKD is of mixed type. It is important

TABLE 15.4. Five Principles of Pain Management in Advanced CKD

Principle	Description	Specific Considerations in Advanced CKD
"By mouth"	- Oral administration is the safest and preferred route of administration. - If ingestion or absorption is uncertain, analgesics should be administered via alternative routes such as transdermal, rectal, or subcutaneous routes.	- Intravenous administration should be avoided to optimize safety and minimize the risk of analgesic abuse and addiction.
"By the clock"	- For continuous or predictable pain, analgesics should be given regularly. Additional "breakthrough" or "rescue" medication should be available on an "as needed" basis.	- Some patients with mild pain may achieve adequate pain relief with analgesic dosing posthemodialysis only. An example would be gabapentin postdialysis for mild neuropathic pain.
"By the ladder"	- A cautious stepwise approach to analgesic therapy is recommended with slow introduction and upward titration, starting with nonopioids then progressing to opioids using the WHO analgesic ladder.	- Careful selection of analgesics taking into account the degree of kidney failure is critical. - Sustained-release preparations are generally not recommended given the higher risk for toxicity.[21]
"For the individual"	- There is large variability in patients' response to analgesics. The "correct" dose is the amount needed to relieve the pain without producing intolerable side effects.	- Chronic pain is often experienced in the context of numerous other physical, psychosocial, and spiritual concerns. Close attention to these other issues is part of the pain management strategy.
"Attention to detail"	- Ongoing reassessment is required as pain changes over time. - Side effects should be explained and actively managed (eg, constipation and nausea).	- There are no studies on the long-term use of analgesics in patients with CKD. Careful attention must be paid to efficacy and safety. - The impact on overall symptom burden, physical, emotional and cognitive function, and QOL should be reassessed routinely.

Abbreviations: CKD, chronic kidney disease; QOL, quality of life; WHO, World Health Organization.

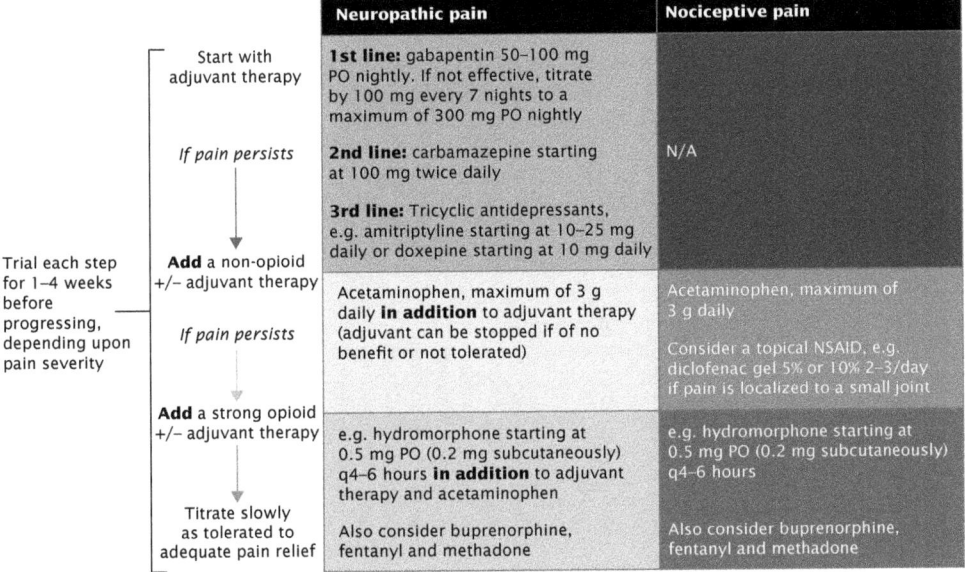

FIGURE 15.2. A stepwise approach to the management of pain in patients with advanced chronic kidney disease. Reproduced with permission from Davison SN. Clinical pharmacology considerations in pain management. *Clin J Am Soc Nephrol.* 2019;14(6):917–931.

Abbreviations: NSAID, nonsteroidal anti-inflammatory drug; PO, per os; TCAs, tricyclic antidepressants.

to target the neuropathic component first with adjuvant therapy to prevent inappropriate use of opioids.

Anticonvulsants such as the gabapentinoids and tricyclic antidepressant (TCA) drugs have the most evidence of efficacy, especially for reducing neuropathic pain due to diabetic peripheral neuropathy and postherpetic neuralgia.[22] The evidence for effectiveness for other causes of neuropathic pain is limited; a small study in patients on hemodialysis showed improvement in pain and QOL scores for diverse causes of neuropathic pain using gabapentin.[23] Since gabapentin is cleared by the kidneys, a substantial dose reduction is required to avoid toxicity in patients with CKD (see Table 15.5). Adverse effects include somnolence, dizziness, peripheral edema, and gait disturbances. For ESKD patients being medically managed without dialysis, older or frail patients, or those with moderate rather than severe neuropathic pain, it may be reasonable to start with doses as low as 100 mg postdialysis or 100 mg every second night. Pregabalin is structurally very similar to gabapentin. Substantial dose reductions are also required as follows: estimated glomerular filtration rate (eGFR) >30 to 60 mL/min, 150 mg twice per day; eGFR 15 to 30 mL/min, 150 mg once per day; and eGFR <15 mL/min, 75 mg once per day.

Other options for adjuvant therapy are outlined in Table 15.5. Evidence suggests carbamazepine may be as effective as gabapentin for treating neuropathic pain. Unlike gabapentin, it requires no dose adjustment in CKD. TCAs such as amitriptyline are effective in the management of neuropathic pain but may be less well tolerated than the gabapentinoids in patients with CKD because of the anticholinergic, histaminergic, and adrenergic adverse effects such as dry mouth, orthostatic hypotension, and somnolence. Ketamine has been poorly

TABLE 15.5. The Pharmacokinetics of Adjuvants Recommended for the Treatment of Neuropathic Pain in Patients With Advanced CKD

Adjuvant	Clinical Description	Oral Bioavailability	Peak plasma Concentration	Route of Clearance	Removal by HD	Maximum Dosing Recommendations
Gabapentin	Analogue of the neurotransmitter GABA with high affinity binding to $\alpha_2\delta$ proteins. It reduces the release of excitatory neurotransmitters from the brain (although does not have activity at GABA receptors) and has analgesic and anticonvulsant activities.	High-moderate: ~80%-90%	~3 hours	Not appreciably metabolized, and >95% is excreted unchanged by the kidneys. Plasma half-life therefore is greatly prolonged with advanced CKD	Highly water soluble and not bound to serum proteins so is well dialyzed. ~50% of serum drug is removed during a 4-hour HD session. Supplemental dosing postdialysis may be required. It is also slowly removed by CAPD.	- eGFR 50–79 mL/min: 600 mg 3× daily - eGFR 30–49 mL/min: 300 mg 3× daily - eGFR 15–29 mL/min: 300 mg 2× daily - eGFR <15 mL/min: 300 mg 1× daily Dose post HD.
Carbamazepine	Tricyclic compound anticonvulsant that is chemically related to TCAs and also functions as a mood stabilizer.	High: ~89%	~6 hours	Metabolized in the liver via phase 1 metabolism, primarily CYP3A4. Metabolites are excreted via the kidneys with ~20%–30% excreted via the faeces. Only 3%–5% is excreted unchanged by the kidneys. Plasma half-life remains unchanged with ESKD	Highly water soluble but 70%–80% bound to serum proteins. It is partially removed by HD. Supplemental dosing post HD is not required because of the long elimination half-life of 35 hours for carbamazepine compared to a 4-hour HD session.	Start at 100 mg once or twice daily and increase by 100 mg daily to a maximum of 1200 mg daily.
Amitriptyline	A TCA with sedative effects that is used to treat major depressive and anxiety disorders as well as migraines and neuropathic pain.	Low-moderate due to extensive first-pass hepatic metabolism: ~33%–62%	~6 hours	Extensively metabolized on first pass through the liver. It undergoes phase 1 metabolism primarily by CYP2D6 and CYP3A4. Plasma half-life remains unchanged with ESKD.	Highly lipophilic and highly bound to plasma and tissue proteins therefore is not dialyzed with HD or PD.	Although no dose reduction is required, a low starting dose of ~25 mg every night is recommended given the likelihood of anticholinergic adverse effects such as blurred vision, dry mouth, and constipation.

Ketamine	Ketamine is an anesthetic with analgesic, anti-inflammatory and antidepressant properties when used at subanesthetic doses. Its use is typically reserved for intractable neuropathic pain resistant to other adjuvants and opioids such as with calciphylaxis.	Low due to extensive first-pass hepatic metabolism: 16%–29%	Oral: 20–120 minutes IV: <5 minutes	Extensive first pass metabolism through the liver. It is metabolised by both CYP3A4 and CYP2B6 before being further metabolized to mostly inactive DHNK. The kidneys clear metabolites.	Highly water soluble with 10%–50% protein binding. It has not been studied in dialysis.	PO: 0.5 mg/kg 2×daily or 2 mg/kg daily SC: 0.05–0.15 mg/kg per hour for up to 7 days IV: 0.15–0.25 mg/kg To reduce the adverse effects of psychosis and tachycardia, the concurrent administration of haloperidol or midazolam is recommended.

Abbreviations: $\alpha_2\delta$ protein, alpha-2-delta protein; CAPD, continuous ambulatory peritoneal dialysis; CKD, chronic kidney disease; CYP, cytochrome P450; DHNK, dehydronorketamine; eGFR, estimated glomerular filtration rate; ESKD, end stage kidney disease; GABA, gamma-aminobutyric acid; HD, hemodialysis; HNKs, hydroxynorketamines; NMDA, N-methyl-D-aspartate; PD, peritoneal dialysis; TCA, tricyclic antidepressant.

studied in patients with advanced CKD and is reserved for intractable neuropathic pain resistant to other adjuvants and opioids. Although there is no need for dose adjustment in CKD, adverse events such as tachycardia and psychosis may limit its use. There are insufficient data or clinical experience with selective serotonin reuptake inhibitors and selective serotonin norepinephrine reuptake inhibitors for neuropathic pain in CKD to make a recommendation. In the general population, they tend to be less effective than anticonvulsants and TCAs but have fewer adverse effects.[22] If neuropathic pain remains inadequately controlled despite maximum adjuvant therapy, analgesics should be used as described in the following discussion for nociceptive pain, starting with the nonopioid analgesic acetaminophen.

Pharmacologic Approach to Nociceptive Pain

The pharmacologic management of nociceptive pain is initiated with acetaminophen (see Figure 15.2). Recent evidence suggests that lifetime cumulative doses of acetaminophen do not have an adverse effect on CKD progression.

The use of NSAIDs should generally be avoided in patients with advanced CKD due to increased risks of bleeding, cardiovascular events, psychiatric events (eg, agitation, depression, anxiety, paranoia, delirium, and hallucinations), and kidney-related complications in those with residual kidney function. Geriatric and rheumatologic societies also recommend that the chronic (>21 days) use of all oral NSAIDs be avoided, especially in the elderly patients over the age of 75 years, for these same concerns.[24] Therefore, the use of NSAIDs at the lowest effective dose for the shortest duration is best reserved for specific indications of acute inflammatory pain. Topical NSAIDs can provide effective pain relief without the systemic adverse events associated with oral NSAIDs. When pain is present in joints or nonulcerated skin, they may be a useful alternative to oral administration.

The Use Opioids for Patients with CKD

Opioids should only be considered if nonpharmacologic and nonopioid approaches have proven to be insufficient to meet treatment goals. Prior to commencing opioids, patients should be screened for substance use disorder. There is no single test or instrument that absolutely predicts this risk, but several risk factors should be considered such as current or past illicit drug or alcohol abuse; a family history of alcohol or drug abuse; and/or a history of sexual abuse, psychiatric disorder, or posttraumatic stress disorder. Patients deemed at high risk of substance use disorder should be prescribed naloxone and be followed by a pain specialist. A prescription monitoring program should be used for all patients prescribed opioids, where available. All patients should be fully informed regarding the potential risks and benefits of opioid therapy with an emphasis on how to keep medications secure at home. Patients should start with a trial of opioid therapy with regular reassessment by their healthcare provider.

Metabolism of Opioids and CKD

Patients with CKD are at increased risk for adverse effects of opioids due to the reduced elimination and increased accumulation of the parent analgesic and/or active metabolites.

Opioids may also be removed by dialysis, leading to uncertain analgesic effects during treatment.

The risks of opioid toxicity, poor analgesic response, and drug interactions for patients with CKD are determined largely by which enzyme systems metabolize the opioid and the patient's genetic factors. Opioid metabolism primarily takes place in the liver, with inactive and active metabolites (and varying degrees of the parent drug) excreted by the kidneys. These will accumulate to various degrees in patients with CKD. Careful selection of opioids is essential and understanding opioid metabolism is important in this determination.

There are 2 forms of metabolism that occur in the liver. Phase 1 metabolism involves primarily the cytochrome P450 2D6 (CYP2D6 gene) and cytochrome P450 3A4 (CYP3A4 gene) enzymes, and phase 2, glucuronidation. Opioids that undergo predominantly phase 1 metabolism are generally to be avoided in patients with advanced CKD. Because the CYP3A4 enzyme metabolizes more than 50% of drugs, there is a high risk of drug–drug interactions when opioids metabolized by this enzyme are used. Concomitant use of CYP3A4 substrates and inhibitors can increase the parent opioid concentration, thereby prolonging the analgesic effect or resulting in toxicity. CYP3A4 inducers can reduce opioid levels and therefore reduce analgesic effect. Oxycodone, a semisynthetic opioid, is metabolized primarily by CYP3A4 to the active metabolite noroxycodone. The potential for drug interactions with oxycodone is relatively high. The CYP2D6 enzyme metabolizes approximately 25% of drugs so is still associated with a risk of drug–drug interactions, although lower than with CYP3A4 metabolism. Drugs that are metabolized by phase 2 glucuronidation, such hydromorphone, have minimal drug interaction potential.

Drugs that undergo predominantly phase 1 metabolism involving CYP2DP enzymes have additional concerns of unpredictable, highly variable responses due to the many genetic polymorphisms of the CYP2D6 gene. Individuals who have 3 or more active copies of the CYP2D6 gene are described as "ultra-rapid metabolizers." Conversely, those who carry inactive copies of the CYP2D6 gene are termed "poor metabolizers." This can result in unpredictable toxicity with trivial doses or poor analgesic response with standard doses. Several opioids are metabolized via this pathway, and this can be particularly problematic for patients with advanced CKD given the narrow therapeutic window between analgesia and toxicity. Examples include codeine, a weak opioid that is metabolized by CYP2D6 to its active metabolite morphine and the weak synthetic opioid, tramadol, which is related to codeine. Tramadol also undergoes CYP3A4-mediated metabolism and is subject to numerous drug interactions. Hydrocodone is primarily metabolized via CYP2D6 to the active metabolite of hydromorphone. The production of hydromorphone is reduced in CYP2D6 "poor metabolizers," but there is little evidence of a difference in analgesic effect. Ultra-rapid CYP2D6 metabolizers may have an increased response to hydrocodone with an increased risk of overdose. Given the lack of studies in patients with CKD, it is not possible to make a recommendation. Oxycodone also undergoes a small amount of metabolism via CYP2D6 enzymes. The ability to remove oxycodone and noroxycodone by dialysis is very limited given oxycodone is nearly 50% protein bound, is only moderately water soluble, and has a relatively high volume of distribution. While genetic variability of phase 2 glucuronidation exists, the clinical relevance is unknown. Drugs metabolized via phase 2 glucuronidation do not appear to have the same risk for unpredictable toxicity as seen with CYP2D6 mediated metabolism.

Although morphine is metabolized via phase 2 glucuronidation, it is metabolized to the active metabolites morphine-3-glucuronide (M3G) and small amounts (~10%) of morphine-6-glucuronide (M6G). Both M3G and M6G accumulate in patients with advanced CKD. Although M3G lacks analgesic effect, it may contribute to adverse effects such as allodynia, myoclonus, and seizures. M6G has a more potent analgesic effect than morphine. Although morphine is removed by dialysis, slow diffusion out of the central nervous system means that complete removal may not occur with a single dialysis treatment. There are many reports in the literature of profound toxicity associated with morphine use in patients with advanced CKD. The use of morphine in patients with CKD is therefore not recommended, especially for patients with stage 5 CKD.

Opioids Recommended for Cautious Use in Patients With Advanced CKD

Table 15.6 describes the pharmacokinetics of the opioids that appear to be the safest for use in patients with advanced (eGFR stages 4 and 5) CKD. Hydromorphone, fentanyl, methadone, and buprenorphine all have minimal changes in pharmacokinetics in advanced CKD. They also appear to have a stable analgesic affect during hemodialysis. Hydromorphone has the advantage of not undergoing phase 1 metabolism, thereby avoiding the complications of the unpredictable toxicity and drug–drug interactions seen with opioids metabolized via the CYP2D6 and CYP34A enzymes. However, it does have the active metabolite hydromorphone-3-glucuronide (H3G), which accumulates in CKD with the potential to cause toxicity if not monitored carefully. This is particularly important for patients with eGFR stage 5 CKD who have yet to start dialysis or have chosen medical management without dialysis. Fentanyl does not produce active metabolites. Although methadone does not produce active metabolites, its metabolism relies on several CYP enzymes in addition to CYP3A4 resulting in the potential for drug–drug interactions. Methadone can also prolong Q-T intervals. It is generally recommended to limit the use of methadone to experienced prescribers. Caution is required when using buprenorphine as the reversal of buprenorphine-induced respiratory depression with naloxone may be delayed, and large doses of naloxone may be required Furthermore, buprenorphine is not removed by dialysis.

Adverse effects of opioids are common, and patients require ongoing reassessment for safety and efficacy. Constipation is nearly universal, and patients should have a bowel regimen prescribed pre-emptively. Nausea and vomiting occur in about 50% of people, wearing off in most cases after 7 to 10 days. Central nervous system effects, such as somnolence, occur most frequently during the initiation of opioids and when increasing the dose, hence the need to start low and titrate slow. Respiratory depression is uncommon if oral, short-acting preparations are used and the dose is titrated against pain and toxicity. Pain is said to be the physiological antagonist of opioids. When pain is stable, opioids can be used in long-acting preparations such as transdermal fentanyl or methadone.

TABLE 15.6. The Pharmacokinetics of Opioids Recommended for Use in Patients With Stages 4 and 5 CKD

Opioid	Clinical Description	Oral Bioavailability	Route of Clearance	Removal by Dialysis
Hydromorphone	A potent μ receptor agonist that is 5–7 times more potent than morphine following oral administration and ~3 times more potent following intravenous administration.	Low-moderate: 5%–35%	Extensive first-pass hepatic metabolism with rapid conversion to H3G. Therefore, the pharmacokinetics of the active parent drug are not altered substantially by CKD. The primary active metabolite, H3G, has no analgesic activity but possibly causes neuro-excitation, agitation, confusion, and hallucinations. Unlike morphine, which has an active analgesic 6-glucuronide metabolite, H6G is only present in trace amounts with hydromorphone.	H3G appears to be removed effectively during HD.[25]
Fentanyl	A potent synthetic opioid that is 50–100 times more potent than morphine. It causes less histamine release, has a lower incidence of constipation, and affords greater cardiovascular stability than morphine.	Low: usually administered intravenously or transdermally	Hepatic metabolism with 10%–20% excreted by the kidneys. Metabolites are inactive.	Lipophilic with a high volume of distribution and high serum protein binding. It is not removed to any significant degree by HD.
Methadone	A potent synthetic opioid with μ receptor activity. It also appears to function as an NMDA receptor antagonist and therefore may be more effective for neuropathic pain than other strong opioids, although evidence to support this remains limited.	High: > 80%	Hepatic metabolism into inactive metabolites with ~20% excreted unchanged in the urine. In anuric patients, methadone is excreted exclusively in faeces with no significant accumulation in plasma.	Lipophilic with a high volume of distribution and high serum protein binding. Neither the parent drug nor metabolites appear to be removed by HD.
Buprenorphine	A potent semisynthetic opioid. It is a partial μ receptor agonist and a κ receptor antagonist.	Low: administered effectively sublingually or transdermally.	Extensive first-pass hepatic metabolism with two major metabolites, B3G and norbuprenorphine, excreted fecally. Only 10%–30% is excreted in the urine. B3G is inactive. Norbuprenorphine is a less potent analgesic than buprenorphine; its clinical relevance is thought to be limited as it does not cross the blood brain barrier readily. A study of 10 patients on HD receiving transdermal buprenorphine (median dose 52.5 mcg/hr) for at least 1 week showed no elevated buprenorphine or norbuprenorphine plasma levels.[26]	Water soluble but very high volume of distribution and serum protein binding. Plasma levels do not appear to be affected by HD.[26]

Abbreviations: CKD, chronic kidney disease; B3G, buprenorphine-3-glucuronide; H3G, hydromorphone-3-glucuronide; H6G, hydromorphone-6-glucuronide; NMDA, N-methyl-D-aspartate; HD, hemodialysis.

Pain Management Near the End of Life for Patients With Advanced CKD

Figure 15.3 depicts an algorithm for terminal pain management for patients with advanced CKD. As a patient's condition deteriorates toward the end of life, swallowing becomes compromised and alternate routes of analgesic administration are required. Parenteral opioids are preferred with fentanyl being the medication of choice. If pain is solely or predominantly

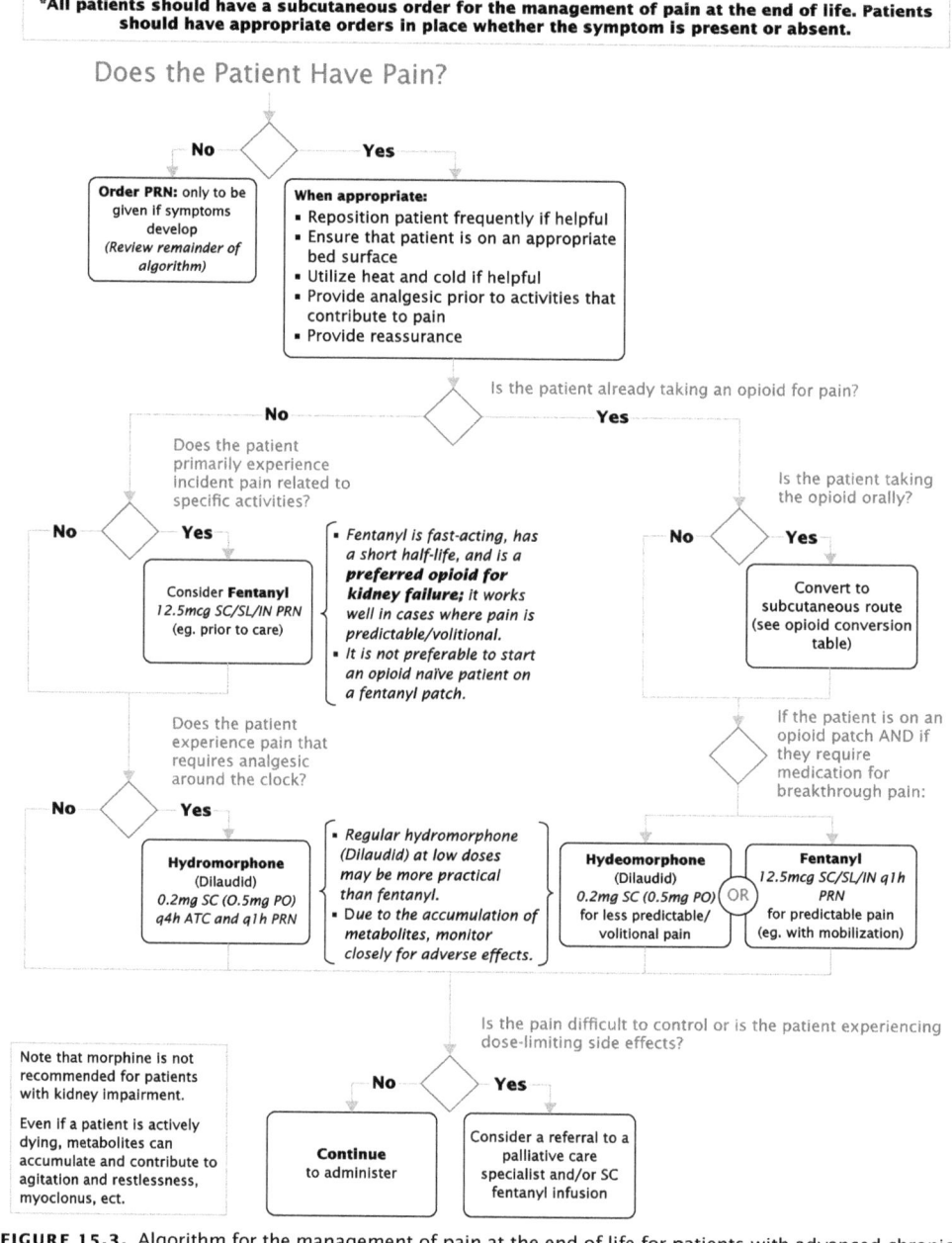

FIGURE 15.3. Algorithm for the management of pain at the end of life for patients with advanced chronic kidney disease. Reproduced with permission from Davison SN. Kidney Supportive Care Research Group. www.CKMCare.com.

neuropathic in nature and the patient is no longer able to swallow, there is good evidence in the general population for the use of parenteral lidocaine.[27] Hallucinations and agitation are very distressing adverse effects of opioids, which may occur. These should be managed by opioid dose reduction, switching to an alternative opioid, or with the approach outlined in Figure 15.4. The co-administration of low dose haloperidol (eg, 0.5 mg) may be very effective.

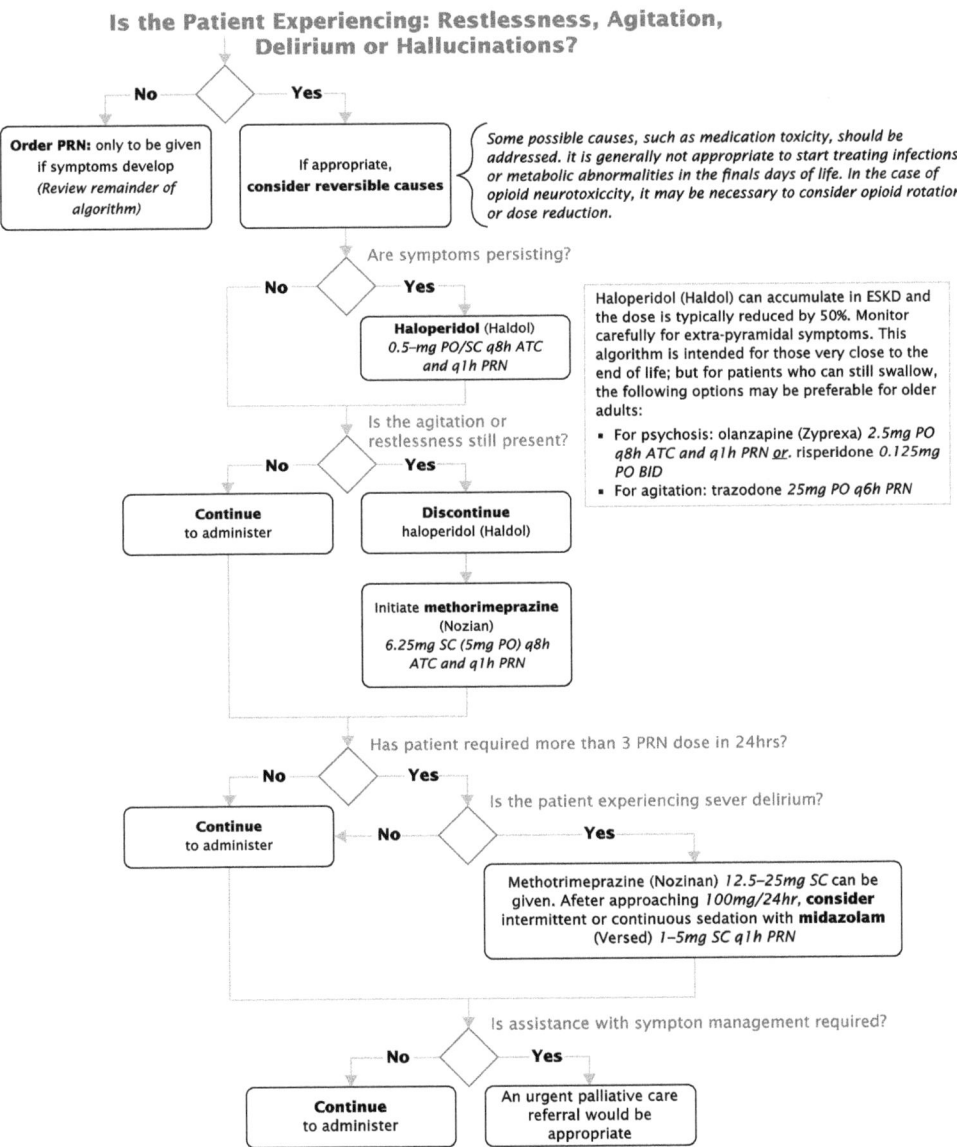

FIGURE 15.4. Algorithm for the management of restlessness, agitation, delirium or hallucinations at the end of life for patients with advanced chronic kidney disease. Reproduced with permission from Davison SN. Kidney Supportive Care Research Group. www.CKMCare.com.

Summary

Pain is a highly complex, multidimensional, and personal phenomenon with far-reaching physical and psychosocial consequences if the pain progresses to become a chronic disorder. Systematic integration of global symptom screening needs to be incorporated into routine kidney care, followed by a comprehensive pain assessment for those with clinically significant pain. Acute pain should be addressed expeditiously to decrease the likelihood of becoming a progressive disorder. The first-line management of chronic pain is a nonpharmacologic approach that may include patient education, exercise, weight reduction, yoga, acupuncture, and cognitive-behavioral therapy as appropriate along with a clear understanding of the patient's goals and expectations for therapy. In the context of advanced CKD and the multimorbidity experienced by many patients, there are numerous reasons for ongoing pain, and many patients will likely require some analgesic treatment to augment nonpharmacologic therapies to meet their treatment goals. There are no studies examining the efficacy and safety of chronic analgesic therapy, including adjuvant or opioid therapy, in patients with advanced CKD. There is a clear need for these studies to help guide safe and effective treatment. In the meantime, the careful selection of analgesics is required along with very close attention to efficacy and safety, keeping in mind the overall goal is to promote functionality and QOL and not to necessarily completely resolve the pain. A multidisciplinary pain team is best positioned to manage chronic pain that is resistant to standard interventions.

Practice Pointers

- Pain assessment and treatment requires close attention to the physical, psychosocial, and spiritual components of pain. Chronic pain is best managed by a multidisciplinary pain team if resistat to simple interventions.
- Analgesics should not be the sole focus of treatment. Nonpharmacological therapies are first-line treatment for chronic nonmalignant pain. Target the neuropathic component of pain first with adjuvant therapy to prevent inappropriate opioid use.
- Complete relief of chronic pain is generally not possible: the goal of therapy is to relive the pain to a tolerable level, allowing for acceptable function and QOL. For most patients this is a target of ≤3/10.

Practice Improvement Opportunities

- The nephrology community needs to develop the skills and comfort required to assess and manage pain, including chronic pain.
- Systematic integration of global symptom screening that includes pain into routine kidney care is needed, followed by a comprehensive pain assessment for those with clinically significant pain.

References

1. Davison SN, Koncicki H, Brennan F. Pain in chronic kidney disease: a scoping review. *Semin Dial*. 2014;27(2):188–204.
2. Brkovic T, Burilovic E, Puljak L. Prevalence and severity of pain in adult end-stage renal disease patients on chronic intermittent hemodialysis: a systematic review. *Patient preference and adherence*. 2016;10:1131–1150.
3. Andersen LN, Kohberg M, Juul-Kristensen B, Herborg LG, Søgaard K, Roessler KK. Psychosocial aspects of everyday life with chronic musculoskeletal pain: a systematic review. *Scand J Pain*. 2017;5(2):131–148.
4. Davison SN, Jhangri GS. Impact of pain and symptom burden on the health-related quality of life of hemodialysis patients. *J Pain Symptom Manag*. 2010;39(3):477–485.
5. Manns B, Hemmelgarn B, Lillie E, et al. Setting research priorities for patients on or nearing dialysis. *Clin J Am Soc Nephrol*. 2014;9(10):1813–1821.
6. Davison SN, Rathwell S, George C, Hussain ST, Grundy K. Analgesic prevalence in advanced CKD: a meta-analysis of analgesics, opioids, NSAIDs and acetaminophen use. Unpublished manuscript; 2018.
7. Merskey H, Bogduk N. *Classification of Chronic Pain*. Seattle, WA: International Association for the Study of Pain Press; 1994.
8. Davison SN, Levin A, Moss AH, et al. Executive summary of the KDIGO Controversies Conference on Supportive Care in Chronic Kidney Disease: developing a roadmap to improving quality care. *Kidney Int*. 2015;88(3):447–459.
9. Dowell D, Haegerich TM, Chou R. CDC guideline for prescribing opioids for chronic pain: United States, 2016. *JAMA*. 2016;315(15):1624–1645.
10. Manchikanti L, Kaye AM, Knezevic NN, et al. Responsible, safe, and effective prescription of opioids for chronic non-cancer pain: American Society of Interventional Pain Physicians (ASIPP) guidelines. *Pain Physician*. 2017;20(2s):S3–s92.
11. Larmer PJ, Reay ND, Aubert ER, Kersten P. Systematic review of guidelines for the physical management of osteoarthritis. *Arch Phys Med Rehabil*. 2014;95(2):375–389.
12. Wewege M, Booth J, Parmenter B. Aerobic vs. resistance exercise for chronic non-specific low back pain: a systematic review and meta-analysis. *J Back Musculoskelet Rehabilitation*. 2018;31(5):889–899.
13. Yurtkuran M, Alp A, Dilek K. A modified yoga-based exercise program in hemodialysis patients: a randomized controlled study. *Complement Ther Med*. 2007;15(3):164–171.
14. Qaseem A, Wilt TJ, McLean RM, Forciea MA. Noninvasive treatments for acute, subacute, and chronic low back pain: a clinical practice guideline from the American College of Physicians. *Ann Intern Med*. 2017;166(7):514–530.
15. Geenen R, Overman CL, Christensen R, et al. EULAR recommendations for the health professional's approach to pain management in inflammatory arthritis and osteoarthritis. *Ann Rheum Dis*. 2018;77(6):797–807.
16. Vickers AJ, Cronin AM, Maschino AC, et al. Acupuncture for chronic pain: individual patient data meta-analysis. *Arch Intern Med*. 2012;172(19):1444–1453.
17. Ju ZY, Wang K, Cui HS, et al. Acupuncture for neuropathic pain in adults. *Cochrane Database Syst Rev*. 2017(12):CD012057.
18. Dimitrova A, Murchison C, Oken B. Acupuncture for the treatment of peripheral neuropathy: a systematic review and meta-analysis. *J Altern Complement Med*. 2017;23(3):164–179.
19. Williams AC, Eccleston C, Morley S. Psychological therapies for the management of chronic pain (excluding headache) in adults. *Cochrane Database Syst Rev*. 2012;11:Cd007407.
20. Davison SN. Clinical pharmacology considerations in pain management. *Clin J Am Soc Nephrol*. 2019;14(6):917–931.
21. Ray WA, Chung CP, Murray KT, Hall K, Stein CM. Prescription of long-acting opioids and mortality in patients with chronic noncancer pain. *JAMA*. 2016;315(22):2415–2423.
22. McQuay HJ, Tramer M, Nye BA, Carroll D, Wiffen PJ, Moore RA. A systematic review of antidepressants in neuropathic pain. *Pain*. 1996;68(2-3):217–227.

23. Atalay H, Solak Y, Biyik Z, Gaipov A, Guney F, Turk S. Cross-over, open-label trial of the effects of gabapentin versus pregabalin on painful peripheral neuropathy and health-related quality of life in haemodialysis patients. *Clin Drug Investigat.* 2013;33(6):401–408.
24. Wongrakpanich S, Wongrakpanich A, Melhado K, Rangaswami J. A comprehensive review of non-steroidal anti-inflammatory drug use in the elderly. *Aging Dis.* 2018;9(1):143–150.
25. Davison SN, Mayo P. Pain management in chronic kidney disease: the pharmacokinetics and pharmacodynamics of hydromorphone and hydromorphone-3-glucuronide in hemodialysis patients. *J Opioid Manage.* 2008;4(6):335, 339–336, 344.
26. Filitz J, Griessinger N, Sittl R, Likar R, Schuttler J, Koppert W. Effects of intermittent hemodialysis on buprenorphine and norbuprenorphine plasma concentrations in chronic pain patients treated with transdermal buprenorphine. *Eur J Pain.* 2006;10(8):743–748.
27. Tremont-Lukats IW, Challapalli V, McNicol ED, Lau J, Carr DB. Systemic administration of local anesthetics to relieve neuropathic pain: a systematic review and meta-analysis. *Anesth Analg.* 2005;101(6):1738–1749.

16

Systematic Nonpain Symptom Assessment and Management

Hana Yu and Jennifer S. Scherer

Patients with advanced chronic kidney disease (CKD) suffer from a substantial burden of physical and emotional symptoms that adversely affect their health-related quality of life. Their number of symptoms when systematically evaluated is comparable to cancer patients. Overall symptom burden and severity are correlated directly with impaired quality of life and depression. Among the most frequent are fatigue, pain, pruritus, sleep disturbances and poor appetite. This chapter highlights one of the most common and troublesome of these symptoms affecting advanced CKD patients, particularly those with end-stage kidney disease: uremic pruritus. The epidemiology, pathophysiology, and current evidence-based treatments are discussed as a way to provide a practical guide for diagnosis and treatment. Lastly, areas for future research to improve symptom management in this growing, chronically ill population are identified.

Case

A 69-year-old Chinese male with a history of end-stage kidney disease (ESKD) on hemodialysis (HD) for 5 years, uncontrolled diabetes, coronary artery disease, and congestive heart failure is admitted to the hospital for pneumonia. The nurse taking care of him reports that the patient is very restless at night. His neighbor in his shared hospital room also complains to the staff that the patient fidgets at night to the point that it is disrupting his own personal sleep. The nurse asks the nephrology consultant, "Is there anything you can prescribe to calm him down at night?"

On history, the patient reports many symptoms including fatigue and poor sleep at night. He reveals that his restlessness is attributed to constant itching. His itch began 1 year ago and has progressively become more intense. It is predominantly located in his upper arms and back and worsens at night. He denies any associated rash, new medication, or fever. No one at home is experiencing the same symptoms. He is seen repetitively scratching himself around his arms during the interview. Patient appears exhausted with noticeable sunken eyes. His exam is significant for multiple excoriations on his upper extremities bilaterally with no obvious rash. He reports he has been given antihistamines in his dialysis unit without any noticeable change in his symptoms.

After a detailed assessment, you realize the patient is experiencing severe uremic pruritus (UP), which is impacting his quality of sleep and energy. You initially recommend a regimen of aggressive skin hydration with 3 times daily application of a high water-containing emollient and a trial of gabapentin 100 mg 3 times a week to be given after dialysis. You follow up in 2 weeks for close monitoring for any adverse effects, and he reports slow improvements in itching. Four weeks later, patient is noticeable in better spirits and reports overall improvement in his mood, pruritus, and sleep.

Introduction

Patients with advanced chronic kidney disease (CKD) suffer from a substantial burden of physical and emotional symptoms. Studies show that the average number of symptoms per patient ranges between 6 to 20, with fatigue, pain, pruritus, sleep disturbances, and poor appetite the most commonly reported.[1,2] This elevated symptom burden is not only physically debilitating for a patient, but also negatively impacts quality of life (QoL) and can affect treatment adherence.[3-5] Therefore, attention to symptom management has the potential to improve the overall patient experience with serious CKD as well as compliance with its treatments.

A majority of research on the topic of symptoms in CKD focuses on those with ESKD undergoing dialysis. Although examination in other populations with serious kidney disease (CKD stages 4 and 5, peritoneal dialysis (PD) patients, and those who choose medical management without dialysis defined as treatment focus on QoL without dialysis initiation) is limited, patients with advanced CKD not on renal replacement therapy and patients with ESKD on HD appear to experience comparable symptom burden and overall low QoL.[6] In general, studies have shown that most patients with kidney disease of all stages do experience a significant level of symptom burden that can impact overall function.[7-9] Figure 16.1 illustrates the prevalence of common symptoms in those with CKD and with stage 5 CKD managed medically without dialysis.

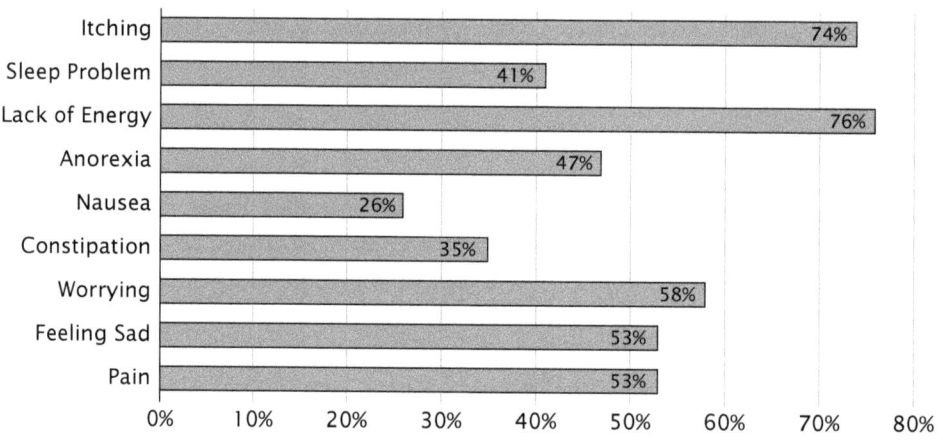

FIGURE 16.1. Prevalence of symptoms in medical management without dialysis patients (*n* = 66). Murtagh F, Addington-Hall JM, Edmonds PM, et al. Symptoms in advanced renal disease: a cross-sectional survey of symptom prevalence in stage 5 chronic kidney disease managed without dialysis. *J Palliat Med.* 2007;10(6)1266–1276.

Due to the complexity of symptoms in CKD, the clinical approach to symptom management should be methodical with consideration of the physiologic impact of kidney disease itself, consequences of dialysis, and the presence of other comorbid conditions. The purpose of the chapter is to provide a framework to help clinicians recognize, understand, and treat UP as an example of an approach to symptom assessment and management in patients with advanced kidney disease.

Symptom Assessment in CKD

Despite the significant prevalence of symptoms in the CKD population, nephrology providers often underrecognize this aspect of the disease and, consequently, undertreat symptoms.[10,11] Multiple factors can explain this, including a belief that symptom management falls outside the scope of the nephrologist, lack of knowledge of potential therapeutic agents, and failure to routinely assess symptom burden.[10,12] As outlined in chapter 5 of this volume, there are several kidney disease-specific validated symptom assessment tools. Integration of these tools into routine care not only gives the clinician data about the patient's most troublesome symptoms and overall symptom burden but can also inform clinical decision-making through a discussion of quality of life goals.

Uremic Pruritus

Epidemiology/Prevalence

Pruritus is defined as an unrestricted and uncomfortable sensation that elicits the desire to scratch.[13] UP, or CKD-associated pruritus, is a common distressing symptom in patients with advanced CKD. The Dialysis Outcomes and Practice Patterns Study (DOPPS), a large international study of prevalent dialysis patients in several countries, has published 2 papers on pruritus, 1 in 2006 and 1 in 2017. The more recent evaluation reports that 18% of patients ($n = 35,452$) experience moderate to severe pruritus, a decrease from 28% in 1996.[14] Significantly, the study shows an association of UP with poor QoL, impaired sleep, and depression.[14] Beyond QoL, the earlier paper describes an increased risk of mortality by 17% in patients with UP, although this may be largely explained by UP leading to sleep disturbances as this significance was lost when adjusting for sleep quality.[15]

The data on the prevalence of UP in patients undergoing PD and those with stage 5 CKD managed medically without dialysis are rather limited. The few studies that have compared the prevalence of UP between HD and PD patients have mixed results, which are likely due to varied study populations and different tools used to measure UP.[16-19] A literature review on symptom prevalence in CKD that included 6 studies of patients with stage 5 CKD managed medically without dialysis found that 67% of this patient population reported pruritus.[1]

Clinical Presentation

The presentation of pruritus in CKD is variable but is most commonly described as a daily or near daily occurrence of itch that worsens at night. It is typically generalized itch that can affect the back, face, and access arm and can persist for months to years if not addressed.[20,21] Importantly, UP is not associated with primary skin lesions or specific dermatomal regions;

however, due to intense scratching activity, excoriations, keratosis papules, lichen simplex, and prurigo nodularis can be seen as secondary skin changes.[21,22] Nonuremic etiologies of pruritus should always be consider in evaluating itch (outlined in Box 16.1). These alternative diagnoses should be considered especially in those patients whose itch is refractory to trial of treatment (described in the following text) or whose itch presents as largely asymmetric.

BOX 16.1. Nonuremic Causes of Itch

Primary Dermatologic Conditions
1. Drug-induced hypersensitivity and other allergies
2. Contact dermatitis
3. Psoriasis
4. Xerosis
5. Urticaria
6. Dermatophytosis (tinea crusis, tinea pedis, tinea corporis)
7. Bullous pemphigoid
8. Kyrle disease (acquired perforating dermatitis)
9. Lichen simplex chronicus
10. Infestation
    - Bed bugs
    - Scabies
    - Lice

Systemic Conditions
1. Hypercalcemic states
2. Cholestasis
   - Viral hepatitis
   - Primary biliary cirrhosis
   - Drug-induced cholestasis
3. Hematologic malignancy
   - Hodgkin lymphoma
   - Cutaneous T-cell lymphoma
   - Multiple myeloma
   - Polycythemia vera
   - Solid tumors with paraneoplastic syndrome
4. Postherpetic neuralgia
5. Human immunodeficiency virus

Reprinted with permission from Scherer JS, Combs SA, Brennan F. Sleep disorders, restless legs syndrome, and uremic pruritus: diagnosis and treatment of common symptoms in dialysis patients. *Am J Kidney Dis*. 2017;69(1):117-128.

Pathophysiology

The pathophysiology of UP is poorly understood. In contrast to other etiologies of itch, UP is believed not to be mediated by histamine.[23] Several etiologies are hypothesized including physiological consequences of CKD and dialysis, immune mechanisms,[24,25] dysregulation of the opioid system,[26] and neuropathic processes.[27,28] A consensus on the pathophysiology of UP remains elusive due to conflicting evidence.

Xerosis, dry scaly skin, is commonly described in patients with renal failure and pruritus.

Skin dehydration and reduced sebum and sweat excretion may contribute to the rough and scaly skin appearances commonly seen in patients on maintenance HD. It is likely that xerosis is a major contributor to UP severity but is not the primary cause of itching.[29]

The immune hypothesis of UP builds upon the pro-inflammatory state of CKD.[30] Studies have shown correlation between high levels of systemic inflammation including elevated levels of C-reactive protein,[31,32] interleukin-6,[24] interleukin-2,[33] and white blood cell counts[15] with severity of itch in dialysis patients.

Neuropathy from nonkidney disease (eg, diabetic neuropathy) is also common in dialysis patients, and it is thought there is a neuropathic component to UP.[34] Newer evidence based upon therapeutic success of neuropathic agents suggests that direct nerve damage may have a role in the pathogenesis of UP.[35] The observed clinical benefit of gabapentin (discussed more in the following text) on UP may work by affecting voltage-dependent calcium-ion channels. These drugs inhibit ectopic discharge activity from injured nerves by blocking neuronal calcium influx and ultimately interrupting the pathway that leads to pruritus sensation. Nerve fiber damage can eventually lead to diminished threshold of perception causing a higher itch perception.[27]

Imbalance in the endogenous opioidergic system may also play a role in causing pruritus.[26] The mu-opioid receptors stimulate itch whereas the kappa-opioid receptors suppress itch.[36] It is believed that μ-opioid receptors are associated with pruritus by disinhibiting the central itch response through their anti-nociceptive properties.[30] HD patients are noted to have elevated levels of β-endorphin, a μ-opioid receptor agonist, compared to healthy controls and with the higher the level correlating with the severity of pruritus.[37]

Treatment

Overview
Given that the pathophysiology of UP is not completely understood, it is a difficult symptom to manage. Various treatments have been proposed, however, each with limited effectiveness and evidence to date. Outlined next are the most common available therapies for UP.

Adequacy of Dialysis Prescription
The first step in UP management is to ensure the patient is optimally dialyzed. It has been suggested that higher dialysis adequacy with a good nutritional state reduces the prevalence and degree of pruritus in hemodialyzed patients.[38] Attention to dialysis adequacy should be

done concurrently with consideration of initiating pharmacological and nonpharmacological treatments as discussed in the following text.

Topical Therapies

Because xerosis is frequently seen with CKD and may aggravate pruritus, emollients with high water content should be used as first-line treatment especially when a component of dry skin is found on examination. Both aqueous cream emollients[39] and baby oil[40,41] when applied liberally 2 to 4 times daily have been shown to decrease itch and may even improve QoL in HD patients. Concurrent and preventative measures such as nail care (keeping nails short) and keeping cool (light clothing, lukewarm baths/showers) may also be useful.[34]

In addition to adequate skin hydration, other topical agents have been used to treat pruritus. The use of neuropathic agent capsaicin to treat UP has been studied, but currently there is insufficient evidence to support its use.[42,43] Gamma-linoleic acid–enriched cream and 1% pramoxine lotion have also been shown in small studies to be effective in treatment of UP.[36] Topical treatment may be preferred in patients with mild or localized symptoms, but more severe or generalized itching may require systemic treatment.

Systemic Medical Treatment

γ-Amionbutyric Acid Analogs

Based on the neuropathic hypothesis of UP, gabapentin and pregabalin have been tried as treatment for UP and currently have the most evidence, albeit limited, to support their use. In a small randomized trial of HD patients ($n = 25$) with UP comparing 300 mg of gabapentin treatment postdialysis to placebo for 4 weeks, the gabapentin group showed a significant decrease in UP severity.[27] There have been other small-scale studies that have shown similar improvements in pruritus with gabapentin doses of 100 to 400 mg postdialysis with the largest effect in those with known neuropathy.[28,44,45] Overall, the starting recommendation is 100 mg after each HD session under close surveillance with slow upward titration to decrease the risk of gabapentin-induced neurotoxicity in patients with decreased renal function (side effects discussed further in the following text).[28,46]

The safety and efficacy of gabapentin for treatment of UP (as well as restless legs syndrome) was assessed in a single-center retrospective cohort study in patients managed medically without dialysis with CKD and ESKD (mean glomerular filtration rate of 18 mL/min/1.73m^2).[47] They found that a median daily dose of 100 mg of gabapentin significantly reduced pruritus in the 34 patients managed medically without dialysis.[47] However, 47% of patients experienced 1 or more side effects (such as dizziness, drowsiness, fatigue), which lead to 17% rate of treatment discontinuation.[47]

Pregabalin has also been studied for UP in several uncontrolled, small prospective studies of HD patients and has been shown to be effective when given in doses of 25 mg or 75 mg at nighttime.[48-50] Dosing adjustments for both gabapentin and pregabalin are required for patients with kidney disease since both are renally excreted with increased half-life with decreasing kidney function. Because gabapentin for UP is an off-label use and is readily cleared by dialysis, it is recommended that gabapentin be given after each session (100–300 mg) and be closely monitored for adverse effects (as previously discussed). Pregabalin can be considered for patients who are unable to tolerate gabapentin.[49]

Opiate Receptor Modulators

The opioidergic system may have an important role in the pathophysiology of UP. Both naltrexone, a μ-receptor antagonist, and nalfurafine, a κ-receptor agonist, have been shown in randomized controlled trials (RCT) to significantly decreased UP.[51,52] In 2 multicenter, RCT including 144 HD patients with UP, 5 μg IV nalfurafine given postdialysis was found to significantly improve itching intensity ($p = .0410$) and sleep disturbances ($p = .0003$) compared to placebo at 4 weeks using meta-analysis approach.[51]

A subsequent trial of 337 HD patients with UP resistant to antihistamines and anti-allergy drugs found that 2.5 or 5 μg of oral nalfurafine reduced itch when compared with placebo.[37] The most common adverse effect reported was insomnia and constipation.[37,51] However, nalfurafine is not currently widely available. Naltrexone (oral, 50 mg/day) was compared with placebo and loratadine and showed no difference in efficacy in patients with ESKD on dialysis.[53,54] Recently, nalbuphine ER, a μ-receptor antagonist and a κ-receptor agonist was found in a multicenter, randomized controlled study including 373 HD patients to significantly reduce itch at a dose of 120 mg twice daily compared to placebo at 7 weeks ($p = .017$).[55] Opioid receptors modulators may be promising future therapies, but further studies are needed.

Phototherapy

Since 1977, ultraviolent B light (UVB) has consistently been shown to be effective in treatment of UP.[56] UVB is thought to alleviate pruritus by reducing cytokine production by lymphocytes[16] as well as inducing mast cell apoptosis.[57,58] According to a meta-analysis of RCT by Tan et al,[59] UVB therapy was a promising mode of phototherapy treatment; however, newer studies testing UVB therapy failed to show any benefits.[60]

The role of UVB phototherapy has also been assessed in the PD population. A recent study evaluated the effectiveness of narrow band UVB therapy as an add-on therapy to standard treatment in 29 PD patients with refractory UP.[58] After completion of a 12-week course of narrow band UVB therapy, 90.4% of the patients showed improvements in pruritus severity.[58] However, poor patient compliance was noted due to the high frequency of visits to the hospital for treatment and relapse occurred in nearly a third of the patients after discontinuation of the phototherapy.[58]

Due to unknown effects of long-term exposure to UV radiation and concerns for risk for skin malignancies, initiation of UVB therapy should be carefully considered, especially in transplant candidates and chronically immunosuppressed patients.

Acupuncture

Acupuncture has been used most commonly as adjunct or alternative treatment for variety of symptoms. It is hypothesized that acupuncture works by blocking spinal cord release of opioid-like substances.[61] A meta-analysis of 6 prospective clinical studies on the effectiveness of needle acupuncture for UP in patients with ESKD found that although all trials reported benefits of acupuncture, the authors ultimately concluded there was insufficient evidence to support the use of acupuncture for UP.[62]

Practice Pointer

- UP is one of the most troubling symptoms CKD and dialysis patients report, and it is typically underrecognized by nephrologists.

Practice Improvement Opportunities

- Because management of UP can be challenging, a step-wise approach with validated assessment tools and nonpharmacologic and pharmacologic approaches should be utilized for treatment.
    - Step 1: All advanced CKD patients with UP should initially have a careful history and physical exam to rule out nonuremic causes for pruritus such as urticaria, atopic dermatitis, occult malignancies, other organ failure, and skin infections.
    - Step 2: If none of these are present, UP treatment should focus on general strategies that include assessing dialysis adequacy, calcium and phosphorus levels, degree of xerosis, and nutrition.
    - Step 3: If a component of dry skin is noted on clinical examination, good skin care and moisturizer are first-line treatment. A glycerol or high-water containing emollient should be considered first.
    - Step 4: For persistent symptoms, pharmacologic and nonpharmacologic therapies can be offered with treatments individualized by incorporating patient's preference, available resources, adverse drug reactions, and drug-drug interaction.
        a. If UP localized, consider topical therapies:
            i. Capsaicin 0.025% or 0.03% ointment. Apply sparingly 2 to 4 times a day to affected areas (may initially cause burning).
            ii. Gamma-linolenic acid 2.2% cream. Can be applied twice daily to identified dry skin.
        b. If pruritus is generalized or topical therapies unsuccessful,
            i. Gabapentin should be started at 100 mg oral every other day (taken after dialysis on dialysis days for dialysis patients). If not effective, it can be further titrated by 100 mg every 7 nights to a maximum of 300 mg oral nightly. It should be taken 1 to 2 hours before bedtime. Monitor closely for side effects such as drowsiness, dizziness, confusion, and fatigue. Peripheral edema can also occur.
            ii. Pregabalin initiated at 25 mg orally every other night and titrated by 25 mg every 7 nights to a maximum of 75 mg PO every other night. It should be taken 1 to 2 hours before bedtime. Potential side effects are similar to those of gabapentin
            iii. Phototherapy or acupuncture can also be considered.
    - Step 5: A clear plan of management, regular close follow-up, and treatment adherence is crucial to helping patients cope with the heavy burden of this symptom.

Summary

As the dialysis population and the number of older ESKD patients continue to grow, understanding symptoms is increasingly important. Symptoms in the advanced CKD population are typically more complex and can be attributed to the impact of renal disease itself, a consequence of dialysis, and/or from other comorbid conditions. This symptom burden can adversely affect QoL and is associated with poorer outcomes. In general, healthcare providers under recognize the prevalence, severity, and negative impact of bothersome symptoms in this chronically ill patient group. To counter this, we recommend routine symptom screening as an integral part of clinical practices. Screening only, however, does not improve patient outcome unless providers respond appropriately to these assessments. Treatments should be considered if the symptoms are severe and are affecting patients' QoL or daily function. This chapter highlights some of the known evidence on management of UP in advanced CKD patients. Despite the high prevalence of these symptoms, there is a dearth of evidence-based treatment guidelines currently available. Additional studies with a larger number of subjects are needed to identify appropriate treatments and management of these symptoms.

References

1. Almutary H, Bonner A, Douglas C. Symptom burden in chronic kidney disease: a review of recent literature. *J Renal Care*. 2013;39(3):140–150.
2. Murtagh FE, Addington-Hall J, Higginson IJ. The prevalence of symptoms in end-stage renal disease: a systematic review. *Adv Chronic Kidney Dis*. 2007;14(1):82–99.
3. Davison SN, Jhangri GS. The impact of chronic pain on depression, sleep, and the desire to withdraw from dialysis in hemodialysis patients. *J Pain Symptom Manage*. 2005;30(5):465–473.
4. Kimmel PL, Emont SL, Newmann JM, Danko H, Moss AH. ESRD patient quality of life: symptoms, spiritual beliefs, psychosocial factors, and ethnicity. *Am J Kidney Dis*.2003;42(4):713–721.
5. Weisbord S, F Fried L, M Arnold R, et al. Prevalence, severity, and importance of physical and emotional symptoms in chronic hemodialysis patients. *J Am Soc Nephrol*. 2005;16(8):2487–2494.
6. Abdel-Kader K, Unruh ML, Weisbord SD. Symptom burden, depression, and quality of life in chronic and end-stage kidney disease. *Clin J Am Soc Nephrol*. 2009;4(6):1057–1064.
7. Brown SA, Tyrer FC, Clarke AL, et al. Symptom burden in patients with chronic kidney disease not requiring renal replacement therapy. *Clin Kidney J*. 2017;10(6):788–796.
8. Almutary H, Bonner A, Douglas C. Which patients with chronic kidney disease have the greatest symptom burden? A comparative study of advanced CKD stage and dialysis modality. *J Renal Care*. 2016;42(2):73–82.
9. Brown MA, Collett GK, Josland EA, Foote C, Li Q, Brennan FP. CKD in elderly patients managed without dialysis: survival, symptoms, and quality of life. *Clin J Am Soc Nephrol*. 2015;10(2):260–268.
10. Weisbord SD, Fried LF, Mor MK, et al. Renal provider recognition of symptoms in patients on maintenance hemodialysis. *Clin J Am Soc Nephrol*. 2007;2(5):960–967.
11. Weisshaar E, Matterne U, Mettang T. How do nephrologists in haemodialysis units consider the symptom of itch? Results of a survey in Germany. *Nephrol, Dial, Transplant*. 2009;24(4):1328–1330.
12. Moledina DG, Perry Wilson F. Pharmacologic treatment of common symptoms in dialysis patients: a narrative review. *Sem Dial*. 2015;28(4):377–383.
13. Han L, Dong X. Itch mechanisms and circuits. *Annu Rev Biophys*. 2014;43:331–355.
14. Rayner HC, Larkina M, Wang M, et al. International comparisons of prevalence, awareness, and treatment of pruritus in people on hemodialysis. *Clin J Am Soc Nephrol*. 2017;12(12):2000–2007.

15. Pisoni RL, Wikstrom B, Elder SJ, et al. Pruritus in haemodialysis patients: International results from the Dialysis Outcomes and Practice Patterns Study (DOPPS). *Nephrol, Dial, Transplant.* 2006;21(12):3495–3505.
16. Mettang T, Fritz P, Weber J, Machleidt C, Hubel E, Kuhlmann U. Uremic pruritus in patients on hemodialysis or continuous ambulatory peritoneal dialysis (CAPD): the role of plasma histamine and skin mast cells. *Clin Nephrol.* 1990;34(3):136–141.
17. Tessari G, Dalle Vedove C, Loschiavo C, et al. The impact of pruritus on the quality of life of patients undergoing dialysis: a single centre cohort study. *J Nephrol.* 2009;22(2):241–248.
18. Min JW, Kim SH, Kim YO, et al. Comparison of uremic pruritus between patients undergoing hemodialysis and peritoneal dialysis. *Kidney Res Clin Pract.* 2016;35(2):107–113.
19. Wu HY, Peng YS, Chen HY, et al. A comparison of uremic pruritus in patients receiving peritoneal dialysis and hemodialysis. *Medicine.* 2016;95(9):e2935.
20. Mathur VS, Lindberg J, Germain M, et al. A longitudinal study of uremic pruritus in hemodialysis patients. *Clin J Am Soc Nephrol.* 2010;5(8):1410–1419.
21. Mettang T, Kremer AE. Uremic pruritus. *Kidney Int.* 2015;87(4):685–691.
22. Combs SA, Teixeira JP, Germain MJ. Pruritus in kidney disease. *Sem Nephrol.* 2015;35(4):383–391.
23. Papoiu AD, Emerson NM, Patel TS, et al. Voxel-based morphometry and arterial spin labeling fMRI reveal neuropathic and neuroplastic features of brain processing of itch in end-stage renal disease. *J Neurophysiol.* 2014;112(7):1729–1738.
24. Kimmel M, Alscher DM, Dunst R, et al. The role of micro-inflammation in the pathogenesis of uraemic pruritus in haemodialysis patients. *Nephrol Dial Transplant.* 2006;21(3):749–755.
25. Mettang T, Pauli-Magnus C, Alscher DM. Uraemic pruritus—new perspectives and insights from recent trials. *Nephrol Dial Transplant.* 2002;17(9):1558–1563.
26. Yosipovitch G, Greaves MW, Schmelz M. Itch. *Lancet.* 2003;361(9358):690–694.
27. Gunal AI, Ozalp G, Yoldas TK, Gunal SY, Kirciman E, Celiker H. Gabapentin therapy for pruritus in haemodialysis patients: a randomized, placebo-controlled, double-blind trial. *Nephrol Dial Transplant.* 2004;19(12):3137–3139.
28. Manenti L, Vaglio A, Costantino E, et al. Gabapentin in the treatment of uremic itch: an index case and a pilot evaluation. *J Nephrol.* 2005;18(1):86–91.
29. Szepietowski JC, Reich A, Schwartz RA. Uraemic xerosis. *Nephrol Dial Transplant.* 2004;19(11):2709–2712.
30. Patel TS, Freedman BI, Yosipovitch G. An update on pruritus associated with CKD. *Am J Kidney Dis.* 2007;50(1):11–20.
31. Chiu YL, Chen HY, Chuang YF, et al. Association of uraemic pruritus with inflammation and hepatitis infection in haemodialysis patients. *Nephrol Dial Transplant.* 2008;23(11):3685–3689.
32. Virga G, Visentin I, La Milia V, Bonadonna A. Inflammation and pruritus in haemodialysis patients. *Nephrol Dial Transplant.* 2002;17(12):2164–2169.
33. Fallahzadeh MK, Roozbeh J, Geramizadeh B, Namazi MR. Interleukin-2 serum levels are elevated in patients with uremic pruritus: a novel finding with practical implications. *Nephrol Dial Transplant.* 2011;26(10):3338–3344.
34. Murtagh F, Weisbord SD. Symptoms in renal disease; their epidemiology, assessment, and management. In: Chambers J, Germain M, Brown E, eds. *Supportive Care for the Renal Patient.* 2nd ed. Oxford, UK: Oxford University Press; 2010: 108–110, 116–123.
35. Blaha T, Nigwekar S, Combs S, Kaw U, Krishnappa V, Raina R. Dermatologic manifestations in end stage renal disease. *Hemodial Int.* 2019;23(1):3–18.
36. Simonsen E, Komenda P, Lerner B, et al. Treatment of uremic pruritus: a systematic review. *Am J Kidney Dis.* 2017;70(5):638–655.
37. Kumagai H, Ebata T, Takamori K, Muramatsu T, Nakamoto H, Suzuki H. Effect of a novel kappa-receptor agonist, nalfurafine hydrochloride, on severe itch in 337 haemodialysis patients: a Phase III, randomized, double-blind, placebo-controlled study. *Nephrol Dial Transplant.* 2010;25(4):1251–1257.
38. Hiroshige K, Kabashima N, Takasugi M, Kuroiwa A. Optimal dialysis improves uremic pruritus. *Am J Kidney Dis.* 1995;25(3):413–419.

39. Morton CA, Lafferty M, Hau C, Henderson I, Jones M, Lowe JG. Pruritus and skin hydration during dialysis. *Nephrol Dial Transplant*. 1996;11(10):2031–2036.
40. Karadag E, Kilic SP, Karatay G, Metin O. Effect of baby oil on pruritus, sleep quality, and quality of life in hemodialysis patients: pretest–post-test model with control groups. *Japan J Nurs Sci*. 2014;11(3):180–189.
41. Lin TC, Lai YH, Guo SE, et al. Baby oil therapy for uremic pruritus in haemodialysis patients. *J Clin Nurs*. 2012;21(1-2):139–148.
42. Gooding SM, Canter PH, Coelho HF, Boddy K, Ernst E. Systematic review of topical capsaicin in the treatment of pruritus. *Int J Dermatol*. 2010;49(8):858–865.
43. Makhlough A, Ala S, Haj-Heydari Z, Kashi Z, Bari A. Topical capsaicin therapy for uremic pruritus in patients on hemodialysis. *Iranian J Kidney Dis*. 2010;4(2):137–140.
44. Razeghi E, Eskandari D, Ganji MR, Meysamie AP, Togha M, Khashayar P. Gabapentin and uremic pruritus in hemodialysis patients. *Renal Fail*. 2009;31(2):85–90.
45. Naini AE, Harandi AA, Khanbabapour S, Shahidi S, Seirafiyan S, Mohseni M. Gabapentin: a promising drug for the treatment of uremic pruritus. *Saudi J Kidney Dis Transplant*. 2007;18(3):378–381.
46. Lau T, Leung S, Lau W. Gabapentin for uremic pruritus in hemodialysis patients: a qualitative systematic review. *Canadian J Kidney Health Dis*. 2016;3:14.
47. Cheikh Hassan HI, Brennan F, Collett G, Josland EA, Brown MA. Efficacy and safety of gabapentin for uremic pruritus and restless legs syndrome in conservatively managed patients with chronic kidney disease. *J Pain Symptom Manage*. 2015;49(4):782–789.
48. Solak Y, Biyik Z, Atalay H, et al. Pregabalin versus gabapentin in the treatment of neuropathic pruritus in maintenance haemodialysis patients: a prospective, crossover study. *Nephrology (Carlton, Vic)*. 2012;17(8):710–717.
49. Rayner H, Baharani J, Smith S, Suresh V, Dasgupta I. Uraemic pruritus: relief of itching by gabapentin and pregabalin. *Nephron Clin Pract*. 2012;122(3-4):75–79.
50. Shavit L, Grenader T, Lifschitz M, Slotki I. Use of pregabalin in the management of chronic uremic pruritus. *J Pain Symptom Manage*. 2013;45(4):776–781.
51. Wikstrom B, Gellert R, Ladefoged SD, et al. Kappa-opioid system in uremic pruritus: multicenter, randomized, double-blind, placebo-controlled clinical studies. *J Am Soc Nephrol*. 2005;16(12):3742–3747.
52. Peer G, Kivity S, Agami O, et al. Randomised crossover trial of naltrexone in uraemic pruritus. *Lancet*. 1996;348(9041):1552–1554.
53. Pauli-Magnus C, Mikus G, Alscher DM, et al. Naltrexone does not relieve uremic pruritus: results of a randomized, double-blind, placebo-controlled crossover study. *J Am Soc Nephrol*. 2000;11(3):514–519.
54. Legroux-Crespel E, Cledes J, Misery L. A comparative study on the effects of naltrexone and loratadine on uremic pruritus. *Dermatology*. 2004;208(4):326–330.
55. Mathur VS, Kumar J, Crawford PW, Hait H, Sciascia T. A multicenter, randomized, double-blind, placebo-controlled trial of nalbuphine ER tablets for uremic pruritus. *Am J Nephrol*. 2017;46(6):450–458.
56. Gilchrest BA, Rowe JW, Brown RS, Steinman TI, Arndt KA. Relief of uremic pruritus with ultraviolet phototherapy. *N Engl J Med*. 1977;297(3):136–138.
57. Szepietowski JC, Morita A, Tsuji T. Ultraviolet B induces mast cell apoptosis: a hypothetical mechanism of ultraviolet B treatment for uraemic pruritus. *Med Hypotheses*. 2002;58(2):167–170.
58. Sapam R, Waikhom R. Role of narrow band ultra violet radiation as an add-on therapy in peritoneal dialysis patients with refractory uremic pruritus. *World J Nephrol*. 2018;7(4):84–89.
59. Tan JK, Haberman HF, Coldman AJ. Identifying effective treatments for uremic pruritus. *J Am Acad Dermatol*. 1991;25(5 Pt 1):811–818.
60. Ko MJ, Yang JY, Wu HY, et al. Narrowband ultraviolet B phototherapy for patients with refractory uraemic pruritus: a randomized controlled trial. *Brit J Dermatol*. 2011;165(3):633–639.
61. Che-Yi C, Wen CY, Min-Tsung K, Chiu-Ching H. Acupuncture in haemodialysis patients at the Quchi (LI11) acupoint for refractory uraemic pruritus. *Nephrol, Dial, Transplant*. 2005;20(9):1912–1915.
62. Kim KH, Lee MS, Choi SM. Acupuncture for treating uremic pruritus in patients with end-stage renal disease: a systematic review. *J Pain Symptom Manage*. 2010;40(1):117–125.

17

Systematic Psychosocial and Spiritual Needs Assessment and Management

Daniel Cukor and Elissa Kozlov

The mental healthcare and spirituality of patients is an important and often undermanaged aspect of holistic palliative care for patients with end-stage kidney disease (ESKD). Assessment for psychological problems should be a standard part of dialysis patient care. Studies show that some form of depression is prevalent in about 30-% to 40% of ESKD patients being treated with hemodialysis, with about 10-% to 20% with a major depressive disorder. Anxiety is also prevalent in dialysis, but it is less well studied. Treatment for both entails both pharmacologic and non-pharmacologic approaches with cognitive behavioral therapy being one of the most effective of the latter. The goals of this chapter are to outline the major psychological and spiritual reactions to living with ESKD, to suggest an approach to a systematic assessment strategy, and to summarize treatment issues in the management of common comorbid psychiatric disorders.

Case

Jeremy (an amalgam of cases) was a 68-year-old white male with end-stage kidney disease (ESKD) on dialysis for 10 years. He consistently scored in the elevated range on his depression screens but refused referral for further evaluation. He was the primary caregiver to his 65-year-old wife who had serious mental health issues as well as physical issues that limited her mobility. Jeremy reported to his nephrologist that he has had thoughts that life was not worth living and that he was considering discontinuing dialysis treatment. Given the context of Jeremy's possible depression, his desire to explore discontinuing dialysis was regarded as potentially part of a suicide plan. The nephrologist referred Jeremy for further psychiatric evaluation.

During the assessment, Jeremy was found to have moderate to severe depression according to the nine-question version of the Patient Health Questionnaire as well as need for support managing his wife's recent mental health exacerbation and additional help around the house. He refused an antidepressant because he was afraid of the side effects he had witnessed in his wife, but he began cognitive behavioral therapy (CBT) and accepted the addition of a home aid for his wife.

Current Evidence—Psychological Assessment and Management

There is growing evidence and recognition that to provide comprehensive care to the advanced chronic kidney disease (CKD) patient, the care team must focus on the patient's emotional state. Figure 17.1 shows the actionable steps in the process for identifying and treating psychiatric needs in CKD and ESKD treatment settings. In addition to the multifactorial ways that a patient's mental health can complicate the patient's medical course, psychological symptoms are also a substantive burden on the patient and family and therefore require clinical attention.[1] Table 17.1 shows the overlap between uremia, depression, anxiety, and spiritual needs, which necessitates careful assessment and differential diagnosis.

Depression

Depression is the most studied psychiatric comorbidity in patients with ESKD. It is important for the clinician to distinguish between normal low mood and a formal diagnosis of depression. The presentation of depression can be quite varied, but it is a mood state characterized by a sense of sadness with related emotional, cognitive, and behavioral symptoms. Depression can be identified through clinical interview, self-report measures, or structured clinical interview (Table 17.1).

There are a wide range of depression screening instruments utilized in CKD populations.[2] Recently, the two-question version of the Patient Health Questionnaire[3] has become an unofficial industry standard for screening in the dialysis centers. However, the purpose of any screening instrument is to identify who would benefit from a more comprehensive assessment, not to serve as the basis of treatment or diagnosis. A clinical interview conducted by a mental health professional encompasses more than identifying particular symptoms; it also tries to create a biopsychosocial formulation to understand how risk factors, the current situation, and the person's premorbid functioning are synergizing at the moment to create the observed presentation.

Despite the heterogeneous methods of assessment and the great diversity in ESKD populations, a rough estimate suggests that 10% to 20% of patients may have a diagnosable major depression and upwards of 30% to 40% may have significantly elevated levels of depressive affect.[4] Because depressive symptoms naturally wax and wane and often present in response to increased challenges in a person's health or social life, the lifetime prevalence of depression in ESKD patients is considerably higher.

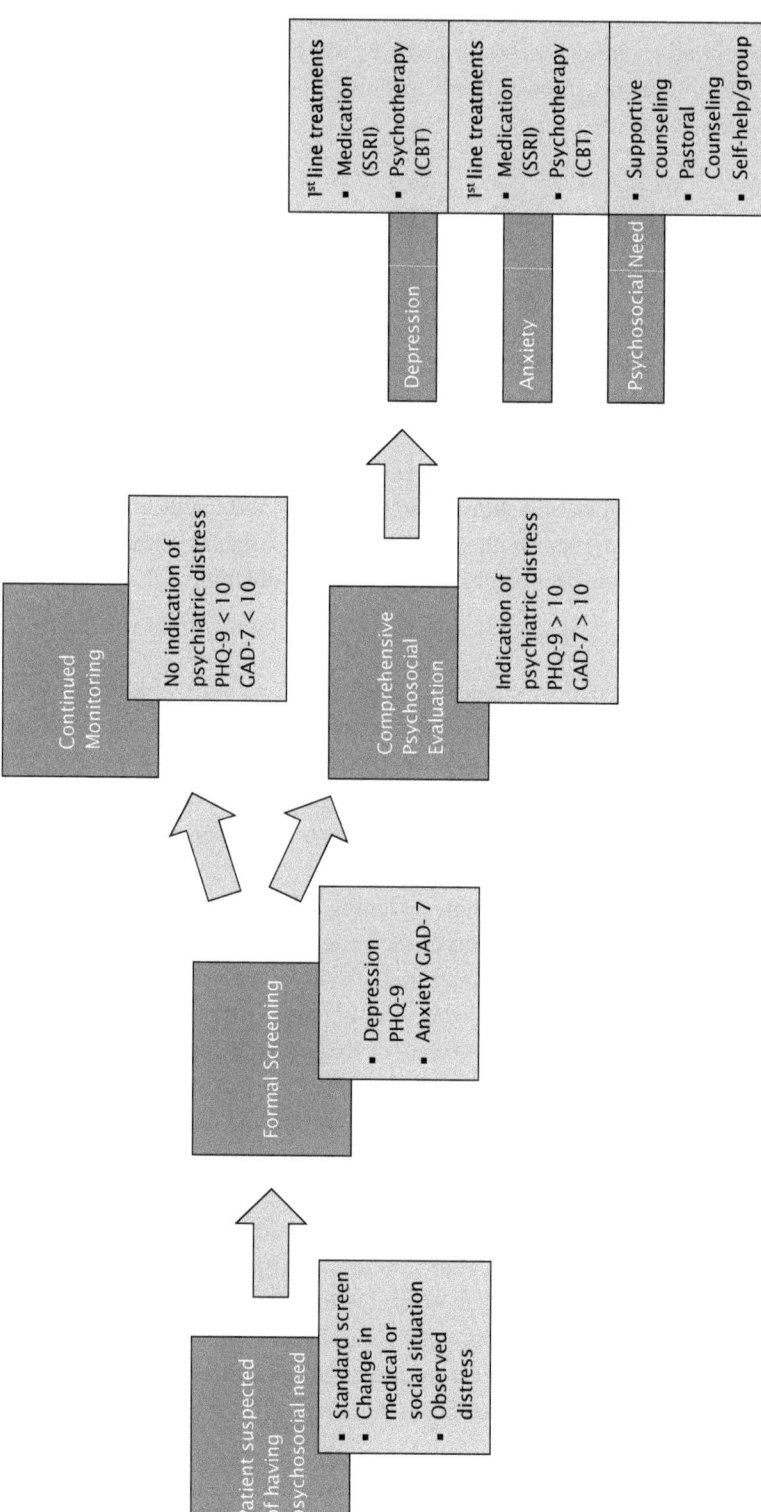

FIGURE 17.1. Actionable steps in identifying and treating psychiatric need. Abbreviations: CBT, cognitive behavioral therapy; GAD-7, Generalized Anxiety Disorder 7-item scale; PHQ-9, Patient Health Questionnaire 9-item scale; SSRI, selective serotonin reuptake inhibitor.

TABLE 17.1. Complex Differential Diagnosis: Symptom Overlap Between Uremia, Depression, Anxiety and Spiritual Need

Symptom	Uremia	Depression	Anxiety	Spiritual Need
Angst		✓	✓	✓
Anhedonia	✓	✓	✓	✓
Appetite and/or weight changes	✓	✓	✓	
Asking why this situation occurred		✓	✓	✓
Body pain	✓	✓	✓	
Difficulty thinking clearly	✓	✓	✓	✓
Guilt, worthlessness, or helplessness		✓		✓
Restlessness	✓	✓	✓	✓
Hopelessness		✓		✓
Irritability	✓	✓	✓	✓
Itching			✓	✓
Low energy or fatigue	✓	✓	✓	✓
Moving or talking more slowly	✓	✓		
Muscle tension	✓		✓	
Feeling abandoned by God		✓		✓
Questioning one's beliefs		✓	✓	✓
Questioning the meaning of life		✓	✓	✓
Sleep Difficulty	✓	✓	✓	✓
Sad or anxious mood	✓	✓	✓	✓
Sexual dysfunction	✓	✓	✓	✓
Thoughts of death or suicide		✓	✓	✓

Treatment

In treating depression, a stepped-approach is universally recommended (Table 17.2). Depending on patient presentation, treatment history, available resources, and patient preference, different strategies should be considered. Treatment for depression in general populations may take the form of psychotherapy, antidepressant medication, or their combination.

Early evidence of antidepressant management of depression in patients with ESKD has consistently found both selective serotonin re-uptake inhibitors (SSRIs) and tricyclic antidepressants to be beneficial. Tricyclic antidepressants as antidepressants have largely been supplanted by the newer generation of drugs, but imipramine and amitriptyline continue to be used for analgesia in neuropathic pain, and trazodone is commonly used in low doses as a sedative for insomnia.

Even though SSRIs are commonly used in ESKD, there has been little systematic research evaluating their efficacy. Fluoxetine and sertraline are commonly used, as they are metabolized hepatically. A recent important study, the Chronic Kidney Disease Antidepressant Sertraline Trial (CAST)[5] was a well-designed study with over 200 nondialysis-dependent CKD patients. Participants were randomized to sertraline or matching placebo. Surprisingly, treatment with sertraline for 12 weeks did not significantly improve depressive symptoms

TABLE 17.2. Treatment Options for Depression

Treatment	Options/Key Components
Pharmacological interventions[a]	Citalopram
	Escitalopram
	Fluoxetine
	Sertraline
Cognitive behavioral therapy	
Psychoeducation	Socialization to treatment, motivational interviewing
Behavioral activation	Promote positive activity scheduling
Cognitive restructuring	Reframe negative beliefs into more adaptive perspectives
Healthy living	Adherence promotion, fluid compliance, sleep hygiene
Anxiety management	Somatic symptom management, existential threat

[a]Tested in clinical trials in dialysis populations.[17]

when compared with placebo. More studies are required to place this study in context. When ESKD patients are being initiated on a new SSRI, it is often advisable to start at the recommended initiation dose and then titrate up slowly.

The most studied form of psychotherapeutic intervention for depression is CBT. CBT focuses on identifying and then changing the behavioral patterns and thought processes that contribute to depression. There is a strong evidence base that CBT is effective for treating depression in a variety of patient populations. The evidence supporting CBT in CKD and ESKD patients in particular is encouraging.[6] The greatest challenges to providing CBT to patients with CKD are the high illness burden, preventing patients from seeking additional appointments, and the relative scarcity of trained CBT therapists with familiarity with CKD. As depression assessment and treatment are becoming part of standard nephrology care, novel models of providing access to this care will need to be developed.

Case Continued

While in psychotherapy, Jeremy identified feeling tremendous stress at home due to his caregiving responsibilities, as well as high symptom burden including fatigue and muscle aches following dialysis. His depression was moderate to severe, but he was still able to perform his everyday functions and provide adequate care to his wife. His psychotherapy focused on alleviating his depression through finding time in his schedule to include pleasurable activities that were focused on his enjoyment (behavioral activation) and finding opportunities to reframe his negative thoughts related to illness and caregiving (cognitive restructuring).

Anxiety

Some anxiety or concern is a common and normative response to chronic illness. Like other medical patients, patients with ESKD are concerned about the severity and progression of their symptoms and the impending restrictions the condition imposes on their life and plans for their future. Worry is a part of the human response to an unknown future course and is not pathological. In fact, it is likely that the majority of dialysis patients will experience episodes of anxiety and stress at some stage in their treatment. Some studies report that about one-third of patients experience episodes of moderate anxiety in their first year of treatment.[7] Excessive anxiety that interferes with a patient's quality of life, however, often goes unrecognized and may require clinical intervention. There are less data on anxiety prevalence in hemodialysis (HD) populations than depression, but 1 study[8] assessed psychiatric diagnoses in a sample of 70 predominantly black ESKD patients and found that about 45% had at least 1 anxiety disorder. The prevalence of panic disorder, characterized by repeated episodes of sudden and intense onset of physical and cognitive symptoms of anxiety such as shortness of breath, elevated pulse, and catastrophic thoughts was much higher than community samples and may be related to overawareness of the bodily sensations associated with HD. Little is known about the natural history of anxiety disorders in HD patients, but for many patients, the symptoms can be mild or transient. There is also a significant minority who have persistent and severe symptoms that warrant assessment and treatment.

Treatment

There is a shortage of literature relating to the psychological treatment of anxiety in patients with ESKD, but interventions should aim to reduce the stress associated with ESKD and increase the patients' coping abilities. There are no clinical trials of psychotherapeutic intervention in ESKD samples, but there is a significant literature highlighting the efficacy of cognitive behavioral interventions in treating the full gamut of anxiety disorders in other populations.[9] Aerobic exercise training, mental imagery, and social support enrichment are also thought to be useful techniques for managing the anxiety/stress experience.

Pharmacological management is typically either directed at acute episodes of anxiety and panic or at more generalized nervousness. SSRIs are widely considered the first-line treatment for chronic worry and formal anxiety disorders. Acute transient anxiety can be treated with limited use of benzodiazepines. Since benzodiazepines are metabolized in the liver, dosage reduction is generally not necessary in ESKD. Exceptions include midazolam and chlordiazepoxide. Many patients receive ordinary doses of diazepam, lorazepam, alprazolam, and clonazepam before or during dialysis sessions to manage symptoms of anxiety related to dialysis.[10]

Case Continued

One of the themes that emerged in Jeremy's psychotherapy was the concern that as his health deteriorated, he would be unable to care for his wife properly. He ruminated about how distressing it would be for him to watch helplessly if his wife needed more assistance than he could provide. He was able to acknowledge that this fear was so profound that he would prefer dying first, and jeopardizing her care, to spare himself the anguish of watching impotently. Once he was able to articulate the core of his fear and discuss it, he identified ways of advocating for his wife's care that would be within his limited physical resources. Knowing that he could still care for his wife, despite lacking the physical strength to do it on his own, brought him a sense of calm.

Current Evidence—Spirituality

Spirituality can be defined as a part of the human experience that gives individuals a sense of transcendent meaning and purpose. Distinct from religiosity and religion, spirituality exists both independent of and within the context of traditional religious systems and can include the way individuals make connections with nature, others, himself/herself/themselves and with sacred realms. Spirituality is a key component of how many people cope with advanced illness and other stressors in their lives.

Increasingly, spirituality is recognized as being a factor related to quality of life and how people cope with illness, suffering, and death. One study of ESKD patients found that strong religious and spiritual beliefs were associated with reduced perception of burden of the illness, fewer depressive symptoms, increased perception of social support, increased satisfaction with life, and higher perceive quality of life.[11] Spirituality can even influence the course of serious illness and treatment decisions, as it can provide a framework for how people conceptualize their illness and its associated challenges.[12,13] One study of ESKD patients found an association between high scores on a spirituality questionnaire and survival rates,[14] suggesting the powerful potential impact of spirituality on patients' health outcomes. Indeed, for individuals with ESKD, spirituality appears to play a role in quality of life and psychological well-being, and patients with ESKD are interested in their nephrology and palliative care team addressing these concerns.

Spiritual care is a key element of palliative care, and good spiritual assessment of ESKD patients can facilitate improved quality of life. Because of the large impact spiritual care can have on a patient's quality of life, the World Health Organization advocates for early identification of unmet spiritual needs, and hospitals in the United States are required to document spiritual assessments of patients to receive and maintain accreditation. Recent research has discovered that individuals with ESKD often have unmet spiritual needs including needing help finding hope and meaning in life, concerns around death and dying, and assistance finding spiritual resources. Having more spiritual needs is not associated with age, gender, race, marital status, dialysis modality, time on dialysis, or comorbidity.[15] Thus, all dialysis patients' spiritual needs should be evaluated and considered as part of a holistic treatment approach.

Case Conclusion

One of the pleasurable activities Jeremy identified for himself was returning to church after a several year hiatus. With help in the home, Jeremy was able to attend services more regularly and developed relationships with new friends and the pastor. Jeremy was supported by the church community and felt reconnected to religion and God, finding new purpose in his life. The psychotherapy, tangible help in the home, and renewed passion for a spiritual life synergistically combined to give Jeremy not only the emotional energy to continue with his demanding treatments and home life, but to see his life as still having potential for growth and meaning.

Research Challenges in Behavioral and Spiritual Care Domains

While the psychological challenges of living with chronic illness have long been known, the field of psychonephrology is in its infancy. The relative lack of epidemiological data and dearth of psychiatric intervention literature are likely due to many factors. First, the focus of the field of nephrology has been on improving dialysis and developing novel technologies for renal replacement, not on coping with current-day dialysis treatment. Second, beyond the mandated social workers at each clinical site, there is relatively little behavioral health expertise integrated into dialysis treatment centers. Finding psychiatric treatment for dialysis patients can be very challenging. Between issues related to stigma, fatigue, and treatment burden, it is often difficult for patients to commit to regular attendance with a mental health provider. Furthermore, well-trained mental health professionals with experience working with renal populations are difficult to find and often have long wait lists and out-of-pocket costs associated. Third, psychiatric clinical trials are more complex and costly than standard randomized clinical trials, and the dialysis population is a relatively small market in US healthcare. Fourth, as academic centers rarely have large dialysis populations, multi-institution cooperation is required to secure a significant sample size. This cooperation is not easily supported by funding agencies and represents a substantial logistical burden. Despite these challenges, there is tremendous opportunity for significant work as many of the basic questions are yet unanswered.

Regarding spiritual care, while the research literature is not robust, spiritual care has long been considered an integral component of comprehensive palliative care. According to the national consensus project for quality palliative care,[16] it is the responsibility of the palliative care team to address spiritual, religious, and existential needs to provide compassionate, dignified, and patient-centered care to patients with serious and life-limiting illnesses. To do this, they recommend standardized assessments of spiritual care as part of routine care, and they promote engagement with a variety of spiritual resources including referrals to community-based faith leaders, discussions with family members, and meditation. Additional research regarding best practices in spiritual care within nephrology are warranted to ensure that CKD and ESKD patients are receiving holistic palliative care that considers spiritual needs.

Summary

- Depression and excessive anxiety are both common, but often undiagnosed in this population. Some form of depression is prevalent in about 30% to 40% of ESKD patients being treated with HD, with about 10% to 20% with a major depressive disorder.
- If treating depression psychopharmacologically, SSRIs are commonly used, but understudied. It is typical to start at a low initiation dose and titrate up slowly, but unless the patient reaches a therapeutic dose, the medication is unlikely to be helpful. Cognitive behavioral therapy for depression seems to be effective in HD populations.

- The palliative care team should consider the spiritual, religious, and existential needs of a patient to provide comprehensive, compassionate care to patients with serious and life limiting illnesses.
- The study of psychonephrology is in its early stages, and despite systematic challenges, there is tremendous opportunity for research and clinical innovation to substantively impact the lives of ESRD patients being treated with HD.

Practice Pointers

- Psychiatric assessment should be a standard component of all medical care. Each site needs to create a workflow that identifies key times for screening, thresholds for further evaluation, and treatment strategies. (See Figure 17.1 for actionable steps for a possible workflow.)
- There is a considerable amount of overlap between diagnostic categories, and it can be difficult to properly identify individual symptoms (see Table 17.1). To minimize misdiagnosis, an interdisciplinary team approach to identifying etiology can be helpful.
- Spiritual care is a key element of palliative care, and good spiritual assessment of ESKD patients can facilitate improved quality of life.

Practice Improvement Opportunities

- Widespread adoption of known antidepressant treatments into standard clinical care.
- More behavioral health expertise integrated into dialysis care organizations.
- Incorporation of spiritual needs into standard palliative care assessments and treatment recommendations

References

1. Cukor D, Cohen SD, Peterson RA, Kimmel PL. Psychosocial aspects of chronic disease: ESRD as a paradigmatic illness. *J Am Soc Nephrol*. 2007;18(12):3042–3055. doi:10.1681/asn.2007030345
2. Hedayati SS, Bosworth HB, Kuchibhatla M, Kimmel PL, Szczech LA. The predictive value of self-report scales compared with physician diagnosis of depression in hemodialysis patients. *Kidney Int*. 2006;69(9):1662–1668. doi:10.1038/sj.ki.5000308
3. Kroenke K, Spitzer RL, Williams JBW. The Patient Health Questionnaire-2: validity of a two-item depression screener. *Med Care*. 2003;41(11):1284–1292. doi:10.1097/01.MLR.0000093487.78664.3C
4. Kimmel PL, Peterson RA. Depression in end-stage renal disease patients treated with hemodialysis: tools, correlates, outcomes, and needs. *Semin Dial*. 2008;18(2):91–97. doi:10.1111/j.1525-139X.2005.18209.x
5. Hedayati SS, Gregg LP, Carmody T, et al. Effect of sertraline on depressive symptoms in patients with chronic kidney disease without dialysis dependence: The CAST randomized clinical trial. *JAM*. 2017;318(19):1876–1890. doi:10.1001/jama.2017.17131
6. Cukor D, Saggi SJ, Asher DR, et al. Psychosocial intervention improves depression, quality of life, and fluid adherence in hemodialysis. *J Am Soc Nephrol*. 2014;25(1):196–206. doi:10.1681/asn.2012111134
7. Nichols KA, Springford V. The psycho-social stressors associated with survival by dialysis. *Behav Res Ther*. 1984;22(5):563–574.

8. Cukor D, Coplan J, Brown C, Peterson RA, Kimmel PL. Course of depression and anxiety diagnosis in patients treated with hemodialysis: a 16-month follow-up. *Clin J Am Soc Nephrol.* 2008;3(6):1752–1758. doi:10.2215/CJN.01120308
9. Rachman S. Psychological treatment of anxiety: the evolution of behavior therapy and cognitive behavior therapy. *Annu Rev Clin Psychol.* 2009;5(1):97–119. doi:10.1146/annurev.clinpsy.032408.153635
10. Cohen SD, Cukor D, Kimmel PL. Anxiety in patients treated with hemodialysis. *Clin J Am Soc Nephrol.* 2016;11(12):2250–2255. doi:10.2215/CJN.02590316
11. Patel SS, Shah VS, Peterson RA, Kimmel PL. Psychosocial variables, quality of life, and religious beliefs in ESRD patients treated with hemodialysis. *Am J Kidney Dis.* 2002;40(5):1013–1022. doi:10.1053/ajkd.2002.36336
12. Breitbart W. Spirituality and meaning in supportive care: spirituality-and meaning-centered group psychotherapy interventions in advanced cancer. *Support Care Cancer.* 2002;10(4):272–280. doi:10.1007/s005200100289
13. Puchalski C, Romer AL. Taking a spiritual history allows clinicians to understand patients more fully. *J Palliat Med.* 2000;3(1):129–137.
14. Spinale J, Cohen SD, Khetpal P, et al. Spirituality, social support, and survival in hemodialysis patients. *Clin J Am Soc Nephrol.* 2008;3:1620–1627. doi:10.2215/CJN.01790408
15. Davison SN, Jhangri GS. Existential and religious dimensions of spirituality and their relationship with health-related quality of life in chronic kidney disease. *Clin J Am Soc Nephrol.* 2010;5(11):1969–1976. doi:10.2215/CJN.01890310
16. National Consensus Project for Quality Palliative Care. *Clinical Practice Guidelines for Quality Palliative Care.* 3rd ed. Pittsburgh, PA: National Consensus Project for Quality Palliative Care; 2013.
17. Palmer SC, Natale P, Ruospo M, et al. Antidepressants for treating depression in adults with end-stage kidney disease treated with dialysis. *Cochrane Database Syst Rev.* 2016;(5):CD004541. doi:10.1002/14651858.CD004541.pub3

18

Geriatric Nephrology Syndromes and Assessment and Management of Cognitive Impairment

Edwina A. Brown and Osasuyi Iyasere

The demographics of the renal population have evolved, such that the elderly are the fastest growing group. Consequently, the multidisciplinary renal team often encounters clinical issues associated with advancing age. In this chapter, frailty, falls, and cognitive impairment are discussed as underrecognized geriatric syndromes in patients with chronic kidney disease. A case history illustrates how these syndromes tend to co-exist and affect quality of life and survival. The risk factors, management strategies, and future research priorities are discussed, recognizing the importance of a multidisciplinary approach to the management of elderly patients with kidney disease.

Case

Mr. B is a 78-year-old man with end-stage kidney disease (ESKD) of unknown cause. He lives with his son and his family. Over the last few months, he has needed more help from his family with daily activities and has had a couple of falls. He does not go out of the house on his own because of fear of falling. He is clear that he does not want hemodialysis (HD), but he will consider peritoneal dialysis (PD) at home. The PD nurses, however, find that he cannot be trained to do his own PD as he does not retain information from one training session to the next. Cognitive function screening is done, and this shows an abbreviated mental test score of 9/10 but impaired executive function (clock drawing test score 3/15). At the subsequent discussion with the family, they agreed to carry out PD themselves. A future planning meeting was held with Mr. B, son, and granddaughter a few months later; Mr. B was clear the he would not want HD, wanted to avoid being admitted to hospital, and wanted to die at home. It was felt that he had capacity to make these decisions. After 18 months, he was admitted with peritonitis and delirium. The peritonitis resolved after prolonged antibiotics. During a subsequent visit by the community PD nurse, Mr. B stated that he never wanted to go back to the hospital. He has now been at home for over a year following this episode with no further episodes of infection.

He is visited by the community palliative care team for pain control (back pain related to arthritis) and by the community PD team. His son and granddaughter continue to do the PD. He needs full support for activities of daily living. Dialysis withdrawal has been mentioned to the family, but they do not want to consider this further until the next crisis.

This case history illustrates many of the features associated with aging, namely, impaired physical function, impaired cognitive function, falls, and delirium. The overarching syndrome encompassing these various features is frailty.

Frailty

In the absence of a global consensus on an operational definition of frailty, the World Health Organization Clinical Consortium on Healthy Aging recently concluded that "frailty may be conceptually defined as a clinically recognizable state in older people who have increased vulnerability, resulting from age-associated declines in physiological reserve and function across multiple organ systems, such that the ability to cope with every day or acute stressors is compromised."[1] Clinically, frailty presents as a composite of poor physical function, exhaustion, low physical activity, and weight loss and is associated with an increased risk of falls, cognitive impairment, hospitalization, and death.[2] The Frail Elderly Patient Outcomes on Dialysis study has also shown that frailty is the principal factor associated with worse quality-of-life outcomes for older people on both HD and assisted PD.[3]

How "frail" a person is before commencing and while on dialysis is important to know, assess, and intervene on. Assessments for frailty have been developed in the general population and are now used routinely in practice.[4] Most involve questionnaires or scales administered in healthcare settings and can range from a solely functional assessment such as the Clinical Frailty Scale[5] to ones that involve more formal measures of physical aspects of frailty such as gait speed, weight loss, and cognitive dysfunction.[4] Several studies have found that the incidence and prevalence of frailty in the dialysis population is greater than in the general population.[6-9] The Frail Elderly Patient Outcomes on Dialysis study compared patients on assisted PD and HD and showed that frailty is the principal association with patient outcomes for older people and not dialysis modality.[3]

The Comprehensive Geriatric Assessment (CGA) is recognized as an international gold standard for assessments (including frailty) of older people in clinical practice, both in secondary and primary care.[2] The CGA involves a multidisciplinary assessment of physical, psychological, and functional ability from which an individualized plan can be made. Its applicability in chronic kidney disease (CKD) has not been studied in detail, but there is some indication that its relevance is vital to individualize rehabilitation and supportive services and to improved quality of life.[9] A recent systematic review identified a need for further research in evaluating the role of a geriatric assessment in the advanced CKD population.[10] This was further supported by the European Renal Best Practice Working Group emphasizing the need "to identify those who would benefit from more in-depth geriatric assessment and rehabilitation" and recommending further research in this area (p. 13).[11] The key is not only to apply the principles of CGA to patients with kidney disease but also to work toward collaborating with other services so patients can access the specialist input required to support them. These include complementary medicine, geriatric psychiatry, geriatricians, community, and rehabilitation teams.[12] An approach to frailty is summarized in Box 18.1.

> **BOX 18.1. Frailty and Its Assessment**
>
> - Frailty is commonly found in older patients with advanced CKD.
> - Routine frailty screening should be part of assessment of patients with advanced CKD (before starting or on maintenance dialysis).
> - Identification of frailty syndromes should initiate a comprehensive geriatric assessment (CGA).
> - The CGA is a gold standard assessment to develop individualized plans but requires a multidisciplinary team approach and expertise from geriatricians.
> - Evidence is needed on optimizing use of CGA, determining key interventions and their impact on outcomes for CKD.
>
> Abbreviations: CGA, Comprehensive Geriatric Assessment; CKD, chronic kidney disease.

Falls

Falls are thought to be one of the leading causes of injury and death among older people. It is also a herald for frailty. In the United States, nearly a third of those who are 65 years and above fall every year.[13] Fifty percent of those over the age of 80 fall at least once a year. They are also estimated to cost about $2.3 billion every year.[14] Falls are associated with poor outcomes including fragility fractures and injuries, loss of confidence and independence, and increased mortality.

CKD is a risk factor for falls. Older people with CKD are more likely to fall and sustain fall-related injuries compared to those without CKD.[15] Falls are no less common in the dialysis population with a falls rate of between 1.2 to 1.8 falls per patient year. Interestingly, the falls rate is similar between HD and PD patients.[16]

Falls tend to be multifactorial in nature. The traditional risk factors for falls in the general population such as frailty, polypharmacy, and cognitive impairment are also common in the renal population. There are, however, additional contributory risk factors attributable to ESKD and dialysis (Box 18.2) The postdialysis initiation period is potentially a high-risk period for serious fall-related injuries.[17]

The UK National Institute for Health and Care Excellence recommends that the older person presenting with falls should undergo a multifactorial assessment, ranging from a functional assessment to medication review.[14] Taking a falls history in the nephrology clinic could unmask significant fall-related morbidity. An individualized multifactorial intervention should be considered in recurrent fallers. This often includes strength and balance training, home hazard assessment, vision assessment, and medication review and withdrawal.[14] For HD patients, such interventions may be challenging to deliver. Nonetheless, targeted interventions including staff education and environmental modifications have been shown to reduce the risk of falls in an outpatient HD unit.[20] In addition, careful consideration should be given to target weight assessment and ultrafiltration rates in older frail HD patients, especially in the postinitiation period when the risk of falls is high.

> **BOX 18.2. Renal-Specific Risk Factors for Falls**
>
> Chronic kidney disease
> - Predisposing causes such as diabetes, hypertension and vascular disease
> - Anemia
> - Malnutrition
> - Sleep disorders
> - Cardiovascular disease
> - Sarcopenia
> - Postural hypotension due to drug interactions/adverse effects
>
> Dialysis
> - Fluid and electrolyte shifts
> - Hypotensive episodes
> - Arrythmias
>
> Sources: Abdel-Rahman, Turgut, Turkmen, and Balogun[18]; Rossier, Pruijm, Hannane, Burnie, and Teta[19]; and Heung, Adamowski, Segal, Malani.[20]

The falls prevention strategies may also be warranted in CKD patients at risk of falls. Tools that enable falls risk assessment are a research priority. One such tool is the Dialysis Falls Risk Index, which has been developed to predict falls but requires further validation.[21] The role of exercise as a falls prevention strategy also requires further study.

Cognitive Impairment

Cognition is the mental process of acquiring knowledge and understanding through thought, experience, and the senses. These mental processes or domains include memory, language, executive function, intellect, emotion, attention, visuospatial abilities, and processing speed.

Global cognitive function is thought to be preserved with healthy aging. However, there are subtle changes in some cognitive domains such as processing speed[22] and working memory[23] that decline with increasing age (cognitive aging). Mild cognitive impairment (MCI) occurs when cognitive function declines beyond what is expected for chronological age. It is an intermediate phase in cognitive decline, with dementia being the severe end of the spectrum. Dementia is defined as a progressive clinical syndrome that encompasses difficulties in memory, language, and behavior that leads to impairments in activities of daily living.[24,25] MCI does not invariably progress to dementia. However, patients with MCI have a higher risk of dementia compared with healthy controls.[26]

Cognitive impairment and dementia are prevalent in patients with CKD. In the Reasons for Geographic and Racial Differences in Stroke study, there was an 11% increase in the risk of cognitive impairment for every 10 mL decrease in estimated glomerular filtration rate (eGFR) below 60 mL/min/1.73m^2 [27] with a 20% prevalence in those with eGFR <20 mL/min/

1.73m². A recent meta-analysis showed that patients with CKD were at a higher risk of cognitive impairment when compared to those without CKD, more so in those with moderate to severe renal impairment.[28] In the ESKD population, the prevalence of cognitive impairment of up to 70% was reported in 1 cross-sectional study. However, only 2.9% of the studied population had a clinical diagnosis.[29,30] As demonstrated in the previously presented case history, executive function is often affected in patients with CKD and may present before global cognitive impairment becomes apparent.[31]

Dementia is also common in patients with renal disease, with reported prevalence of at least 30% in the dialysis population.[32] While Alzheimer's dementia is the most common subtype of dementia in the general population,[25] the affected cognitive domains (particularly executive function) in patients with CKD are similar to that of vascular dementia. A population cohort study of 7839 participants over 65 years reported an association between declining renal function and a higher risk of dementia with a vascular component.[33]

Cognitive impairment is associated with adverse clinical outcomes. It has been linked with increased mortality,[34,35] sleep disorders, increased length of hospital stay, poor nutrition, dialysis withdrawal, and impaired physical function.[24] Cognitive impairment may also impact on a patient's ability to make decisions, as demonstrated in the presented case.[24,36]

Cerebrovascular disease underpins the pathogenesis of cognitive impairment in patients with advanced CKD. This is supported by the similarities in affected cognitive domains in patients with vascular dementia and those with renal impairment.[24] The brain and kidney are prone to microvascular injury, as they possess low vascular resistance systems. Dialysis patients have been shown to have a higher burden of silent cerebral infarcts, micro bleeds, cerebral atrophy, and subclinical ischemic white matter changes on magnetic resonance imaging, compared to the healthy controls.[37-39] These findings have also been reported in patients with moderate to severe CKD not on dialysis.[40] CKD-related cognitive impairment is not driven solely by traditional vascular risk factors, however. There is a complex interplay with nephrogenic and dialysis related risk factors, some of which are directly neurotoxic (Figure 18.1).[24]

Cognitive impairment, as with the other geriatric syndromes, is often underdiagnosed in renal patients and yet linked to adverse outcomes. Routine screening may therefore be warranted. While the use of the neuropsychological battery remains the gold standard for cognitive assessment, it is often not feasible in busy clinical practice. The Montreal Cognitive Assessment tool is a brief screening tool that has been validated in dialysis patients, with a suggested cut off value of 24 out of 30.[41,42] It is increasingly considered to be the preferred assessment tool in renal patients, especially as it evaluates executive function. Other assessment tools that have been used commonly in this population include the Mini-Mental State Examination; the Modified Mini-Mental State Examination, the Trails Making Tests, Forms A and B; and components of the Wechsler Adult Intelligence Scale: Digit Span and Digit Symbol.[43] Consideration should be given to the timing of cognitive testing in HD patients, as cognition fluctuates during dialysis.[44] A nondialysis day is preferred.

A suspected diagnosis of cognitive impairment based on cognitive screening should prompt history-taking from the patient and caregiver as to the duration and severity of behavioral symptoms. Other generic interventions are summarized in Box 18.3. Where cognitive impairment affects daily living and reversible causes have been excluded, a referral to a specialist dementia diagnostic service (such as a memory clinic) should be considered.[45]

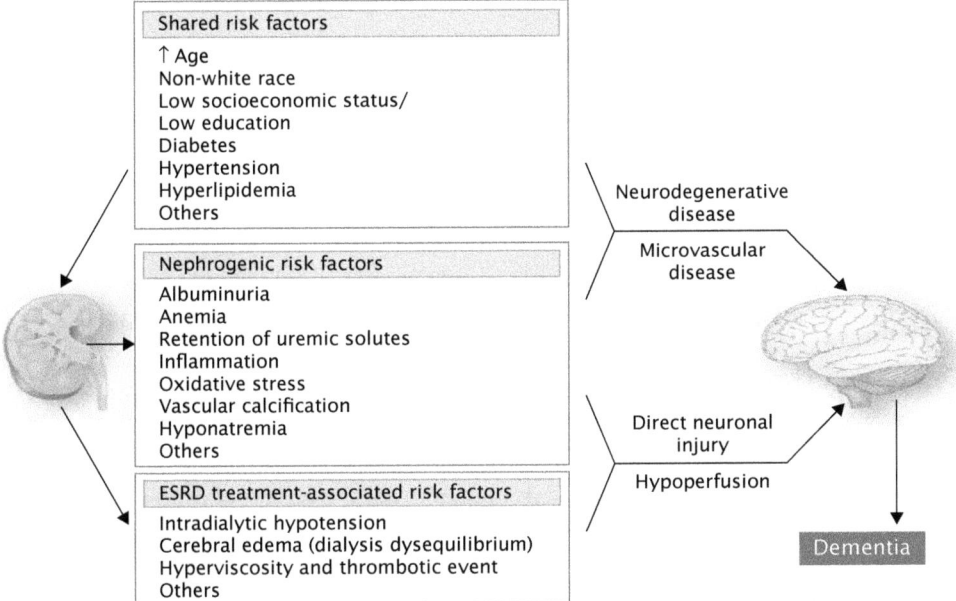

FIGURE 18.1. Complex interplay of risk factors for cognitive impairment in patients with advanced chronic kidney disease.

Evidence-based strategies for managing cognitive impairment and dementia in patients with CKD are lacking. Pharmacotherapy such as acetylcholinesterase inhibitors or memantine may be indicated in patients with Alzheimer's dementia or vascular dementia with co-existing Alzheimer's disease, Parkinson's disease, or Lewy body dementia.[45] Dose adjustment is not required with renal impairment.[46] There is currently no specific pharmacotherapy for vascular dementia, a variant of dementia that is more likely in the renal population. In addition to managing vascular risk factors, dialysate cooling may be protective against cognitive impairment in dialysis patients.[47]

As in the case, there are other nonpharmacological interventions that should be considered when cognitive impairment is recognized (Box 18.4). The diagnosis of dementia is

---

BOX 18.3. Interventions in Cases of Suspected Cognitive Impairment

- Collateral history
- Physical examination
- Medication review with focus on anticholinergics and antihistamines
- Formal test of cognition using a test such as the MoCA
- Screen for depression
- Blood and urine tests to exclude reversible causes of cognitive impairment
- Refer to memory clinic where appropriate

Abbreviation: MoCA, Montreal Cognitive Assessment.

> **BOX 18.4. Management Strategies in CKD Patients with Cognitive Impairment**
>
> - Tailored dialysis education and training
> - Decision making capacity assessment
> - Behavioral symptom management
> - Caregiver support
> - Advance care planning
> - Dialysis withdrawal and responsive medical management without dialysis
>
> Abbreviation: CKD, chronic kidney disease.

not an absolute contraindication to dialysis initiation, nor is it an absolute indication to withdraw dialysis. Concurrent liaison with palliative care and geriatric services could be helpful in symptom management and advance care planning.

Research has focused predominantly on the prevalence, risk factors, and pathogenetic mechanisms of cognitive impairment in CKD. Future research is required on specific therapeutic interventions that ameliorate cognitive impairment in renal patients. The evidence base for how, when, and how often cognitive function is assessed is limited and warrants attention. Finally, further research is required into optimal models of care that promote liaison between nephrology, geriatrics, and palliative care for renal patients with geriatric syndromes including cognitive impairment.

Practice Pointers

- Frailty, cognitive impairment, and falls are common yet underrecognized geriatric syndromes in older people with CKD, and each has been associated with increased mortality and morbidity, indicating a need for routine screening in clinical practice.
- It is important to identify these syndromes to inform clinical practice in terms of advance care planning and decision-making around initiation or continuation of renal replacement therapy.
- There is emerging evidence on feasible screening tools to use in the renal population, including the Clinical Frailty Scale and Montreal Cognitive Assessment test.

Practice Improvement Opportunities

- There is need to identify optimal models of care that promote liaison between nephrology, palliative, and geriatric services.
- Further research is required to identify and evaluate the role of evidence-based interventions (such as CGA) for geriatric syndromes in older people with advanced CKD.

References

1. WHO Clinical Consortium on Healthy Ageing. Topic focus: frailty and intrinsic capacity. http://www.who.int/ageing/health-systems/first-CCHA-meeting-report.pdf?ua=1. Published 2017.
2. Clegg A, Young J, Iliffe S, Rikkert MO, Rockwood K. Frailty in elderly people. *Lancet*. 2013;381(9868):752–762.
3. Iyasere OU, Brown EA, Johansson L, et al. Quality of life and physical function in older patients on dialysis: a comparison of assisted peritoneal dialysis with hemodialysis. *Clin J Am Soc Nephrol*. 2016;11(3):423–430.
4. Sternberg SA, Wershof Schwartz A, Karunananthan S, Bergman H, Mark Clarfield A. The identification of frailty: a systematic literature review. *J Am Geriatr Soc*. 2011;59(11):2129–2138.
5. Rockwood K, Song X, MacKnight C, et al. A global clinical measure of fitness and frailty in elderly people. *CMAJ*. 2005;173(5):489–495.
6. Johansen KL, Chertow GM, Jin C, Kutner NG. Significance of frailty among dialysis patients. *J Am Soc Nephrol*. 2007;18(11):2960–2967.
7. Bohm C, Storsley L, Tangri N. The assessment of frailty in older people with chronic kidney disease. *Curr Opin Nephrol Hypertens*. 2015;24(6):498–504.
8. Kutner NG, Zhang R, Huang Y, McClellan WM, Soltow QA, Lea J. Risk factors for frailty in a large prevalent cohort of hemodialysis patients. *Am J Med Sci*. 2014;348(4):277–282.
9. Jassal SV. Geriatric assessment, falls and rehabilitation in patients starting or established on peritoneal dialysis. *Perit Dial Int*. 2015;35(6):630–634.
10. van Loon IN, Wouters TR, Boereboom FT, Bots ML, Verhaar MC, Hamaker ME. The relevance of geriatric impairments in patients starting dialysis: a systematic review. *Clin J Am Soc Nephrol*. 2016;11(7):1245–1259.
11. Farrington K, Covic A, Nistor I, et al. Clinical practice guideline on management of older patients with chronic kidney disease stage 3b or higher (eGFR <45 mL/min/1.73 m2): a summary document from the European Renal Best Practice Group. *Nephrol Dial Transplant*. 2017;32(1):9–16.
12. Cesari M, Marzetti E, Thiem U, et al. The geriatric management of frailty as paradigm of "The end of the disease era." *Eur J Intern Med*. 2016;31:11–14.
13. Tinetti ME, Speechley M, Ginter SF. Risk factors for falls among elderly persons living in the community. *N Engl J Med*. 1988;319(26):1701–1707.
14. National Institute for Health and Care Excellence. Falls in older people: assessing risk and prevention. NICE clinical guideline 161 https://www.nice.org.uk/guidance/cg161. Published 2013.
15. Kistler BM, Khubchandani J, Jakubowicz G, Wilund K, Sosnoff J. Falls and fall-related injuries among us adults aged 65 or older with chronic kidney disease. *Prev Chronic Dis*. 2018;15:E82.
16. Farragher J, Rajan T, Chiu E, et al. Equivalent fall risk in elderly patients on hemodialysis and peritoneal dialysis. *Perit Dial Int*. 2016;36(1):67–70.
17. Plantinga LC, Patzer RE, Franch HA, Bowling CB. Serious fall injuries before and after initiation of hemodialysis among older ESRD patients in the United States: a retrospective cohort study. *Am J Kidney Dis*. 2017;70(1):76–83.
18. Abdel-Rahman EM, Turgut F, Turkmen K, Balogun RA. Falls in elderly hemodialysis patients. *QJM*. 2011;104(10):829–838.
19. Rossier A, Pruijm M, Hannane D, Burnier M, Teta D. Incidence, complications and risk factors for severe falls in patients on maintenance haemodialysis. *Nephrol Dial Transplant*. 2012;27(1):352–357.
20. Heung M, Adamowski T, Segal JH, Malani PN. A successful approach to fall prevention in an outpatient hemodialysis center. *Clin J Am Soc Nephrol*. 2010;5(10):1775–1779.
21. Kono K, Nishida Y, Yabe H, et al. Development and validation of a fall risk assessment index for dialysis patients. *Clin Exp Nephrol*. 2018;22(1):167–172.
22. Salthouse TA, Mitchell DR, Skovronek E, Babcock RL. Effects of adult age and working memory on reasoning and spatial abilities. *J Exp Psychol Learn Mem Cogn*. 1989;15(3):507–516.
23. Lezak M HD, Bigler E, Tranel D. *Neuropsychological Assessment*. New York, NY: Oxford University Press; 2011.

24. Kurella Tamura M, Yaffe K. Dementia and cognitive impairment in ESRD: diagnostic and therapeutic strategies. *Kidney Int.* 2011;79(1):14–22.
25. Robinson L, Tang E, Taylor JP. Dementia: timely diagnosis and early intervention. *BMJ.* 2015;350:h3029.
26. Boyle PA, Wilson RS, Aggarwal NT, Tang Y, Bennett DA. Mild cognitive impairment: risk of Alzheimer disease and rate of cognitive decline. *Neurology.* 2006;67(3):441–445.
27. Kurella Tamura M, Wadley V, Yaffe Kea. Kidney function and cognitive impairment in US adult: the Reasons for Geographic and Racial Differences in stroke (REGARDS) study. *Am J Kidney Dis.* 2008;52(2):227–234.
28. Elias MF, Dore GA, Davey A. Kidney disease and cognitive function. *Contrib Nephrol.* 2013;179:42–57.
29. Murray AM, Tupper DE, Knopman DS, et al. Cognitive impairment in hemodialysis patients is common. *Neurology.* 2006;67(2):216–223.
30. Kalirao P, Pederson S, Foley RN, et al. Cognitive impairment in peritoneal dialysis patients. *Am J Kidney Dis.* 2011;57(4):612–620.
31. Sarnak MJ, Tighiouart H, Scott TM, et al. Frequency of and risk factors for poor cognitive performance in hemodialysis patients. *Neurology.* 2013;80(5):471–480.
32. Ying I, Levitt Z, Jassal SV. Should an elderly patient with stage V CKD and dementia be started on dialysis? *Clin J Am Soc Nephrol.* 2014;9(5):971–977.
33. Helmer C, Stengel B, Metzger M, et al. Chronic kidney disease, cognitive decline, and incident dementia: the 3C Study. *Neurology.* 2011;77(23):2043–2051.
34. Griva K, Stygall J, Hankins M, Davenport A, Harrison M, Newman SP. Cognitive impairment and 7-year mortality in dialysis patients. *Am J Kidney Dis.* 2010;56(4):693–703.
35. Drew DA, Weiner DE, Tighiouart H, et al. Cognitive function and all-cause mortality in maintenance hemodialysis patients. *Am J Kidney Dis.* 2015;65(2):303–311.
36. Iyasere O, Okai D, Brown E. Cognitive function and advanced kidney disease: longitudinal trends and impact on decision-making. *Clin Kidney J.* 2017;10(1):89–94.
37. Drew DA, Bhadelia R, Tighiouart H, al e. Anatomic brain disease in haemodialysis patients: a cross-sectional study. *Am J Kidney Dis.* 2013;61(2):271–278.
38. Kim HS, Park JW, Bai DS, al e. Diffusion tensor imaging findings in neurologically asymptomatic patients with end stage renal disease. *NeuroRehabilitation.* 2011;29(1):111–116.
39. Griva K, Newman SP, Harrison MJ, et al. Acute neuropsychological changes in hemodialysis and peritoneal dialysis patients. *Health Psychol.* 2003;22(6):570–578.
40. Khatri M, Wright CB, Nickolas TL, et al. Chronic kidney disease is associated with white matter hyperintensity volume: the Northern Manhattan Study (NOMAS). *Stroke.* 2007;38(12):3121–3126.
41. Tiffin-Richards FE, Costa AS, Holschbach B, et al. The Montreal Cognitive Assessment (MoCA): a sensitive screening instrument for detecting cognitive impairment in chronic hemodialysis patients. *PLoS One.* 2014;9(10):e106700.
42. Angermann S, Baumann M, Steubl D, et al. Cognitive impairment in hemodialysis patients: Implementation of cut-off values for the Montreal Cognitive Assessment (MoCA) test for feasible screening. *PLoS One.* 2017;12(10):e0184589.
43. Vanderlinden JA, Ross-White A, Holden R, Shamseddin MK, Day A, Boyd JG. Quantifying cognitive dysfunction across the spectrum of end-stage kidney disease: a systematic review and meta-analysis. *Nephrology (Carlton).* 2019;24(1):5–16.
44. Costa AS, Tiffin-Richards FE, Holschbach B, et al. Clinical predictors of individual cognitive fluctuations in patients undergoing hemodialysis. *Am J Kidney Dis.* 2014;64(3):434–442.
45. National Institute for Health and Care Excellence. Dementia: assessment, management and support for people living with dementia and their carers. NICE guideline NG97. https://www.nice.org.uk/guidance/ng97. Published 2018.
46. Lefèvre G, Callegari F, Gsteiger S, Xiong Y. Effects of renal impairment on steady-state plasma concentrations of rivastigmine: a population pharmacokinetic analysis of capsule and patch formulations in patients with Alzheimer's disease. *Drugs Aging.* 2016;33(10):725–736.
47. Eldehni MT, Odudu A, McIntyre CW. Randomized clinical trial of dialysate cooling and effects on brain white matter. *J Am Soc Nephrol.* 2015;26(4):957–965.

19

Palliative Considerations for the Patient With Acute Kidney Injury in the Intensive Care Unit

Tamara Rubenzik and Alvin H. Moss

Acute kidney injury is a common occurrence in the intensive care unit and one that is associated with a high morbidity and mortality. One role for palliative care is to guide medical decision-making regarding management of patients with acute kidney injury. This role can be fulfilled as part of primary palliative care by the intensive care unit and nephrology teams or by specialist palliative care clinicians if there is a need for assistance with conflict resolution. In such discussions, it is important to understand the patient's prognosis and values, preferences, and goals to inform the shared decision-making discussion about whether to initiate or continue renal replacement therapy. This chapter reviews the literature and guideline recommendations on a palliative care approach to managing critically ill patients with acute kidney injury.

Case

LM was 51-year-old woman with a neuroendocrine tumor (insulinoma) with resection 7 years prior with recurrent metastatic disease who presented to the hospital with altered mental status and right upper quadrant abdominal pain. The patient's husband reported that over the last few weeks she had been spending most of the day sleeping in bed, only waking up to eat meals (Palliative Performance Score, 30%; ECOG, 3). She was found to have multiorgan failure, including acute liver failure, acute kidney injury (AKI), and acute respiratory failure requiring emergent intubation. She was admitted to the intensive care unit (ICU) where she required fluid resuscitation and initiation of vasopressors to maintain an adequate blood pressure. Despite these interventions, the patient remained anuric, prompting nephrology consultation for initiation of renal replacement therapy (RRT). Her laboratory studies were notable for a serum creatinine of 5.74 mg/dL (baseline 0.9 mg/dL), a serum bicarbonate of 15 mmol/L, and a potassium of 5.5 mmol/L. She had transaminitis with an AST:ALT elevation of 2:1 and an elevated total bilirubin of 2.63 mg/dL. Imaging was notable for confirmation of multiple liver metastases on abdominal ultrasound. She lacked decision-making capacity. She had completed an advance directive and appointed her husband as her durable power of attorney for health care. She had no children.

The etiology of the patient's shock and multiorgan failure were unclear; in the 12 hours since admission, she was without evidence of an infectious process. Hepatology was consulted, and they felt her pattern of liver injury was more consistent with shock liver rather than tumor infiltration or drug-related liver injury. The patient's oncologist was contacted to obtain a better understanding of her oncologic prognosis, and he reported a recent rapid progression of her cancer with limited treatment options. If she was well enough, she might be a candidate for a clinical trial at another cancer center. This trial would involve 8 months of treatment and require good functional status, which she did not have prior to admission and which was worse now (ECOG, 4). Aside from this clinical trial, there were no other cancer-directed therapies available.

Current Evidence

Nephrologists are often called upon to help manage critically ill patients in the ICU. AKI is a common occurrence in the ICU, with a reported incidence ranging from 34% to 57% in recent studies, and is associated with increased length of stay, risk of developing chronic kidney disease (CKD) and end-stage kidney disease (ESKD), and hospital mortality ranging from 28% to 75%.[1-6] For these reasons, palliative considerations are imperative for individuals who develop AKI in the ICU. In *Shared Decision-Making in the Appropriate Initiation of and Withdrawal from Dialysis*, the Renal Physicians Association recommended a palliative care approach to critically ill patients with AKI.[7] Using the guideline recommendations as a framework and supplementing them with recent literature, we outline a systematic approach for caring for these patients.

Recommendation 1: Establish a Shared Decision-Making Relationship

Shared decision-making is the recommended process by which providers and patients come to agreement on a specific course of action. It is based on a common understanding of treatment goals and risks and benefits of the chosen course compared with any reasonable alternative. This recommendation emphasizes the need for the physician and patient to make decisions jointly regarding management of AKI in the ICU. In the case of LM, since the patient lacked decision-making capacity, her husband was the designated legal decision maker and the one with whom the shared decision-making discussion should occur. When RRT is considered, the patient/family should be informed of the risks and benefits of this intervention. The physician should ensure that such an intervention is concordant with the patient's values and preferences for medical care. Fortunately, LM had indicated a proxy decision maker should she became unable to make her own medical decisions. In the absence of an advance directive specifying preference for a durable power of attorney for healthcare, a healthcare surrogate should be selected according to state law. While shared decision-making is usually focused on the patient–physician relationship, it should also occur between treatment teams. In the case of LM, the intensive care, hepatology, nephrology, and oncology teams needed to reach agreement if possible on her prognosis with and without dialysis and to decide what treatment options they wanted to recommend as being in her best interest. This involved consideration of the safety and effectiveness of RRT in a patient progressively deteriorating from metastatic cancer and with recent onset multiorgan failure.

Recommendation 2: Fully Inform AKI Patients About Their Diagnosis, Prognosis, and Treatment Options

Patients (and/or their legally designated decision makers) should understand what it means to have AKI in the setting of their critical illness, including that patients in the ICU requiring RRT can have a high mortality.[4] In a multinational study examining more than 29,000 patients admitted to the ICU, 5.5% had severe acute renal failure (oliguria with urine output less than 200 mL in 12 hours and/or a blood urea nitrogen level greater than 84 mg/dL), and 4.2% were treated with RRT. Of those with acute renal failure, there was an in-hospital mortality of 60.3%.[5] Similar mortality rates have been reported elsewhere.[6] When patients do survive, their mortality and quality of life following discharge also need to be considered. In 1 study examining outcomes of ICU patients ages 18 and older requiring RRT, investigators found a lower mortality rate of 45% at 90 days but, noted that 25.1% of survivors remained dialysis-dependent at 90 days.[8] The Veterans Affairs/National Institutes of Health Acute Renal Failure Trial Network study examined intensive versus less intensive RRT in 1,124 critically ill patients, looking at mortality and quality of life at 60 days. This study showed a 60-day mortality of 52.6%, with 27% of survivors who were analyzed reporting a quality of life that was equal to or worse than death.[9] Given these outcomes, patients and their family members should be aware of their treatment options. If dialysis is indicated, then they should understand that they can choose to forego RRT.

Recommendation 3: Give All Patients With AKI an Estimate of Their Prognosis Specific to Their Overall Condition

For patients to make informed decisions, it is important for them to understand their prognosis in the setting of their critical illness. It is difficult to predict outcomes on an individual basis. There are, however, certain populations that are at increased risk of morbidity and mortality following initiation of RRT in the ICU. Zhou and colleagues[1] found that, for patients with AKI, independent risk factors for ICU mortality at 28 days included ICU length of stay, severity of AKI, higher baseline serum creatinine, severe pancreatitis, sepsis, mechanical ventilation, and 3 or more failed organ systems. Uchino and colleagues[5] found some overlapping risk factors, with predictors of in-hospital mortality including septic and cardiogenic shock, liver failure, vasopressor use, and mechanical ventilation. Age is also an important consideration. Some researchers have found age greater than 60 as a predictor of mortality, while others found that age greater than 80 was a predictor of mortality.[6,10] Finally, functional status should also be considered when predicting mortality. There has been little research on the effect of functional status on AKI outcomes in particular, but a small study from Spain examined the prehospital Karnofsky Performance Scale (KPS) in 336 individuals with AKI who were 16 years of age or older. The KPS is used to predict mortality based upon functional status in patients with underlying malignancy, but it also has been studied in patients with ESKD (Table 19.1). Researchers found increasing mortality for decreasing KPS scores, with the latter corresponding to decreasing ability for work, activity, and self-care. Patients with scores of ≤50 presented adjusted odds ratios for in-hospital mortality of 8.87 (95% confidence interval 3.03–25.99) compared with those with scores of ≥80.[11] Decreasing functional status prior to admission in this group of patients (as in LM) corresponded with an increased risk of death in the hospital.

Mortality is not the only consideration when discussing AKI and the need for RRT in the ICU. It is important to think of long-term outcomes, including quality of life and the possibility of dialysis dependence. In a chart review of 1,530 patients receiving RRT in ICUs in Paris, risk of post-AKI chronic dialysis dependence in survivors was 18% for those less than 52 years of age and 30% for those greater than 80 years of age. Only 6% of the patients greater than 80 years of age were living at home without dialysis dependence at 3 months following initial AKI.[10] Although they were not looking at ICU patients specifically, Ishani

TABLE 19.1. Karnofsky Performance Scale.

Able to carry on normal activity and to work; no special care needed.	100	Normal no complaints; no evidence of disease.
	90	Able to carry on normal activity: minor signs or symptoms of disease.
	80	Normal activity with effort; some signs or symptoms of disease.
Unable to work; able to live at home and care for most personal needs; varying amount of assistance needed.	70	Cares for self; unable to carry on normal activity or to do active work.
	60	Requires occasional assistance, but is able to care for most of his personal needs.
	50	Requires considerable assistance and frequent medical care.
Unable to care for self; requires equivalent of institutional or hospital care; disease may be progressing rapidly.	40	Disable; requires special care and assistance.
	30	Severely disabled; hospital admission is indicated although death not imminent.
	20	Very sick; hospital admission necessary; active supportive treatment necessary.
	10	Moribund; fatal processes progressing rapidly.
	0	Dead

Adapted from Karnofsky DA, Burchenal J (eds). *The Clinical Evaluation of Chemotherapeutic Agents in Cancer.* New York, NY: Columbia University Press, 1949.

and colleagues[12] found that the hazard ratio for developing ESKD in patients >65 years of age initiating dialysis was 13 for patients with AKI and 41.2 for patients with AKI superimposed on baseline CKD compared to those without AKI or CKD. This implies that, especially for older individuals with baseline CKD in addition to AKI, the long-term risk of dialysis dependence needs to be taken into account.

Recommendation 4: Institute Advance Care Planning

The purpose of advance care planning is to determine and document how the patient would want to be treated in the future if unable to participate in shared decision-making. This involves patient understanding of the condition and its likely trajectory and the patient expressing wishes for future treatment based upon values, preferences, and goals. Ideally, this is done long before an admission to an ICU, but less than 50% of severely or terminally ill patients have an advance directive in their medical record.[13] In the case of LM, she had documented her preference for who should make decisions when she lost decision-making capacity. There is no indication that she expressed to her husband her values and goals with regard to future treatment.

When managing AKI, it is important for the patient and/or the patient's medical decision makers to understand prognosis as previously discussed to make decisions. The team should be aware if there have been discussions in the past regarding values about aggressive medical care. The team should inquire about an advance directive either in the medical record or elsewhere such as in a registry. If prior conversations or documentation of the patient's wishes are available, these become useful to guide the medical team to make treatment decisions that align with the patient's wishes and enable the team to respect patient autonomy. Communicating information with families and understanding a patient's goals of care are best done using a systematic approach.

Recommendation 5: If Appropriate, Forgo (Withhold Initiating or Withdraw Ongoing) Dialysis in Certain, Well-Defined Situations

The clinical practice guideline lists scenarios in which forgoing dialysis would be appropriate.

- Patients with decision-making capacity, being fully informed and making voluntary choices, refuse dialysis or request dialysis be discontinued.
- Patients who no longer possess decision-making capacity who have previously indicated refusal in an oral or written advance directive.
- Patients who no longer possess decision-making capacity and whose properly appointed legal agents/surrogates refuse dialysis or request that it be discontinued.
- Patients with irreversible, profound neurological impairment such that they lack signs of thought, sensation, purposeful behavior, and awareness of self and environment.[7]

In the case of LM, in the absence of advance directives specifying values with regard to treatment or general values regarding avoiding suffering or living as long as possible, her husband could decide that dialysis is not in her best interest.

Recommendation 6: Consider Forgoing Dialysis in AKI Patients Who Have a Very Poor Prognosis or for Whom Dialysis Cannot Be Provided Safely

Examples provided in the clinical practice guideline include the following:

- Those whose medical condition precludes the technical process of dialysis because the patient is unable to cooperate (eg, advanced dementia patient who pulls out dialysis needles, psychiatric illness causing combativeness) or because the patient's condition is too unstable (eg, profound hypotension limiting dialysis itself or persistent thrombocytopenia with massive edema from marked volume overload precluding safe catheter placement).
- Those who have a terminal illness from nonrenal causes, acknowledging that some in this condition may perceive benefit from and choose to undergo dialysis[7] (eg, metastatic cancer without options for further cancer-directed therapy, end-stage liver disease in a patient who is not a transplant candidate, refractory heart failure in a patient who is not a candidate for heart transplant or ventricular assist device, etc.).

LM is hypotensive, but the case does not indicate that the technical process of dialysis is not possible. A justification for the treating team to recommend forgoing dialysis is that she has a terminal illness from her metastatic cancer without options for further cancer-directed therapy. It could be determined that dialysis would offer no realistic expectation of benefit in terms of prolonging survival.

Recommendation 7: Consider a Time-Limited Trial of Dialysis for Patients Requiring Dialysis but Have an Uncertain Prognosis, or for Whom a Consensus Cannot Be Reached About Dialysis

RRT in the ICU is often viewed as 1 component of general intensive care, including mechanical ventilation and vasopressor support. As a result, a decision to forgo dialysis initiation rarely occurs. Because LM's prognosis is clear, hers would be a case in which it is expected that RRT would not be initiated. There are situations, however, where it is unclear if RRT initiation is appropriate based upon patient prognosis and goals of care. It might be unclear if RRT will be tolerated because of hypotension or if it will benefit the patient in the context of her critical illness. In these situations, a time-limited trial of dialysis should be considered.

Scherer and Holley[14] have reviewed the ethics of and outlined a stepwise approach to a time-limited trial of dialysis for patients with AKI (Figure 19.1). In such a trial, RRT is initiated to achieve predetermined milestones over a certain period of time. Prior to the start of dialysis, the expected milestones are discussed and agreed upon with the ICU team and the patient's family. These might include improvement in hemodynamics, cognitive function, or oxygenation in a patient with respiratory failure. A time period for the trial is agreed upon in advance to ensure all care teams are communicating with each other and the patient's family about the

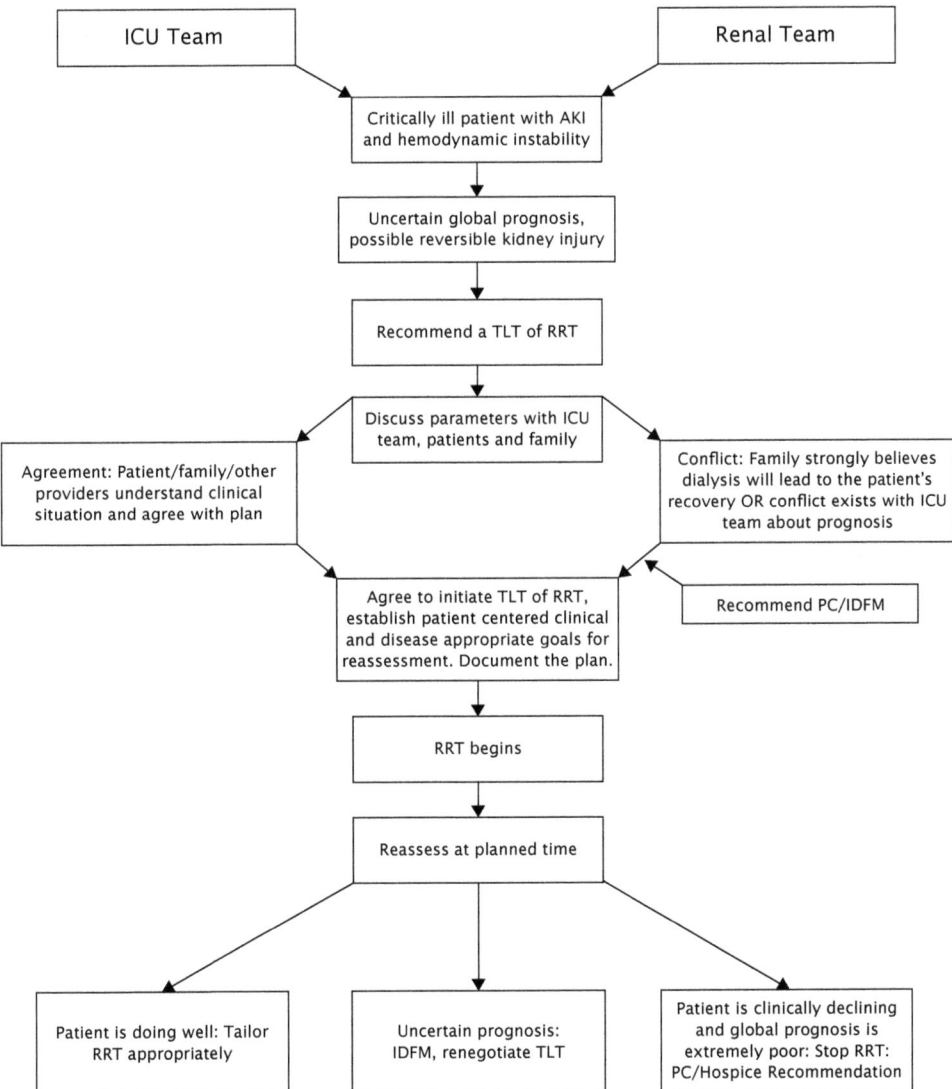

FIGURE 19.1. Approach to time-limited trial for a critically ill patient with acute kidney injury. This figure was previously published in Scherer JS, Holley JL. The role of time-limited trials in dialysis decision making in critically ill patients. *Clin J Am Soc Nephrol.* 2016;11(2):344–353 and is used with permission.

Abbreviations: ICU, intensive care unit; IDFM, interdisciplinary family meeting; PC, palliative care; RRT, renal replacement therapy.

patient's clinical progress. The team and the family should set a time to reconvene to discuss outcomes with dialysis and subsequent treatment. If the patient is improving or the clinical course remains unclear, then the decision might be made to continue RRT. If the patient has continued to decline clinically, then the decision might be made to discontinue RRT and change the focus of care toward comfort care.[14,15]

Case Revisited

Given some uncertainty regarding the etiology of LM's critical illness and her overall prognosis, the decision was made to initiate a time-limited trial of dialysis. An agreement was reached that continuous RRT would be initiated for 3 days to see if, with this support, there would be improvement in LM's neurologic functioning, respiratory failure, liver failure, or hemodynamic compromise. Following 72 hours of RRT, the nephrology team, the ICU team, and the patient's family would reassess whether dialysis remained in the patient's best interest.

Recommendation 8: Establish a Systematic Due Process Approach for Conflict Resolution if There Is Disagreement About What Decision Should Be Made With Regard to Dialysis

Disagreement can occur between the medical teams and the patient or family or between the different medical care teams. Early in the course of a critical illness, families are often hopeful that a loved one might recover even though the medical team believes it is unlikely. Good communication is essential for resolving conflict, and the nephrologist should sit with the patient and/or family members to understand their perspective. The nephrologist should provide prognosis and data to support recommendations that are made in addition to ensuring there are no misunderstandings between the patient/family and the medical teams. When there is ongoing disagreement about treatment approaches, a time-limited trial of dialysis might be a good option for managing such conflict. If this is not enough to resolve the conflict, however, an ethics consultation might be indicated.

Recommendation 9: To Improve Patient-Centered Outcomes, Offer Specialist Palliative Care Services and Interventions to All AKI Patients Who Suffer From Burdens of Their Disease

Specialists palliative care services are appropriate for any AKI patient in the ICU who has uncontrolled symptoms, unclear goals of care, or needs assistance achieving goals of care, regardless of whether or not RRT is initiated. A palliative care team is a multidisciplinary team comprised of variable combinations of physician, nurse, social worker, psychologist, psychiatrist, and spiritual counselor. This interdisciplinary team can help manage uncontrolled symptoms, including pain, constipation, nausea, and shortness of breath. In addition, these care providers can help determine and implement goals of care for patients/families. If a patient is coming to the end of life, then the palliative care team can assist with aggressive symptom management and psychological and spiritual support in the hospital or with transition to hospice if appropriate. Unfortunately, research indicates that palliative care consultations are relatively infrequently requested.[16] Bansal and Schell[17] point out that the nephrologist is often in position to see AKI not as an isolated event, but rather as one component of the critical illness. By pausing to consider a patient's overall prognosis, the nephrologist can play an essential role in identifying a patient's palliative care needs and assuring appropriate use of palliative care services whether or not dialysis initiation is pursued.

Recommendation 10: Use a Systematic Approach to Communicate About Diagnosis, Prognosis, Treatment Options, and Goals of Care

Effective communication is essential when discussing prognosis and treatment options, but it can be challenging to convey information while also trying to align care plans with patient values and to support the patient/family emotionally. It is helpful to use an established, systematic approach to determine the best treatment plan. There are various published approaches for navigating discussions regarding prognosis and goals of care. The SPIKES protocol for breaking bad news is reviewed in the NephroTalk curriculum as outlined by Schell and colleagues,[18] and the PERSON mnemonic for goals of care discussions is reviewed by Edmonds et al.[19] In the SPIKES protocol, nephrologists navigate breaking bad news by obtaining the patient or family's perception of the current illness, providing knowledge to fill any gaps in understanding, and using empathy to provide support (Figure 19.2). The PERSON mnemonic is helpful[19]:

- Perception: obtain patient and family perception of current health status.
- Explore: explore who the individual was before he or she became ill.
- Relate: relate prior level of functioning to current health status, give medical update, use both to guide medical decision-making.
- Sources of worry: inquire about sources of worry following what has been discussed.
- Outline: outline the current plan moving forward, discuss time-limited trial if applicable.
- Notify: inform other care providers of the plan.

For some providers, having such a framework can be helpful for navigating difficult conversations. For others, however, this might seem too complicated. In such a situation, a simple technique that provides medical information while showing empathy is the use of "hope and worry" statements. For example, you can share with LM's family that, although you hope she will recover from her acute illness, you are worried that RRT will not address her

S = "Setting"
Private room, undisturbed conversation, box of tissues.

P = "Perception"
What does the patient and family know?
Ask, "What is your understanding of your illness? and How serious is it?
Follow the principle, "Before you tell, ask."

I = "Invitation"
Ask for permission to give information.
What do they want to know?

K = "Knowledge"
Provide information in an understandable, layperson language.
Avoid medical jargon.
Give a warning shot.

E = "Empathizing and Exploring"
Acknowledge emotions and respond with empathy.

S = "Strategy and Summary"
Make a plan with follow-through.
Summarize main areas.
Agree to time for next meeting.

FIGURE 19.2. Communicating about serious illness: "SPIKES" 6-step protocol. Adapted from Buckman RA. Breaking bad news: the S-P-I-K-E-S strategy. *Communit Oncol.* 2005;2:138–142.

underlying problem. Furthermore, you are worried that she might not survive this hospitalization. Regardless of which strategy a provider uses for guiding difficult conversations, the first step should always include obtaining the patient and family perspective of the patient's clinical condition.

Case Conclusion

Following 3 days of RRT, LM did not improve clinically, but she also did not show any signs of clinical decline. The etiology of her shock remained unclear, and the decision was made to continue RRT. After an additional 36 hours, LM developed an acute worsening of hypotension with rising lactate, potassium, and phosphorous despite being maintained on RRT. She was found to have an ischemic bowel but was determined to be too ill to undergo surgical intervention. A meeting was held with the ICU team and the patient's family, and the decision was made to transition to comfort care. RRT was discontinued, medications were prescribed to ensure her pain and shortness of breath were treated, and she was extubated. She died a few hours later with her family at her side.

Following the recommendations in this chapter, supported by the literature on outcomes of AKI in the ICU, the patient's course could have been predicted earlier than it was and a decision to forgo dialysis or to have undergone a shorter time-limited time trial of dialysis could have been implemented. The authors hope that this review of a systematic approach to the application of palliative care principles to the AKI patient in the ICU will benefit all involved in the care of these critically ill patients and their families who have significant palliative care needs.

Summary

Patients with AKI in the ICU have high morbidity and mortality. Although RRT is often viewed as another component of general ICU care, it should be viewed as a treatment option to be carefully evaluated in each individual patient based on the balance of benefits to burdens rather than an automatic treatment in management of severe AKI. Estimating and communicating prognosis are important steps in determining whether or not RRT should be pursued in the ICU. The guideline recommendations described here provide a framework for these discussions, but there also needs to be emphasis on communicating bad news and having difficult conversations during nephrology and critical care fellowship training. In addition, practicing nephrologists would benefit from skills training in difficult communication. When prognosis is uncertain, benefit from RRT is unclear or when the family is having a particularly hard time accepting the patient's poor prognosis, then a time-limited trial of dialysis can be a good option. Studies looking at outcomes of time-limited trials of RRT for AKI in the ICU would be beneficial to determine satisfaction on the part of care providers and patients/families in addition to patient outcomes following initiation of RRT.

Practice Pointers

- Palliative care consultation for patients with AKI in the ICU can improve patient's quality of life and identify patients' goals of care. The mnemonic PERSON may be particularly helpful to facilitate communication in meetings with the patient/family.
- Primary and/or specialist palliative care can elicit goals of care including preferences for aggressive medical care from patients or family members.

Practice Improvement Opportunities

- Be aware of the clinical practice guideline recommendations and rationale and implement them in the care of patients with AKI in the ICU.
- Institute primary palliative care services in the ICU for patients who have poorly controlled symptoms, unclear goals of care, or need assistance in achieving their goals of care. Consider palliative care consultation for these patients.
- Use a systematic approach for communicating prognosis and determining goals of care:
  - SPIKES protocol for breaking bad news.
  - PERSON mnemonic for goals of care discussions.
  - Hope and worry statements.

References

1. Zhou J, Yang L, Zhang K, Lui Y, Fu P. Risk factors for the prognosis of acute kidney injury under the Acute Kidney Injury Network definition: a retrospective, multicenter study in critically ill patients. *Nephrology*. 2012;17(4):330–337.
2. Hoste EAJ, Bagshaw SM, Bellomo R, et al. Epidemiology of acute kidney injury in critically ill patients: the multinational AKI-EPI study. *Intensive Care Med*. 2015;41(8):1411–1423.
3. Ishani A, Xue J, Himmelfarb J, et al. Acute kidney injury increases incidence of ESRD among elderly. *J Am Soc Nephrol*. 2009;20(1):223–228.
4. Douma CE, Redekop WK, Van der Meulen JH, et al. Predicting mortality in intensive care patients with acute renal failure treated with dialysis. *J Am Soc Nephrol*. 1997;8(1):111–117.
5. Uchino S, Kellum JA, Bellomo R, et al. Acute renal failure in critically ill patients: a multinational, multicenter study. *JAMA*. 2005;294(7):813–818.
6. Allegretti AS, Steele DJ, David-Kasdan JA, et al. Continuous renal replacement therapy outcomes in acute kidney injury and end-stage renal disease: a cohort study. *Critical Care*. 2013;17(3):R109
7. Moss, AH. Revised dialysis clinical practice guideline promotes more informed decision-making. *CJASN*. 2010;5(12): 2380–2383.
8. Wald R, McArthur E, Adhikari N, et al. Changing incidence and outcomes following dialysis-requiring acute kidney injury among critically ill adults: a population-based cohort study. *Am J Kidney Dis*. 2015;65(6):870–877.
9. Johansen KL, Smith MW, Unruh ML, et al. Predictors of health utility among 60-day survivors of acute kidney injury in the Veterans Affairs/National Institutes of Health Acute Renal Failure Trial Network Study. *Clin J Am Soc Nephrol*. 2010;5(8):1366–1372.
10. Commereuc M, Guerot E, Charles-Nelson A et al. ICU patients requiring renal replacement therapy initiation: fewer survivors and more dialysis dependents from 80 years old. *Crit Care Med*. 2017;45(8):e722–e781.
11. Perez Valdivieso JR, Bes-Rastrollo M, Mondereo P, De Irala J, Lavilla FJ. Karnofsky performance score in acute renal failure as a predictor of short-term survival. *Nephrology (Carlton)*. 2007;12(6):533–538.
12. Ishani A, Xue JL, Himmelfarb J et al. Acute kidney injury increases risk of ESRD among elderly. *J Am Soc Nephrol*. 2009;20(1):223–228.
13. Benson WF and Aldrich N. Advance care planning: ensuring your wishes are known and honored if you are unable to speak for yourself, critical issue brief. *Centers for Disease Control and Prevention*. https://www.cdc.gov/aging/pdf/advanced-care-planning-critical-issue-brief.pdf. Published 2012.
14. Scherer J, Holley J. The role of time–limited trials in dialysis decision making in critically ill patients. *Clin J Am Soc Nephrol*. 2016;11(2):344–353.
15. Renal Physicians Association. *Clinical Practice Guideline: Shared Decision-Making in the Appropriate Initiation of and Withdrawal From Dialysis*. 2nd ed. Rockville, MD, Renal Physicians Association, 2010.
16. Chong K, Silver S, Long J, et al. Infrequent provision of palliative care to patients with dialysis-requiring AKI. *Clin J Am Soc Nephrol*. 2017;12(11):1744–1752.
17. Bansal A and Schell JO. Recognizing the elephant in the room: palliative care needs in acute kidney injury. *Clin J Am Soc Nephrol*. 2017;12(11):1721–1722
18. Schell JO, Cohen RA, Green JA, et al. NephroTalk: evaluation of a palliative care communication curriculum for nephrology fellows. *J Pain Symptom Manage*. 2018;56(5):767–773.
19. Edmonds KP, Toluwalase AA, Cain J, Yeung HN, and Thornberry K. Establishing goals of care at any stage of illness: the PERSON mnemonic. *J Palliat Med*. 2014;17(10):1087.

SECTION V

Throughout the Continuum—Enhanced Support at the End of Life

20

Coordination of Care and Care Transitions With Primary Care Clinicians, Specialty Palliative Care, and Hospice

Areeba Jawed and Joseph D. Rotella

Patients with chronic kidney disease typically have needs that cut across a range of services, including nephrology, other specialties, primary care, and palliative care. This chapter proposes a model of integrated supportive care from diagnosis to end of life that coordinates the efforts and maximizes the benefits of different healthcare teams. Supportive care teams can learn primary kidney supportive care skills to manage symptoms, provide emotional support, and facilitate conversations that focus on what matters most to patients and families. Applying best practices of care coordination, they can facilitate seamless transitions as the patient's condition evolves.

Case

After a long history of chronic kidney disease (CKD) due to diabetes, a year on hemodialysis, and a recent diagnosis of multiple myeloma, Ms. S was admitted to the intensive care unit for septic shock and acute respiratory failure following a major debridement of her infected diabetic foot ulcers. Although she saw her nephrologist and hematologist regularly, she remained attached to the primary care physician (PCP) she had known for 10 years. She had consulted her PCP when making the decision to go on dialysis and later to pursue chemotherapy and stem cell transplant, which failed to induce a remission. With volume resuscitation and antibiotics, she improved enough that her hematologist was hopeful that she might recover and pursue second-line chemotherapy. After weaning from ventilator support, though, she had limited mobility due to severe deconditioning and required frequent trips to the operating room for debridement.

The hospital palliative care team collaborated with the critical care and consulting services and provided symptom management and spiritual support. They learned that her only close family member was a son living in Portugal with a newborn grandson whom she had her heart set on visiting. It was clear that Ms. S was too sick for an overseas trip, so her son made plans to bring her grandson to her. The palliative care, nephrology, and hematology teams discussed her preferences and treatment options, but she didn't want to decide without consulting her PCP, who attended a care planning meeting where Ms. S said she would not want to be dependent on machines but needed to live to see her son and grandson. She decided not to pursue further chemotherapy and enrolled in hospice. Since multiple myeloma was determined to be her terminal diagnosis and deemed unrelated to her diabetic nephropathy, she continued to use her ESRD benefit for twice weekly palliative dialysis while awaiting her family's visit. At her request, her PCP accepted the role of hospice attending physician. After a wonderful visit with her son and grandson, her condition deteriorated, and she stopped dialysis and died peacefully in her home.

In this chapter, we will describe models of care coordination involving nephrology, supportive care, primary care, and specialty palliative care throughout the continuum of CKD and principles for providing safe and compassionate transitions of care.

Coordinating Primary Care, Nephrology Care, Supportive Care and Specialty Palliative Care Throughout the Course of Chronic Kidney Disease

As patients with serious illness progress from diagnosis to death, there is a complex interplay of needs for both disease management, kidney supportive care, and palliative care. Models of palliative care integration beginning at diagnosis can enhance the care of patients with CKD.

Integrated Supportive Care Model

Patients with advanced CKD often have multiple comorbidities, high symptom burden, and limited life expectancy, and kidney supportive care should complement their routine nephrology care.[1,2] Supportive care addresses patients' and families' palliative needs, but may be provided at a "generalist" or "primary" level by clinicians who are not necessarily trained and certified as palliative care specialists. Supportive care teams sometimes require additional assistance from specialty-level palliative care for complex problems.[3] In an integrated supportive care model, an interdisciplinary team trained in essential skills of palliative care is anchored in the dialysis center or nephrology clinic and adds another layer of symptom management, enhanced communication, care coordination, and psychosocial and spiritual support to the efforts of the nephrology team directed at managing the kidney disease and its complications.

Figure 20.1 depicts the typical shifting of roles of primary care, nephrology with integrated supportive care, and specialty palliative care or hospice teams as CKD progresses.

These different teams each bring unique knowledge and skills to the care of people living with CKD. In an ideal scenario, they seamlessly co-manage renal and nonrenal conditions, quality of life concerns and critical conversations, always centered on the needs and preferences of the patient and family, with different teams taking or sharing the lead as CKD progresses through its expected stages.

Shifting Focus of Care and Ideal Provider Roles as CKD Progresses in an Integrated Supportive Care Model					
Focus of Care / Provider Role	Diagnose and Manage Early-Mid Stage CKD	Decide -Transplant -Dialysis -Neither and Support	Manage -Late Stage CKD -Symptoms -Non-renal Conditions	Address -↓QOL -Shifting Treatment Benefits/ Burdens	-Decide on Stopping Dialysis -Provide End-of-Life Care
Primary Care	Co-Manage	Consult	Consult	Consult	Consult
Nephrology and Integrated Supportive Care	Co-Manage	Manage	Manage	Manage	Co-Manage
Specialty Palliative Care and Hospice	Consult	Consult	Consult	Consult	Co-Manage

FIGURE 20.1. Shifting focus of care and ideal provider roles as chronic kidney disease progresses in an integrated supportive care model. Source: Joe Rotella. Used with permission.
Abbreviations: CKD, chronic kidney disease; QOL, quality of life.

Earlier Stages of CKD (Stages 1 to 3)

In earlier stages of CKD, the focus is on diagnosing CKD and its underlying causes, controlling risk factors, and monitoring progression. Although this would also be an ideal time for advance care planning, particularly regarding circumstances in which dialysis would or would not be acceptable, in practice, most patients do not have these conversations.[4] Primary care teams most frequently lead the management of early stage CKD. A nephrologist may not be consulted unless the underlying cause is unclear, progression is more rapid than expected, the patient is hospitalized or CKD advances to stage 4 or 5.[5] PCPs, though, are less likely than nephrologists to recognize CKD or adhere to clinical management guidelines and often make inappropriately late referrals for specialty care.[6,7] When guidelines are not followed and nephrologists are not involved appropriately, markers of CKD progress more quickly, monitoring is inadequate and important clinical targets such as blood pressure control are missed.[8,9] Moreover, a Cochrane Review found that CKD patients referred to a nephrologist at earlier stages had better outcomes, including decreased mortality, decreased hospital length of stay, and higher proportion of peritoneal dialysis.[10] For these reasons, many experts call for primary care and nephrology providers to co-manage the earlier stages of CKD.[11] If a palliative care specialist is involved, it is usually to manage symptoms of comorbidities, such as diabetic neuropathy.

Deciding on Transplant, Dialysis, or Medical Management Without Dialysis

The decision point regarding whether, when, and how to initiate renal replacement therapy is a critical juncture. Shared decision-making is recommended as a best practice, and a nephrologist most frequently leads the discussion.[12,13] Sometimes, a PCP decides not to refer a patient to a nephrologist for consideration of renal replacement therapy due to age, functional or cognitive impairment, or comorbid illnesses.[14] Nephrologists and PCPs alike may feel uncomfortable and ill prepared to have challenging conversations around serious illness and goals of care.[15] Primary care, specialty care, and palliative care providers can bring different perspectives and skills to discussions of treatment options for patients with serious illness. For example, in an exploration of how to discuss goals of care for a patient with advanced cancer featured in a *New England Journal of Medicine* vignette, a primary care physician, cancer specialist, and palliative care specialist each make cogent arguments for why their discipline would best lead the discussion.[16] The PCP argues that her discipline should take the lead because it has a "relationship with continuity" and can put the discussion in the context of the patient's unique history and hearken back to discussions held years earlier in the course of illness. The cancer specialist proposes that he would have the best knowledge of the patient's current condition, expected disease trajectory, and benefits and burdens of treatment options. Finally, the palliative care specialist suggests that the palliative care team has the advantage in "advanced training in pain and symptom management and in skilled communication with patients and families . . . and the ability to provide continuity and coordination across disease stages and settings" (p. 670). Clearly, a collaborative approach that brings these complementary strengths together and aligns everyone with what matters most to the patient and family would yield the best decisions. That is challenging in a fragmented care system marked by workflow constraints and communication barriers but critical to deliver the best patient-centered care.

Discussing Goals of Care and Making Shared Decisions

To determine appropriate goals of care, patients need a good understanding of their condition and prognosis. Research suggests that most patients with CKD welcome such information, but nephrologists do not routinely discuss prognosis.[17,18] In shared decision-making, the physician and patient develop a common understanding of the patient's condition, goals, and possible outcomes and choose the treatment plan that aligns best with what matters most to the patient.[2,19] Along the trajectory of CKD, inflection points that may prompt such discussions include initial diagnosis, progression to end-stage kidney disease (ESKD), new complications, declining function, and imminent end of life. Current evidence suggests that many patients lack the information they need to live well with CKD and plan for end-of-life care.[20]

Later Stages of CKD (Stages 4 and 5)

Once CKD patients embark on a pathway of dialysis or medical management without dialysis, they typically experience a host of symptoms, complications, and problems related and unrelated to their kidney disease and its treatment. The nephrology and supportive care teams usually lead during this phase. There are dwindling benefits to some routine preventive measures such as cancer screening, and primary care providers may take a less active role. When asked about barriers to engaging with dialysis patients, primary care providers identified time constraints, miscommunication, and lack of clarity about appropriate roles.[21] Integrated supportive care is especially helpful for ensuring shared decision-making, managing symptoms, and providing psychosocial support.[22] Prompt recognition of the need for renal supportive care is key as early palliative care referrals alongside routine disease modifying therapy have been found to be beneficial for patients with other chronic diseases such as heart failure and cancer.[23,24] Despite calls for integrated supportive care from key thought leaders, it has not been widely adopted. For example, in a survey of dialysis professionals and administrators, few believed they were providing high-quality supportive and end-of-life care, with unmet needs identified for bereavement and spiritual support, end-of-life discussions and palliative care consultation.[25] CKD patients are sometimes referred to specialty palliative care teams that operate outside the dialysis center or nephrology clinic, especially during hospital stays. One academic inpatient palliative care service found that, although few of its consultations were for patients with ESKD, their outcomes were mostly similar to those with other serious illnesses, including a reduction in full code status by half; they differed, although in having a greater reduction in anxiety and fewer hospice referrals.[26]

Discussing Discontinuation of Dialysis

When quality of life is decreasing and benefits of dialysis are dwindling, it is appropriate to discuss stopping dialysis. Nephrologists may find these discussions to be difficult and uncomfortable. A qualitative study of nephrologists in the United States and England identified a number of system-level barriers and facilitators for foregoing or withdrawing dialysis, including training in how to have end-of-life conversations, public policies, the culture of medicine, societal beliefs, expectations for aggressive care among nonnephrologists and the public, and financial incentives.[27] Although availability may be limited outside the hospital setting, consultation with a specialty palliative care team can be very helpful in navigating a transition in priority from disease management to care that maximizes comfort and quality of life.

Transition to End-of-Life Care

The 5-year mortality rate for dialysis patients is nearly twice that of adults with cancer, congestive heart failure, or stroke.[28] Despite the strong evidence that palliative care improves the quality of life for patients with CKD, its utilization in this patient population remains far below that of other chronic disease populations irrespective of its availability.[29,30] The final transition to end-of-life care may be gradual for patients with ESKD who follow the medical management without dialysis pathway, but it is often abrupt for those on the dialysis pathway, whether they choose to stop dialysis or not. In their last month of life, patients with ESKD are more likely to undergo invasive procedures and die in the intensive care unit and less likely to receive hospice care or die outside the hospital compared to those with other serious illnesses.[31] Only half as many ESKD patients die receiving hospice care as for other Medicare beneficiaries.[32] Although hospice use is higher in patients who withdraw from dialysis, death typically occurs in 7 to 10 days, affording hospice teams little time to develop rapport and provide the full benefits of hospice care.[33,34]

In 2016, 27% of Medicare patients with ESKD had a hospital admission or discharge within 3 days of death, which was virtually unchanged from 2000. There is wide interstate variation in hospice and hospital utilization for CKD patients at the end of life suggesting that systemic factors rather than patient preferences drive utilization patterns.[35]

As disease burden increases, a shift in emphasis from curative to supportive care can be daunting and distressing for patients and providers alike. Such transitions often involve not only shifts in the setting of care and roles of clinical teams, but also fundamental changes in the expectations and experience of patients and families and how they find meaning and support hope.

Strategies for addressing the challenges associated with end-of-life transitions for ESKD patients

Challenge	Strategy
Patient reluctance: patients don't see themselves as ready for end-of-life services or are frightened by prospect of meeting with hospice staff.	Tailor message about early referral to patient/family concerns: • Elicit goals from patients such as "I don't want to be in pain, go to the hospital, or have dialysis." • Respond with "Do you know anyone who has been through that before?" and listen for language that might be about hospice. If patient doesn't reply, "Did you know that hospice is something that can help you with those things?" "You are in charge here. Sometimes someone will come do a home visit just to give you information." "Did you know that hospice often provides a home health aide and pays for all medications related to pain?" "We find it is very helpful to have a plan B in place 'just in case.'" "Meeting palliative care or hospice 'just in case' can take stress off family caregivers. It gives them a back-up plan, so they know who to call if something happens." "Palliative care or hospice is the best way I know to help you stay at home (or whatever other goal patient has expressed)." "Hospice isn't just about dying; it's about helping you have the best quality of life possible."
Financial constraint: concurrent hospice care and dialysis not covered by Medicare for patients whose terminal diagnosis is ESKD.	Work out contractual arrangement with palliative care or hospice service ahead of time to provide concurrent dialysis and hospice care.
Nephrology providers are unfamiliar with the services that local palliative care providers can offer.	Proactively establish relationships and processes with local palliative care and hospice organizations.
Palliative care/hospice providers uncertain about management in face of kidney disease.	Provide joint networking and education opportunities to build collaborative relationships between nephrology and palliative care staff.

Essential Practices for Care Coordination around Care Transitions

In addition to the previously described shifting focus of care and provider roles along the course of CKD, other care transitions can also be distressing and problematic for patients, families, and providers. These include hospitalizations, subacute rehabilitation stays, escalations in caregiving arrangements, and moves to facilities for safety and increased assistance. Whenever a patient moves to a new setting or new providers/caregivers get involved, there is a great risk for disruptions to the care plan, miscommunications, medication errors, and misunderstandings. Meticulous documentation, communication, patient assessment, patient and caregiver education, and medication reconciliation are warranted.

With the focus over the past decade on healthcare innovation to increase value, a variety of care coordination models have emerged along with descriptors and definitions that sometimes overlap, including care management, care navigation, case management, and disease management.[36] The costs of administering these programs are typically justified on the basis of cost savings or avoidance associated with reductions in unnecessary or unwanted healthcare utilization, such as hospital readmissions. Scoping and systematic reviews of transition-of-care interventions support the value of a multimodal approach led by an interdisciplinary team focused on strengthening communication, with key roles for nurse, social worker, and pharmacist.[37] Integrated supportive care teams are ideally positioned to coordinate care with other healthcare teams and manage care transitions. Since crises are not limited to regular working hours, supportive care services should be available on a continuous 24/7 basis and poised to respond quickly to changing needs and circumstances.

Summary

Patient-centered care for CKD calls for coordination of concurrent nephrology, primary care, and palliative care services, ideally using an integrated supportive care model. For effective shared decision-making, a collaborative approach that aligns all the care teams around what matters most to the patient and family is critical. CKD patients are sometimes referred to specialty palliative care teams outside the dialysis unit or nephrology clinic, especially during hospitalizations. Hospice remains underutilized in dialysis patients, due in part to Medicare payment policies that limit concurrent use of dialysis and hospice benefits. A shift in emphasis from disease-oriented to kidney supportive care can be daunting for both patients and clinicians, and compassionate, open communication about fears and concerns of patients can help navigate a smooth transition.

Practice Pointers

- CKD patients have complex supportive care needs, which warrant coordination with primary care, specialty care and nephrology throughout the course of the illness.
- Interdisciplinary teams form the foundation of integrated care, providing and coordinating disease-oriented and palliative treatments in parallel.

Practice Improvement Opportunities

- Early specialty palliative care consultations can be especially helpful when it comes to dialysis discontinuation and increasing hospice utilization among ESKD patients.
- Nephrologists should establish relationship and processes with local palliative care and hospice programs.
- Joint networking and education opportunities should be provided to build relationships between nephrology and palliative care staff.

References

1. Kurella T, Meier, D. Five policies to promote palliative care for patients with ESRD. *Clin J Am Soc Nephrol*. 2013;8(10):1783–1790.
2. O'Hare A, Armistead N, Schrag W, Diamond L, Moss A. Patient-centered care: an opportunity to accomplish the "Three Aims" of the National Quality Strategy in the Medicare ESRD program. *Clin J Am Soc Nephrol*. 2014;9(12):2189–2194.
3. Quill T, Abernethy A. Generalist plus specialist palliative care—creating a more sustainable model. *N Engl J Med*. 2013;368(13):1173–1175.
4. Feely M, Hildebrandt D, Edakkanambeth V, Mueller P. Prevalence and contents of advance directives of patients with ESRD receiving dialysis. *Clin J Am Soc Nephrol*. 2016;11(12):2204–2209.
5. Diamantidis C, Powe N, Jaar B, Greer R, Troll M, Boulware LE. Primary care-specialist collaboration in the care of patients with chronic kidney disease. *Clin J Am Soc Nephrol*. 2011;6(2):334–343.
6. Regan M. Implementing an evidence-based clinical decision support tool to improve the detection, evaluation and referral patterns of adult chronic kidney disease patients in primary care. *J Am Acad Nurse Pract*. 2017;29:741–753.
7. Boulware LE, Troll M, Jaar B, Myers D, Powe N. Identification and referral of patients with progressive CKD: a national study. *Am J Kidney Dis*. 2006;48:192–204.
8. van Dipten C, van Berkel S, van Gelder VA, et al. Adherence to chronic kidney disease guidelines in primary care patients is associated with comorbidity. *Fam Pract*. 2017;34(4):459–466.
9. Schreimer A, Simpson K. Primary care and chronic disease: the intersection of comfort and specialty involvement- a cross-sectional study. *J Eval Clin Pract*. 2017;23:494–497.
10. Smart N, Dieberg G, Ladhani M, Titus T. Early referral to specialist nephrology services for preventing the progression to end-stage kidney disease. *Cochrane Database Syst Rev*. 2014;18(6):CD007333.
11. Sakhuja A, Hyland J, Simon J. Managing advanced chronic kidney disease: a primary care guide. *Cleve Clin J Med*. 2014;81(5):289–299.
12. Galla J. Clinical practice guideline on shared decision-making in the appropriate initiation of and withdrawal from dialysis. *J Am Soc Nephrol*. 2000;11:1340–1342.
13. Moss A. Revised dialysis clinical practice guideline promotes more informed decision making. *Clin J Am Soc Nephrol*. 2010;5:2390–2383.
14. Hunter Campbell K, Dale W, Stankus N, Sachs G. Older adults and chronic kidney disease decision making by primary care physicians: a scholarly review and research agenda. *J Gen Intern Med*. 2007;23(3):329–336.
15. Mandel E, Bernacki R, Block S. Serious Illness conversations in ESRD. *Clin J Am Soc Nephrol*. 2017;12(5):854–863.
16. Tolle S, Back A, Meier D. End-of-life advance directive. *N Engl J Med*. 2015;372(7):667–670.
17. Schell J, Patel V, Steinhauser K, Ammarell N, Tulsky J. Discussions of the kidney disease trajectory by elderly patients and nephrologists: a qualitative study. *Am J Kidney Dis*. 2012;59(4):495–503.
18. Davison S. End-of-life care preferences and needs: perceptions of patients with chronic kidney disease. *Clin J Am Soc Nephrol*. 2010;5(2):195–204.

19. Davison S. Facilitating advance care planning for patients with end-stage renal disease: the patient perspective. *Clin J Am Soc Nephrol*. 2006;1(5):1023–1028.
20. Morton R, Tong A, Howard K, Snelling P, Webster A. The views of patients and carers in treatment decision making for chronic kidney disease: systematic review and thematic synthesis of qualitative studies. *BMJ*. 2010;340:c112.
21. Wang V, Diamantidis C, Wylie J, Greer R. Minding the gap and overlap: a literature review of fragmentation of primary care for chronic dialysis patients. *BMC Nephrol*. 2017;18:274.
22. Moss A. Integrating supportive care principles into dialysis decision making: a primer for palliative medicine providers. *J Pain Symptom Manage*. 2017;53(3):656–662.
23. Parikh R, Kirch R, Smith T, Temel J. Early specialty palliative care: translating data in oncology into practice. *N Engl J Med*. 2013;369(24):2347–2351.
24. Temel, J, Greer J, Muzikansky A, et al. Early palliative care for patients with metastatic non-small-cell lung cancer. *N Engl J Med*. 2010;363(8):733–742.
25. Culp S, Lupu D, Aranella C, Armistead N, Moss A. Unmet supportive care needs in U.S. dialysis centers and lack of knowledge of available resources to address them. *J Pain Symptom Manage*. 2016;51(4):756–761.
26. Grubbs V, O'Riordan D, Pantilat S. Characteristics and outcomes of in-hospital palliative care consultation among patients with renal disease versus other serious illnesses. *Clin J Am Soc Nephrol*. 2017;12(7):1085–1089.
27. Grubbs V, Tuot D, Powe N, O'Donoghue D, Chesla C. System-level barriers and facilitators for foregoing or withdrawing dialysis: a qualitative study of nephrologists in the United States and England. *Am J Kidney Dis*. 2017;70(5):602–610.
28. Saran R, Robinson B, Abbott K, et al. US Renal Data System 2017 annual data report: EPIDEMIOLOGY OF KIDNEY DISEASE In the United States. *Am J Kidney Dis*. 2018;71(3S1):A7.
29. Murray AM, Arko C, Chen SC, Gilbertson DT, Moss AH. Use of hospice in the United States dialysis population. *Clin J Am Soc Nephrol*. 2006;1(6):1248–1255.
30. Green JA, Mor MK, Shields AM, et al. Renal provider perceptions and practice patterns regarding the management of pain, sexual dysfunction, and depression in hemodialysis patients. *J Palliat Med*. 2012;15(2):163–167.
31. Wong SP, Kreuter W, O'Hare A. Treatment intensity at the end of life in older adults receiving long-term dialysis. *Arch Intern Med*. 2012;172(8):661–664.
32. United States Renal Data System. Chapter 12: End-of-life care for patients with end-stage renal disease, 2000–2015. In *2018 Annual Data Report*. Vol. 2, *ESRD in the United States*. https://www.usrds.org/2018/view/v2_12.aspx. Accessed March 9, 2019.
33. Oliver M, Quinn R, Richardson E, Kiss A, Lamping D, Manns B. Home care assistance and the utilization of peritoneal dialysis. *Kidney Int*. 2007;71(7):673–678.
34. Rickerson E, Harrold J, Kapo J, Carroll J, Casarett D. Timing of hospice referral and families' perceptions of services: are earlier hospice referrals better? *J Am Geriatr Soc*. 2005;53(5):819–823.
35. Murtagh FE, Addington-Hall JM, Higginson IJ. End-stage renal disease: a new trajectory of functional decline in the last year of life. *J Am Geriatr Soc*. 2011;59(2):304–308.
36. Ahmed O. Disease management, case management, care management and care coordination: a framework and a brief manual for care programs and staff. *Prof Care Manage*. 2016;21(3):137–146.
37. Rodrigues C, Harrington A, Murdoch N, et al. Effect of pharmacy-supported transition-of-care interventions on 30-day readmissions: a systematic review and meta-analysis. *Ann Pharmacother*. 2017;51(10):866–889.

21

Palliative Dialysis

Vanessa Grubbs

Dialysis is typically thought of as a life-saving treatment for patients with end-stage kidney disease (ESKD), but for a subset of older patients with dementia or ischemic heart disease or other advanced comorbidities it may not confer a survival benefit, stop the ESKD trajectory, and be life-extending despite achieving standard quality metrics. Providers should consider palliative dialysis for patients with ESKD who have a life expectancy of less than one 1 year, symptoms that might be ameliorated by dialysis, and values such that they would consider a trial of dialysis. Offering palliative dialysis should be considered part of a patient-centered approach for some patients with ESKD with a poor prognosis even with dialysis. In this broadened view of choices for patients with ESKD, decision-making need not only include forgoing or withdrawing dialysis as options. Dialysis is a care plan that strives to achieve hopes while minimizing fears. This balance of the positives and negatives of dialysis can be thought of as palliative dialysis.

Case

Mrs. L is an 84-year-old, 40-kilogram woman who presents for initial renal clinic visit after hospitalization for prolonged epistaxis during which she was noted to have an elevated creatinine and potassium. Comorbidities include hypertension and gastroesophageal reflux disease. Her estimated glomerular filtration rate is 5mL/min but she has no uremic signs or symptoms. Family wants to know about dialysis options, so her nephrologist referred her to options education where the patient and family watched videos about modalities followed by a conversation with the dialysis nurse to answer questions and discuss. On return to clinic, neither Mrs. L nor her family felt she would be able to tolerate in-center hemodialysis because they heard it can be painful, and peritoneal dialysis seemed too burdensome, as the nurse explained she would have to do 4 exchanges every day. When asked if she would prefer to forgo dialysis, she only responds that she doesn't want to be in pain and wants to take as few pills as possible. She spends her days with her extended family and goes to the park twice a day to play Mahjong. She ambulates unassisted and can perform all activities of daily living but needs help with independent activities of daily living like grocery shopping.

When Mrs. L develops uremic symptoms, should palliative dialysis be offered? This chapter will discuss what palliative dialysis is, what it entails, and when it should be considered.

Why Palliative Dialysis

Because dialysis temporarily corrects uremia but does not change the trajectory of end-stage kidney disease (ESKD), all dialysis could be considered palliative. Although a set of standard guidelines for dialysis delivery is defined by lowest mortality, dialysis may not be life-extending for older patients with dementia or ischemic heart disease despite achieving standard metrics.[1] Frail patients over the age of 75 can expect less than 6 months of survival after initiating dialysis.[2]

Survival is not the only consideration for older patients approaching ESKD. A national observational study of older Medicare beneficiaries found that 60% of patients initiated dialysis in the hospital and, depending on age, spent up to 37% of the first year after dialysis initiation in a skilled nursing facility. Those with dementia spent roughly 50% of the first year after dialysis initiation in a skilled nursing facility regardless of age. Such outcomes run counter to the priorities of many patients. When asked to prioritize maintaining independence, staying alive, and reducing pain and other symptoms, older patients with CKD stage 4/5 in the southern United States prioritized maintaining independence over staying alive, and nearly half ranked staying alive as third or fourth.[3] In a nominal rank study of hemodialysis patients in Australia and Canada, patients' top 3 priorities were fatigue/energy, dialysis-free time, and the ability to travel.[4]

While dialysis may help achieve some patient priorities, such as surviving to the first grandchild's birth or graduation, dialysis may itself cause symptoms. Physical and emotional symptoms are common, are usually severe and undertreated, and tend to correlate directly with impaired quality of life among maintenance dialysis patients.[5-7] In 1 study using the Edmonton Symptom Assessment System, maintenance dialysis patients reported 7.5 symptoms on average, 4.5 of which they characterized as moderate or severe.[8] In another study using the Dialysis Symptom Index, dialysis patients reported 9 symptoms on average, with more than 50% reporting dry skin, fatigue, itching, and joint/bone pain.[5]

In addition to the burdens of the dialysis procedure itself, initiation often means that patients are committing to intensive patterns of healthcare utilization, in many instances without full understanding and adequate discussion of the implications.[9] In a study of Medicare beneficiaries over age 65 years, dialysis patients were more likely to have a hospital admission, longer hospital stays, more intensive procedures (like mechanical ventilation, feeding tubes, and cardiopulmonary resuscitation), lower hospice use, more intensive care unit admission, and more death in the hospital in the last month of life than those with cancer or heart failure.[10]

Additional burdens of life on dialysis include stringent fluid and dietary restrictions, procedures to maintain vascular access, and time consumed traveling to and from dialysis. While peritoneal dialysis is associated with fewer symptoms and restrictions, only 6% of patients over age 75 years in the United States are managed with this modality.[11] At the same time, many patients, families, and providers may be hesitant to forgo dialysis or stop dialysis abruptly because of concerns about suffering from ESKD-related symptoms or death within the mean 8-day timeframe following dialysis cessation in patients with no residual kidney function.[12] Therefore, there is a role for palliative dialysis—that is, a treatment plan balancing

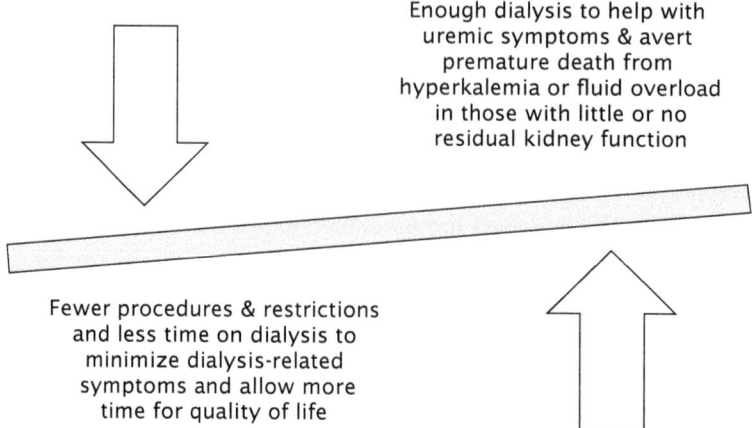

FIGURE 21.1. Palliative dialysis balance.

the amount of dialysis needed to alleviate symptoms of uremia and allow participation in important life events but avoid dialysis-related symptoms and procedures (Figure 21.1).

Current Evidence

The benefits of palliative care for patients with ESKD are clear. Among a cohort study of US hemodialysis patients propensity matched for receipt of inpatient palliative versus usual care, those who received inpatient palliative care were 8 times more likely to have enrolled in hospice and 20% less likely to readmitted within 30 days of hospital discharge.[13] In a study of patients who received palliative care consultation in US hospitals participating in the Palliative Care Quality Network, a national palliative care quality improvement collaborative, patients with renal disease had similar health status, symptom burden, and symptom improvement as patients with other serious illnesses.[14]

Conversely, direct research demonstrating the benefits of palliative dialysis is lacking. The dearth is attributable, at least in part, to the tendency of research to focus on survival rather on the patient priorities. In addition, up to now there has been little written about what truly constitutes palliative dialysis and how to readily identify appropriate patients.

It would be useful to have studies comparing outcomes of patients receiving palliative dialysis to those of patients receiving medical management without dialysis and standard dialysis. Relevant outcomes for palliative dialysis might include symptom improvement, caregiver satisfaction, hospice and/or palliative care utilization, healthcare utilization, provider orders for life-sustaining treatment/advance directives completion, patient self-report of quality of life, and meeting patients' stated goals (goal-concordant care).

Palliative dialysis should be considered for patients with ESKD who have a life expectancy of less than 1 year and have symptoms that might be ameliorated by dialysis. Specific clinical scenarios include the patient with ESKD not yet on dialysis who begins to develop uremic symptoms; the maintenance dialysis patient who develops a severe illness that causes an abrupt decline in life expectancy; and the maintenance dialysis patient with progressive functional or cognitive decline.

The treatment plan for each would begin with a conversation about hopes and fears—how the patient hopes and wants to live out the rest of life and fears about the dying process. Hopes might include maintaining independence, witnessing an event, spending time with family, or, like Mrs. L, minimizing pills and going to the park to play Mahjong. Potential fears of dying from kidney failure might include a quick or a protracted process involving pain or drowning in one's own fluids. Once specific hopes and fears are elicited, the treatment plan can be shaped through clinicians providing a realistic explanation of what role dialysis could play in helping best achieve hopes and avoid fears, when death might be expected, what the dying process might look like, and what besides dialysis can be done to ease its symptoms.

The ESRD Quality Incentive Program measures—that drive standard dialysis care—are not appropriate for a palliative dialysis patient. Rather, an approach incorporating palliative dialysis requires repeated assessment and conversation with patients/families to inform adjustments. The care team must learn what things matter most to patients and what aspects of standard dialysis care impede things that are important. Timing of impeding factors is also critical to determine. For example, if cramping occurs in the last hour of hemodialysis, then providers should consider shortening dialysis time or decreasing ultrafiltration. While such adjustments may result in less than ideal kinetics or mild lower extremity edema, the trade-off is an improved patient experience. The Integrated Palliative care Outcomes Scale for patients with ESRD and the Edmonton Symptom Assessment System–Renal are helpful and widely used tools for assessing symptom burden and quantifying improvement over time. Table 21.1 compares metrics of the existing disease-focused approach of standard dialysis with those preferred as part of a person-centered palliative dialysis approach.

All members of the care team can and should participate in a palliative dialysis care plan. Dialysis technicians, nurses, and social workers invariably spend more time with patients than nephrologists and can provide critical insights into patients' lives and well-being. Specialist palliative care services can help with refractory symptoms and provide psychological and spiritual support. In areas where outpatient palliative care services are limited, renal social workers who are able to provide counseling can help fulfill support needs.

TABLE 21.1. Standard Dialysis Versus Palliative Dialysis Practices

Standard Dialysis Practice	Palliative Dialysis Practice
Disease-focused	Patient-centered
Fistula first, catheter last	Catheter preferred given limited life expectancy to avoid procedures
Increase dialysis prescription to achieve standard kinetics targets	Adjust dialysis prescription to minimize dialysis-related symptoms
Strict fluid and dietary restrictions	Mild edema/hyperkalemia/hyperphosphatemia to allow more food enjoyment
Palliative care often not involved	Palliative care involved
Frequent labs	Minimal labs

For Mrs. L, peritoneal dialysis could be offered and titrated to minimize symptoms, yet allow her the freedom to get the most enjoyment from her remaining time. While Mrs. L has family that could assist with peritoneal dialysis exchanges, many older patients do not. With palliative dialysis, one need not feel that dialysis is a full-time job in itself. An exchange before and/or after the caregiver's outside work or the cycler overnight might be all the patient requires. Further, as the patient begins spending more time asleep instead of awake (ie, approaching death), the notion of allowing the patient to sleep rather than wake them to do an exchange could be more palatable to family as opposed to family possibly fearing a more abrupt death if an in-center hemodialysis treatment or 2 was missed.

The implementation of a plan of care incorporating palliative dialysis is not without barriers. Some providers, patients, and families may be resistant to the concept of palliative dialysis and may characterize palliative dialysis as substandard care. For providers, this characterization is fueled by an allegiance to standard metrics. However, one might argue that a set of metrics that does not incorporate metrics for what matters most for patients is substandard.

For patients and families, the substandard characterization may be driven by false hope or belief that less dialysis would mean earlier death. It is important for providers to be clear when dialysis will not prolong survival and stress importance of quality of life. Minority distrust of the medical system is well established. Poor patients and patients of color may particularly be suspicious of providers giving less treatment or trying to hasten their death. In an effort to build rapport/trust across socioeconomic and racial differences, providers could consider statements like: "If you were my [relative] I would give the same recommendation," as reassurance that the care plan offered is not different from that a provider would recommend to a personal loved one.

In the United States, many providers may perceive significant financial barriers to implementing a palliative dialysis care plan. While federal payment under the ESRD Quality Incentive Program can be reduced up to 2% for dialysis centers not meeting the performance measures, providers should remember that not all patients need to meet the standard quality metrics to avoid financial penalties.

US in-center hemodialysis providers could also be resistant to palliative dialysis due to potentially losing revenue under a fee-for-service payment model if patients dialyze less than 3 times per week. The same could be said for newcomers to dialysis with significant residual function who may benefit from incremental dialysis.[15] This creates an opportunity for a shift from traditional scheduling that could accommodate both incremental dialysis start patients and palliative dialysis patients while minimizing "empty chairs" and lost revenue. That stated, a larger shift to a payment model that incentivizes what is best for patients is needed.

Summary

Even though palliative dialysis is not yet defined by a set of quality metrics, a robust body of literature supporting it, or a payment model accommodating it, providers should consider it as part of a patient-centered treatment plan for some patients with ESKD with a prognosis of 1 year or less to live. Among patients for whom standard dialysis would result in more harm than benefit, the choice need not be dialysis or not, but rather how much dialysis would best help achieve patient goals.

Practice Pointers

- Dialysis may not be life-extending for older patients with dementia or ischemic heart disease despite achieving standard metrics.
- While dialysis may temporarily alleviate some symptoms of uremia and help patients achieve short-term survival priorities, it may also cause symptoms and create substantial burdens including intensive patterns of healthcare utilization, prolonged skilled nursing facility stays, stringent fluid and dietary restrictions, procedures to maintain vascular access, and time consumed traveling to and from dialysis.
- Palliative dialysis is a treatment plan that balances the amount of dialysis needed to alleviate symptoms of uremia and allow participation in important life events but avoid dialysis-related symptoms and procedures.

Practice Improvement Opportunities

- Providers should consider palliative dialysis for patients with ESKD who have a life expectancy of less than 1 year and have symptoms that might be ameliorated by dialysis.
- In developing a palliative dialysis treatment plan, providers must elicit patients' and families' specific hopes and fears and share a realistic explanation of what role dialysis could play in helping best achieve hopes and avoid fears, when death might be expected, what the dying process might look like, and what besides dialysis can be done to ease its symptoms.
- The nephrology community needs to develop a set of quality metrics for palliative dialysis.

References

1. Chandna SM, Da Silva-Gane M, Marshall C, Warwicker P, Greenwood RN, Farrington K. Survival of elderly patients with stage 5 CKD: comparison of conservative management and renal replacement therapy. *Nephrol Dial Transplant.* 2011;26(5):1608–1614.
2. Tamura MK, Tan JC, O'Hare AM. Optimizing renal replacement therapy in older adults: a framework for making individualized decisions. *Kidney Intl.* 2012;82(3):261–269.
3. Ramer SJ, McCall NN, Robinson-Cohen C, et al. Health outcome priorities of older adults with advanced CKD and concordance with their nephrology providers' perceptions. *J Am Soc Nephrol.* 2018;29(12):2870–2878.
4. Urquhart-Secord R, Craig JC, Hemmelgarn B, et al. Patient and caregiver priorities for outcomes in hemodialysis: an international nominal group technique study. *Am J Kidney Dis.* 2016;68(3):444–454.
5. Weisbord SD, Fried LF, Arnold RM, et al. Prevalence, severity, and importance of physical and emotional symptoms in chronic hemodialysis patients. *J Am Soc Nephrol.* 2005;16(8):2487–2494.
6. Feldman R, Berman N, Reid MC, et al. Improving symptom management in hemodialysis patients: identifying barriers and future directions. *J Palliat Med.* 2013;16(12):1528–1533.

7. Cohen LM, Moss AH, Weisbord SD, Germain MJ. Renal palliative care. *J Palliat Med.* 2006;9(4):977–992.
8. Davison SN, Jhangri GS, Johnson JA. Cross-sectional validity of a modified Edmonton symptom assessment system in dialysis patients: a simple assessment of symptom burden. *Kidney Intl.* 2006;69(9):1621–1625.
9. Wong SP, Kreuter W, O'Hare AM. Healthcare intensity at initiation of chronic dialysis among older adults. *J Am Soc Nephrol.* 2014;25(1):143–149.
10. Wong SP, Kreuter W, O'Hare AM. Treatment intensity at the end of life in older adults receiving long-term dialysis. *Arch Intern Med.* 2012;172(8):661–663; discussion 663–664.
11. United States Renal Data System. *USRDS 2018 annual data report: Atlas of chronic kidney disease and end-stage renal disease in the United States.* Bethesda, MD: USRDS; 2018.
12. O'Connor NR, Dougherty M, Harris PS, Casarett DJ. Survival after dialysis discontinuation and hospice enrollment for ESRD. *Clin J Am Soc Nephrol.* 2013;8(12):2117–2122.
13. Chettiar A, Montez-Rath M, Liu S, Hall YN, O'Hare AM, Kurella Tamura M. Association of inpatient palliative care with health care utilization and postdischarge outcomes among medicare beneficiaries with end stage kidney disease. *Clin J Am Soc Nephrol.* 2018;13(8):1180–1187.
14. Grubbs V, O'Riordan D, Pantilat S. Characteristics and outcomes of in-hospital palliative care consultation among patients with renal disease versus other serious illnesses. *Clin J Am Soc Nephrol.* 2017;12(7):1085–1089.
15. Golper TA. Incremental dialysis: review of recent literature. *Curr Opin Nephrol Hypertens.* 2017;26(6):543–547.

22

Process of Dialysis Withdrawal for Patients Failing to Thrive on Dialysis

Daniel Lam and Rebecca J. Schmidt

Dialysis therapy should be aligned with patient goals, values, and preferences. Withdrawal from dialysis is common, requiring kidney care professionals to recognize when the burden of dialytic therapies outweighs its benefit for any given patient. Informing patients early of the option to withdraw as part of periodic advance care planning can ease future conversations around withdrawal. A systematic approach to discussing withdrawal will address patient and family needs and includes assessing decision-making capacity, eliciting values, clarifying preferences, and educating patients and families about the physical, psychosocial, spiritual, and legal aspects of end-of-life care. All are key components of shared decision-making and the process of withdrawing from dialysis.

Case

Mr. P is a 73-year-old man with diabetes, hypertension, hyperlipidemia, peripheral vascular disease, heart failure with reduced ejection fraction, and end-stage kidney disease from diabetes and hypertension, with a dialysis vintage of 5 years. He was previously a long-time owner of a local supermarket before retiring to spend time with his family, including numerous grandchildren. Dialysis treatments have been uneventful, and he dialyzes via a left brachiobasilic arteriovenous fistula that is working well. He was previously living independently but moved into assisted living 2 years ago after it was becoming more difficult to perform instrumental activities of daily living such as grocery shopping, cooking, and cleaning. Since that time, he has been hospitalized for an acute myocardial infarction and developed heart failure, which has been complicated by 2 hospitalizations within the past year. He is now using a walker for ambulation.

Now, he feels "tired of everything." He feels fatigued all the time, whereas before it was only after his treatment on dialysis days. His dialysis days are the most difficult because he spends 8 hours away from his assisted living facility due to transportation. His small molecule adequacy is excellent, as are most of his labs except for his albumin, which is 3.3 g/dL despite oral nutritional supplements. He has tried antidepressant therapy without improvement in his fatigue. His exercise tolerance has worsened, and he worries about his ability to perform basic activities of daily living, such as showering and toileting, on his own.

His nephrologist and dialysis care team recognize that he is declining globally and schedule an appointment to discuss his priorities.

Introduction

Since the advent of Scribner–Quinton shunt, chronic dialysis has afforded patients the possibility of increased longevity. It is not, however, a cure. Dialysis patients have a high physical and psychological burden, in addition to the logistical burden of dialysis. When dialysis no longer provides benefits, a patient's overall goals of care are no longer met, or dialysis is prolonging suffering, discontinuation is reasonable. While there is no standard definition of dialysis withdrawal, dialysis discontinuation is now the second most common cause of death among US dialysis patients[1] and is associated with increasing age, comorbidities, depression, and pain.[2] The unadjusted percentage of known deaths among US dialysis patients attributed to dialysis withdrawal was 18% in 2015; for comparison, cardiovascular, infectious, and malignant causes comprised 54%, 11%, and 4% of deaths in the same year, respectively. Crude mortality rates preceding dialysis withdrawal range widely from 3 to 50 per 1000 person years across studies.[3] The most complete data comes from United States Renal Data System ESRD Death Notification Form, requiring the reason for withdrawal to be specified. Data reported all-cause withdrawal between 2005 and 2010 to be approximately 50 per 1000 person years. Dialysis withdrawal described as "withdrawal from dialysis/uremia" accounted for 42.4% of deaths among those who withdrew from 2008 to 2010.

With such a substantial percentage of the dialysis population opting to withdraw from dialysis, it is imperative that kidney care professionals develop the critical skills needed for preparing patients and families for the prospect that withdrawal will become desired and/or appropriate.[4]

Incorporating the Option for Withdrawal Into Advance Care Planning

Patient-centered communication is paramount to ensuring that patient goals and values drive medical decision-making. This is especially important with any chronic serious illness, where patients, providers, and families routinely contend with some level of uncertainty, even when a shorter prognosis is expected. One tool to help prepare patients/families is advance care planning—discussing the kind of future medical care to be prioritized should the patient become more ill. This process is a series of conversations that elicit important values—values that may shift over time as the patient's medical condition, functional status, and psychosocial situation change. The prioritization of values enable care professionals to act as better guides for patients/families, since these values set the guardrails for the kind of care that may help or harm an individual patient.

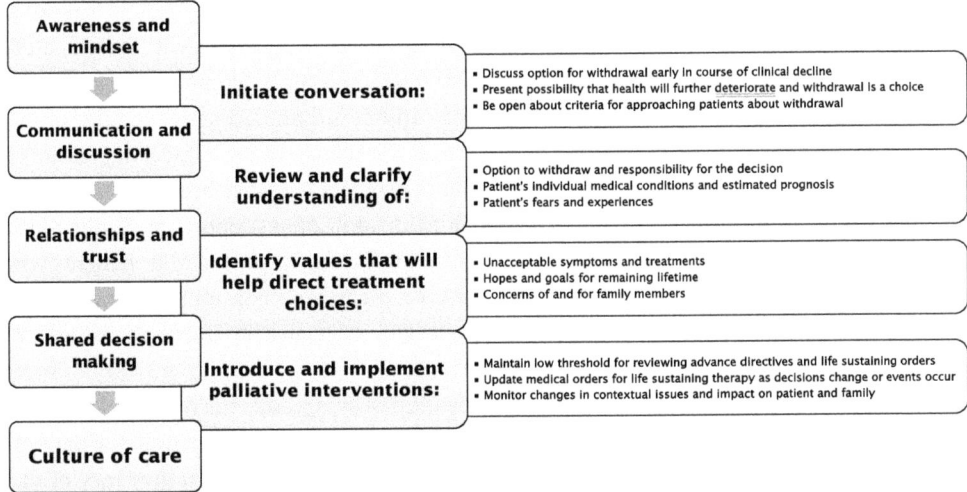

FIGURE 22.1. Incorporating the option of withdrawal into advance care planning.

These same skills of values elicitation and prioritization may be used when discussing the appropriateness of starting, foregoing, continuing, or withdrawing dialysis. Just as advance care planning involves discussion about dialysis modality, it should also address the potential for circumstances to evolve such that dialysis no longer serves the patient's bests interests. Given the limited life expectancy of end-stage kidney disease patients, advance care planning should be ongoing with all patients, taking special care to identify patients who may have a poorer prognosis. Triggers for more urgent advance care planning include the "surprise" question—"Would I be surprised if this patient died in the next year?" There are also prognostic tools that estimate 6-month prognosis for patients on dialysis.[5] In short, incorporating the option of withdrawal into dialysis care is dependent upon awareness, communication, trust, and a culture of care that shares decisions about what is best for any given patient including the option of withdrawal (Figure 22.1).

Reasons and Rationale for Withdrawal

The first step in addressing a request for dialysis withdrawal is formally assessing decision-making capacity. The 4 criteria for decision-making capacity include assessing the patient's understanding of their situation, their appreciation of the downstream consequences of different treatment options on their quality of life, reasoning for their decision-making, and the ability to express a choice. Decision-making capacity is both time-specific and task-specific. For example, a patient may have decision-making capacity to decline a routine lab draw but may not possess decision-making capacity for a complex decision regarding dialysis. Delirious patients may not have decision-making capacity in a period of confusion but could possess decision-making capacity in a period of lucidity. For patients without decision-making capacity, the assessment will need to occur with the surrogate decision maker as well.

In any request for dialysis withdrawal, it is also critical for the kidney care professional to explore the rationale behind this request. In some cases, a request to withdraw is a cry for help—a patient may be suffering from an intractable physical symptom, such as pain. When such symptoms are addressed, dialysis may still afford an acceptable quality of life. Other patients may endorse depression or low mood. Investigating for clinical depression is warranted, and after appropriate treatment, patients may feel that they are achieving an acceptable quality of life. Since patients may benefit from additional support, explicitly asking patients if there are friends or family they wish to be involved is important. For patients who do not have decision-making capacity and whose surrogate decision maker has made the request, the same principles hold true, while keeping in mind that the focus of discussions should center on what their loved one would prioritize.

There will be situations that, despite optimization of symptoms, the burdens of dialysis outweigh the benefit to the patient. This decision often reflects overall changes in the patient's trajectory, including their overall health trajectory as well as the values that they may prioritize. For example, with increasing global frailty and cognitive impairment, a patient may now choose to prioritize comfort and independence over longevity compared to prioritizing longevity when dialysis was initiated. Withdrawal may be desired and appropriate for patients with declining clinical status as depicted in Figure 22.2.

A useful concept when discussing goals of care pertaining to any treatment, including withdrawal of dialysis, is eliciting the patient's acceptable level of better.[6] While patient goals of care focus on their hopes for the future, the acceptable level of better refers to the patient's least acceptable quality of life. This provides a framework for shared decision-making where medical therapies—including dialysis—are viewed from the patient's definition of what "harm" would look like. For example, consider a frail, elderly dialysis patient who is too ill to be transplanted. This patient may have a goal of living long enough to see the birth of a grandchild, and an acceptable level of better that precludes living in a nursing home long-term. This person is continuing dialysis to welcome their new grandchild, but if they became so ill that they would need to live in a nursing facility long-term, they would rather focus

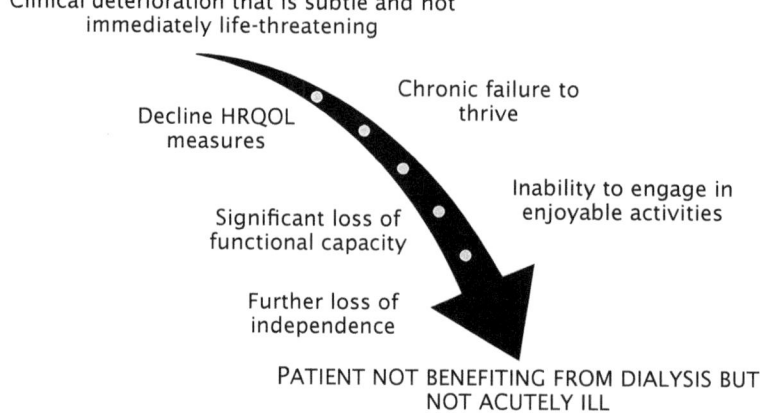

FIGURE 22.2. Withdrawal may be desired and appropriate for patients with declining clinical status.

their care on being comfortable. Shared decision-making in the context of the patient's prognosis, goals, and acceptable level of better empowers kidney care professionals to make recommendations aligned with the patient's values, including decisions regarding withdrawal of dialysis. Explicitly aligning with a patient's decision, when that decision truly reflects their goals, values, and preferences, may help relieve the existential distress that patients and families experience.[7]

Educating Patients and Families About Withdrawal

Once a patient and/or their surrogate decision maker has elected to withdraw from dialysis, the next step is eliciting the patient/family informational needs to tailor the education necessary to well prepare them for dialysis withdrawal. Guiding a patient and family through this decision includes the assessment of and desire for prognostic awareness, the communication of an estimate to the patient and/or appropriate family members, and a description of end-of-life or hospice services that may be available.

Discussing prognosis sets the stage for outlining what patients may expect and what steps and/or decisions about future care may be needed. Residual kidney function will impact prognosis following withdrawal. Studies looking at prognosis after withdrawal suggest that 79% of patients die within 10 days of withdrawal and less than 5% live beyond 1 month.[8] The largest study revealed that mean survival was 7.4 days, although the range was between 0 and 40 days.[9] As a general guide, a range can be provided, and given the data, an expectation that a patient will live days to weeks following dialysis withdrawal is reasonable.

Assessing where the patient would prefer to live out their days and the level of caregiving support that is available is the next step. For many patients, being at home is of utmost importance. Patients will be eligible for hospice services, which provides an interprofessional team support. Importantly, hospice does not provide 24-hour caregiving, and thus, plans for 24-hour caregiving in another care setting such as a nursing home or adult family home may be necessary. If the patient family choose home with hospice services, hospice will provide a social worker, nurse, spiritual care provider, and often home health aides, among other services. A nurse is on call 24/7 and may be reached after hours to guide the patient's caregivers through acute symptom issues or come to the home to address severe symptoms. The hospice on-call number is the new emergency number (replaces 911) for caregivers to call as the hospice nurse is able to address symptoms more efficiently and effectively than medics. If necessary, a hospice nurse will triage a patient for inpatient hospice, either in a freestanding hospice facility or hospital.

Education around end-of-life symptoms is also important. While many patients who stop dialysis slowly become progressively obtunded and "slip away," some have active symptoms. Explaining the dying process, such as expected changes in breathing patterns at the very end of life will prepare family members for physiologic changes and the accompanying symptoms that are unfamiliar to many caregivers and may provoke anxiety. Specific recommendations for supporting patients through withdrawal of dialysis are listed in Box 22.1.

> **BOX 22.1. Recommendations for Supportive Care for Patients Withdrawing From Dialysis**
>
> - Assure patients and families that withdrawal does not mean termination or care or abandonment.
> - Emphasize a plan for maximal medical therapy that is patient-centric and individually focused.
> - Address clinical, emotional and physical symptoms with a focus on pain and "in the moment" suffering.
> - Hospice may provide needed clinical assistance and social support.
> - Work with multidisciplinary team to keep care coordinated.
> - Plan for dealing with nonacute but discomforting symptoms that could occur with dialysis withdrawal.
> - Plan for acute symptom management may pre-empt the need for "heat of the moment" decisions.
> - Assure emotional, spiritual and family support for psychological pain.

Occasionally, a patient or family member may ask whether declining a life-sustaining treatment is tantamount to suicide. Importantly, any competent person has the right to decline any treatment, including life-sustaining treatment. This is rooted in the ethical principle of autonomy, which is the right to self-determination. Each person is best positioned to define what quality of life looks like for them, as well as what is unacceptable suffering. The courts have examined this issue as well; in the case of *Brophy v New England Sinai Hospital, Inc.*, the Supreme Court of Massachusetts ruled in 1983 that a healthcare surrogate could, using substituted judgement, request life-sustaining measures to be stopped given that it was prolonging an unacceptable quality of life.

Recommendations for Supporting Patients Withdrawing From Dialysis

Supportive care for patients withdrawing from dialysis mandates a comprehensive approach that addresses clinical, functional, and physical symptoms as well as the patient's emotional state, spiritual beliefs, and psychosocial context.[10] For patients choosing to withdraw, it is essential to provide reassurance that choosing to do so does not signify termination of care or herald abandonment but rather a proactive and deliberate approach to symptom management and comfort. Key issues to discuss include the specifics of maximal medical management without dialysis including the availability of palliative care and accessibility to hospice.[11] The option to reconsider their decision may provide comfort to patients who struggle with the conviction that they are choosing rather than allowing death to occur.

Contextual considerations are important to assure that care plans are aligned with the needs of each individual patient and provide a patient-centered rather than disease-centered approach. A focus on the "here and now" commands an understanding of a patients' values and goals and the family dynamics that may impact these. Educating patients who wish to withdraw from dialysis may require incremental introduction of palliative interventions. Supportive care commands attention to that which will impact the quality of life at its end.

An explanation of what to expect from the dying process, an estimated time frame for survival, common symptoms to anticipate, and how these can be managed are key components of this dialogue.[12,13,14] Information about both acute and nonacute but discomforting symptoms that could occur after withdrawal should be provided along with a discussion of how acute symptoms can be managed.

Dietary parameters should be clarified with restrictions advised on an individual patient basis and medications chosen to address current or potential uncomfortable symptoms or pain. Patients' desires for comprehensive symptom control (physical, emotional, and spiritual) including palliative sedation should symptoms become refractory to treatment or more than one can bear should be clarified upfront.

Patients may have other professionals involved in their care, particularly if engaging hospice, and assuring that care is coordinated among team members (medical and otherwise) is a priority. For patients who lack decision-making capacity, the designated decision maker must clearly understand the patient's clinical situation, prognosis, and wishes. Engaged family members can provide psychosocial support.

Steps for Withdrawal and Managing Symptoms in Patients Withdrawing From Dialysis

In preparation for dialysis withdrawal, patients with decision-making capacity should be advised to put their affairs in order with an inventory of bank, brokerage, and financial accounts. Patients should ensure that their will, advance directive, and assignment of durable or medical power of attorney are documented and readily available.[12,14] Translating advance directives from the end-of-life care plan into actionable medical orders can be achieved by documentation of specific wishes for medical orders for life-sustaining treatment at the end of life (physician orders for life-sustaining treatment, physician orders for scope of treatment; medical orders for life-sustaining treatment, or medical orders for scope of treatment, depending on US state).[15] A written, audio, or video message to family and/or friends may be desired. The patient's preferred death site should be determined and whether death at the site is feasible should be discussed; documentation of funeral preferences may be appropriate.

Central to the practice of supportive care is the focus on details of importance to the patient with attention to symptom control and psychosocial needs rather than dietary restrictions or blood tests. Emotional, spiritual, and family support for psychological pain should be sensitively addressed. Suggested steps for preparing for and implementing dialysis withdrawal are shown in Figure 22.3. Proactive management of symptoms and anticipatory prescribing may alleviate worry and pre-empt the need for "heat of the moment" decisions. With rapid access to medications, pain, shortness of breath, nausea, and agitation can be swiftly addressed. Specific treatment recommendations are shown in Box 22.2.

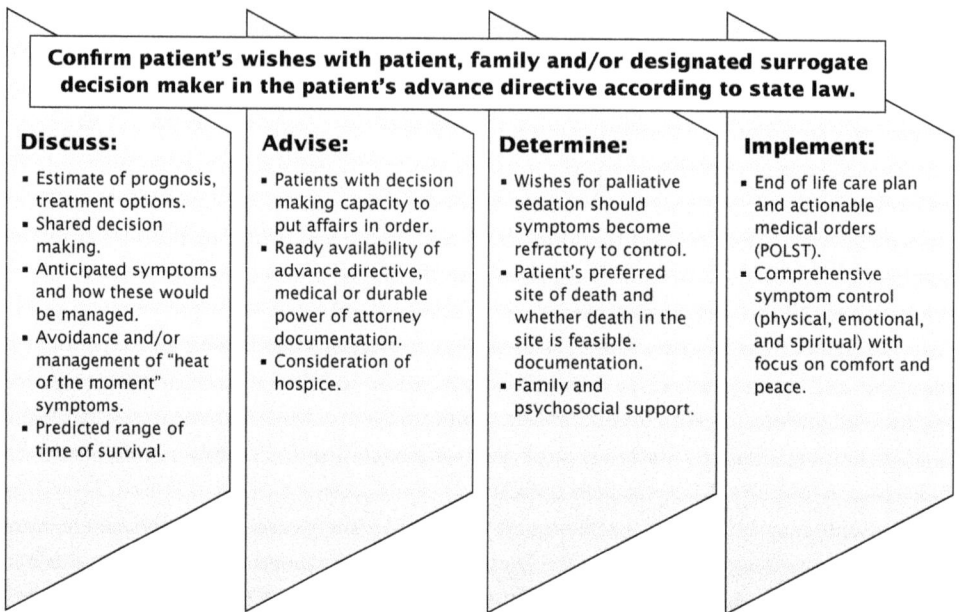

FIGURE 22.3. Suggested steps when preparing for and implementing dialysis withdrawal.

Hospice is a Medicare benefit available to patients with a terminal disease, providing clinical monitoring and support for patients deemed to be near the end of life.[16] In addition to services that address and provide pain relief and symptom management, hospice can provide significant social and emotional support to patients and their families. Hospice promotes sharing the responsibility of caregiving through scheduled visits and education of

---

BOX 22.2. Supportive Symptom Management for Patients Withdrawing From Dialysis

- Anticipate the development of symptoms and prescribe proactively.
- Manage nausea and vomiting with prokinetics (metoclopramide, haloperidol) or, if refractory, methotrimeprazine.
- Minimize breathlessness and edema with diuretics or, if refractory, fentanyl or hydromorphone.
- Manage restlessness, agitation, or delirium with haloperidol or, if refractory, methotrimeprazine; lorazepam or midazolam for anxiety.
- Topical agents, antihistamines, and gabapentin may be needed for pruritis.
- Symptoms of restless leg syndrome may warrant specific therapy.
- Erythropoietin-stimulating agents may be appropriate for anemia-associated fatigue.
- Physical pain may require serious analgesia such as fentanyl or hydromorphone.

loved ones, usually with around-the-clock availability for questions or concerns that may arise after hours.

Case Conclusion

Over several conversations, Mr. P's nephrologist elicits that he has noticed his functional decline and wishes to prioritize his comfort and being with family over longevity, but he is afraid of how his family will process his wishes. He witnessed the decline of his own parents in a nursing facility and does not wish to prolong his life should his level of dependence increase. His main goal is to celebrate the birthday of his daughter one more time, as long as he does not require skilled nursing facility care. He wishes to stop dialysis shortly thereafter. While he views his situation as "mildly depressing," he does not feel depressed and is thankful for the additional time dialysis has afforded him.

To address his concerns, Mr. P's nephrologist leads a family meeting, outlines Mr. P's prognostic trajectory, elicits his concerns and priorities, and involves his family. Together, they plan to enroll in hospice and move Mr. P to his home—a preferred location to his current assisted living facility—a few weeks after he celebrates his daughter's birthday. Mr. P does not suffer any additional setbacks and is able to celebrate his daughter's birthday before enrolling in hospice, where he died 8 days later in his home surrounded by family and friends.

Summary

The goals, values, and preferences of patients should guide and direct medical treatment, including dialysis. When dialysis prolongs suffering, it is important to discuss with the patient and family whether dialysis continues to serve the best interests of the patient. Advance care planning and proactive discussions of what may or may not be acceptable to patients as they contemplate the circumstances impacting the end of life are key to a culture that incorporates the option of withdrawal into dialysis care.

Practice Pointers

- Dialysis withdrawal is the third most common cause of death amongst dialysis patients in the US and may be appropriate for patients with declining clinical status.
- The steps for responding to a request for dialysis withdrawal include: assess decision-making capacity; assess and address reversible reasons for dialysis withdrawal; elicit goals, values and preferences; identify and establish a health care agent; complete actionable advance directives; involve hospice services if appropriate; provide reassurance regarding concerns of non-abandonment; involve social work for assistance with completing wills; and engage the patient in legacy work as desired. Hospice services provide additional support for the patient who elects to stop dialysis.

Practice Improvement Opportunities

- Incorporate conversations about of end-of-life further upstream as part of advance care planning (i.e. during late stage chronic kidney disease).
- Integrate discussions of dialysis withdrawal into advance care planning within the framework of an acceptable level of better (a patient's least acceptable quality of life).
- Address requests for withdrawal with an open stance to better understand the primary reasons for making such a request.

References

1. United States Renal Data System. *2018 USRDS Annual Data Report: Epidemiology of kidney disease in the United States.* Bethesda, MD: National Institutes of Health, National Institute of Diabetes and Digestive and Kidney Diseases; 2017.
2. Bajwa K, Szabo E, Kjellstrand CM. A prospective study of risk factors and decision making in discontinuation of dialysis. *Arch Intern Med.* 1996;156(22):2571.
3. Murphy E, Germain MJ, Cairns H, Higginson IJ, Murtagh FE. International variation in classification of dialysis withdrawal: a systematic review. *Nephrol Dial Transplant.* 2014;29(3):625–635.
4. Schmidt RJ, Moss AH. Dying on dialysis: the case for a dignified withdrawal. *Clin J Am Soc Nephrol.* 2004;9(1):174–180.
5. Cohen LM, Ruthazer R, Moss AH, Germain MJ: Predicting six-month mortality for patients who are on maintenance hemodialysis. *Clin J Am Soc Nephrol.* 2010;5:72–79.
6. Owens D. The role of palliative care in trauma. *Crit Care Nurs Q.* 2012;35(3):223–227.
7. Gramling R, Sanders M, Ladwig S, Norton SA, Epstein R, Alexander SC. Goal communication in palliative care decision-making consultations. *J Pain Symptom Manage.* 2015;50(5):701–706.
8. Fissell RB, Bragg-Gresham JL, Lopes AA, et al. Factors associated with "do not resuscitate" orders and rates of withdrawal from hemodialysis in the international DOPPS. *Kidney Int.* 2005;68(3):1282.
9. O'Connor NR, Dougherty M, Harris PS, Casarett DJ. Survival after dialysis discontinuation and hospice enrollment for ESRD. *Clin J Am Soc Nephrol.* 2013 Dec;8(12):2117–2122.
10. Holley, JL, Schmidt, RJ. Conservative/palliative treatment and end-of-life care in chronic kidney disease. In: Arici M, ed. *Management of Chronic Kidney Disease.* Berlin, Germany: Springer; 2014: 451–461.
11. Holley, JL. Advance care planning in CKD/ESRD: An evolving process. *Clin J Am Soc Nephrol* 2012;7:1033–1038.
12. Renal Physicians Association. *Shared Decision Making in the Appropriate Initiation of and Withdrawal From Dialysis.* 2nd ed. Rockville, Maryland, Renal Physicians Association, 2010.
13. Davison, SN., Levin A, Moss AH, et al. Executive summary of the KDIGO Controversies Conference on Supportive Care in Chronic Kidney Disease: developing a roadmap to improving quality care. *Kidney Int.* 2015;88(3):447–459.
14. Moss, AH. Integrating supportive care principles into dialysis decision making: a primer for palliative medicine providers. *J Pain Symptom Manage.* 2017;53(3):656–662.
15. Citko J, Moss AH, Carley M, Tolle S. The national POLST paradigm initiative. *J Palliat Med.* 2011;14(2):241–242.
16. Medicare hospice benefit. https://www.medicare.gov/Pubs/pdf/02154-Medicare-Hospice-Benefits. Accessed June 15, 2018.

SECTION VI

The Future of Palliative Care Nephrology

23

Ethical Issues in the Supportive Care of Patients With Advanced Kidney Disease

Catherine R. Butler and Alvin H. Moss

Although the benefits of standard dialysis therapy for many older adults with complex comorbid conditions is equivocal, there continues to be substantial moral uncertainty in the practice of withholding and withdrawing dialysis treatment. This chapter reviews several ethical conundrums in palliative care of patients with advanced kidney disease, including uncertainty about the moral status of withholding dialysis and pursuing medical management without dialysis, challenges in decision-making when patients lack capacity to participate, and ethically relevant social and cultural factors influencing practice. Better understanding of the underlying causes of these conundrums reveals opportunities to improve quality of patient care at the individual and system levels by incorporating palliative practices. The chapter also suggests strategies for clinicians to identify and facilitate resolution of ethical conflicts around end-of-life care for patients with advanced kidney disease in clinical practice.

Case

Ms. Wander is a 76-year-old woman, who was formerly a heavy smoker and now has peripheral arterial disease, stage 4 chronic kidney disease (CKD) thought secondary to hypertensive nephrosclerosis, and oxygen-dependent chronic obstructive pulmonary disease. She was hospitalized for sepsis from pneumonia and required a prolonged period of mechanical ventilation in the intensive care unit. Her CKD progressed to end-stage kidney disease (ESKD), and she was started on hemodialysis.

In her young life, she was an avid traveler and journalist, but recently she's been living with family because they had noticed mild cognitive decline thought to be due to early dementia. At the time of presentation, she lacked capacity to make decisions about dialysis initiation. Her family reported that she was someone who always wanted to "think positively" and avoided discussion of specific medical treatment preferences but appeared to have been preparing for dialysis and was actively engaged in medical treatments before her hospitalization. After a 3-week hospital stay, she was discharged to a skilled nursing facility because she continued to be confused, deconditioned, malnourished (serum albumin 2.7 g/dL), and no longer able to care for herself. On discharge, she established dialysis care at an outpatient center. Although she appears to be reasonably comfortable at her nursing facility, dialysis center staff report that she cries and moans throughout treatments. Her family and nephrologist are conflicted about how to proceed with her care.

The Field of Bioethics Has Co-Evolved With Dialysis Technology

When chronic hemodialysis became available in the 1960s, the nephrology community suddenly faced a pressing ethical dilemma about how to ration the scarce supply of dialysis machines among a group of patients with similarly compelling medical indications and who would each die without treatment. In an attempt to include nonmedical perspectives, the Seattle Artificial Kidney Center took a novel approach and delegated the ultimate selection decision to a committee of community members. After much deliberation, this citizen committee chose to select dialysis recipients based on their relative social worth; however, the bias inherent in this selection criterion resulted in an eruption of public controversy and debate that some say triggered the very birth of bioethics.[1]

In response to public distaste over medical rationing practices, the US Congress added an amendment to the Social Security Act in 1972 creating a Medicare coverage entitlement for patients with ESKD, largely eliminating financial pressure to ration dialysis treatment. However, in the following decades, the population of patients initiating dialysis expanded far beyond what Congress members envisioned, both in terms of size and medical complexity. Over the last 3 decades, older adults and those with complex medical comorbidities make up an increasing component of the dialysis population. For this contemporary population of patients with ESKD, the benefits of dialysis are often more limited and the burdens substantial,[2-4] making the appropriate withholding and withdrawing of dialysis treatment a dominant ethical dilemma in nephrology.

Moral Uncertainty and Value Conflicts About Withholding and Withdrawing Dialysis

Moral distress occurs when care providers are constrained from acting in accordance with their moral judgments because of situational or institutional pressures.[5] Commonly identified sources of moral distress include the withdrawal of dialysis and other life-sustaining treatments and provision of intensive therapies in medical contexts that renders them "futile"—that is, when treatment offers no discernable benefit. Patients and family members also struggle with competing priorities when dialysis offers life prolongation at the cost of concurrent values such as comfort, dignity, and independence.

Concern That Withholding Dialysis Is "No Care"

Recent work suggests that for many nephrologists, not providing dialysis feels akin to "no care," and they may avoid discussion of palliative options out of concern that it would jeopardize therapeutic relationships or destroy hope.[6] Nephrologists are more confident in their ability to control symptoms of advanced kidney disease with dialysis and struggle to define their role when renal replacement therapy is declined.[6,7] Similarly, family members often prefer therapy couched in terms of active rather than passive treatment. Family members in situations such as Ms. Wander's may see aggressive medical intervention as a way of demonstrating love and respect.[8] Further, patients offered the dichotomous choice of "dialysis or death" may understandably discount the second option as disingenuous.[9,10] Cultural attitudes and practices may differ in other countries—for instance, up to 15% to 20% of patients with ESKD in Australia, Canada, and the United Kingdom opt for medical management without dialysis.

Collectively, these observations identify a need to develop a medical culture and infrastructure that supports a range of active therapeutic options that account for the diverse preferences of patients with advanced kidney disease who may or may not accept the quality of life afforded by standard dialysis treatment[11] but also may not wish to focus only on comfort to the exclusion of other therapies. Clinicians need to be educated and feel confident providing a range of treatment options as well as facilitating complex end-of-life decisions.

Concern That Dialysis Withdrawal Is Actively Causing Death

Patients, their surrogates and family members, and clinicians may feel that they are in some way responsible for causing or hastening death when deciding to withhold dialysis. One family member explained the decision to continue dialysis for her mother despite an exceedingly poor prognosis, saying "At least I don't have to feel guilty."[12] The principle of double effect states that a person is not morally accountable for an unintended (although potentially anticipated) secondary effect of an action (ie, hastening death) in pursuit of a laudable primary goal (ie, promoting patient comfort).[13] Despite this philosophical claim, it may be difficult to shake a sense of personal responsibility when a patient with ESKD quickly succumbs after withdrawal of dialysis.

Institution of palliative measures early in a patients' course allows for treatment that is responsive to evolving goals of care as a patient approaches the end of life and may also alleviate the sense of abrupt change in health trajectory when dialysis treatment is stopped.[14] For example, palliative dialysis focused on patient-centered goals (eg, prioritizing time with family, minimizing pain) rather than disease-centered goals (eg, dialysis adequacy, achieving biomarker targets) for patients thought to have less than 1 year to live—may include shorter and/or less frequent sessions.

Decisions About Withholding and Withdrawing Dialysis When Patients Lack Decisional Capacity

Decision-making around initiating, withholding, and withdrawing dialysis is complex and ideally takes place over time in the context of a therapeutic patient–provider relationship with early family involvement. However, decisions are often made urgently in settings where patients have impaired cognitive capacity. As in the case of Mrs. Wander, as many as 75% of patients initiate dialysis therapy during an acute hospitalization when medical illness and progressive uremia may limit patients' capacity to participate in discussion.[9,15] Further, as the dialysis population ages, comorbidities affecting cognition, including dementia, are increasingly common. A default toward intensive therapies when patient preferences are unclear makes it especially challenging to withhold or withdraw dialysis in these settings.[16]

Decision-Making When Patients Do Not Have Capacity: Advance Directives and Substituted Judgment

Capacity for medical decision-making is composed of 4 elements: ability to (i) understand relevant information, (ii) appreciate one's medical condition and the personal consequences of treatment options, (iii) rationally weigh alternative options, and (iv) express choice.[17] Decision-making capacity is not all or nothing, and the degree to which a patient is expected to express these capabilities varies by situation, but the threshold is often especially high for life-or-death decisions such as withholding or withdrawing dialysis.[18] When patients lose decision-making capacity, they do not lose their right to autonomous choice. The Patient Self-Determination Act of 1991 requires medical facilities to advise patients of their right to document treatment preferences as advance directives. When advance directives are not in place or do not adequately address the clinical circumstances, a surrogate decision maker—either previously identified by a patient or legally designated—is instructed to support a patient's previously expressed autonomy by using "substituted judgment" to decide on treatment as the patient would have done if he or she had capacity to do so. This substituted judgment standard of decision-making is contrasted with the "best interest" standard (which is foundational in pediatric decision-making) under which the designated decision maker acts according to what they feel is in the patient's best interest.

Limitations to Advance Directives and Substituted Judgment

Although Ms. Wander's family reported that she previously sought life-prolonging therapies, there were no specific discussions about dialysis, and regardless of her prior preferences, they were concerned that dialysis treatment might not be in her best interest. These uncertainties suggest that advance directives and the narrow role of surrogates in making substituted judgments may be insufficient to account for the complexities of decision-making in cases of patient incapacity.

Studies following the Patient Self-Determination Act suggested that the legislation did not greatly increase the number of people with advance directives, and most patients with ESKD still have not documented preferences or assigned a preferred surrogate decision maker.[19,20] Surrogates have rarely specifically discussed patients' preferences about end-of-life therapies—especially dialysis—in advance of serious illness, and even when they do have a sense of patient preferences, they act not only according to the substituted judgment standard but also consider their sense of a patient's best interest.[21] Seriously ill patients affirm this practice, reporting in surveys that they would give substantial leeway to surrogates and medical providers to override their advance directives when it is deemed to be in their best interest.[22] Collectively, these observations suggest that advance care planning is most effective as an ongoing discussion of broad patient values with early involvement of family and that surrogate decision-making involves weighing multiple value considerations including both patient preference and their best interest.[4,23,24]

System-Level Ethical Concerns

The traditional model of medical decision-making focuses on the relationship between a patient with a medical problem and a provider who seeks to help him or her resolve it. However, medical practice is embedded in institutions and communities each with processes, requirements, and values that may or may not align with patient preferences. Recognition of these contextual features and influences is critical to support patient decision-making as well as to identify opportunities for system improvement.

System-Level Barriers to Withdrawal of Dialysis

In a recent interview-based study, nephrologists identified multiple system-level barriers to medical management without dialysis as a therapeutic option for patients with advanced kidney disease.[6] First, nephrologists struggle to incorporate discussion about patient values and goals into brief clinic visits already strained by the need to cover numerous biomedical issues. Second, they note that while patients starting dialysis are supported by an established interdisciplinary team (eg, nurses, social workers, nutritionists, and care coordinators), no parallel network exists to support equally complex care for patients who prefer a medical approach without dialysis. Further, the current structure of healthcare financial compensation is based on dialysis initiation and continuation, and many question the economic viability of providing interdisciplinary care to patients deciding to forgo dialysis.

Disparity in Access to High-Quality Palliative Care and Hospice Services

Opportunity and access to high-quality end-of-life care varies throughout the United States, leading to ethically relevant differences in patients' end-of-life experiences. Patients with ESKD who live in regions of the United States that exhibit patterns of higher intensity end-of-life care (eg, intensive care unit admission, mechanical ventilation) are less likely to discontinue dialysis before death, less likely to receive hospice services, and more likely to die in a hospital.[25] These outcomes are concerning because they do not align with the preferences of the majority of seriously ill patients.[26,27] Individual nephrologists vary greatly in their own practice and education around withdrawal of dialysis and palliative options for ESKD.[7,28] Further, the current structure of the Medicare hospice benefit precludes concurrent payments for hospice and dialysis for patients whose terminal diagnosis is kidney disease or its complications, despite evidence for the financial efficacy of palliative dialysis.[29,30]

In an attempt to improve and standardize care, the Renal Physicians Association published clinical practice guidelines on shared decision-making in withholding and withdrawing dialysis.[4] Unfortunately, few nephrologists report being aware of or using this valuable resource.[7]

Professional Practice and Conflicts of Interest in Palliative Care Nephrology

Over the last 3 decades, the ownership of most dialysis centers has shifted from individual physicians or hospitals to large corporate dialysis organizations. Free enterprise environments are governed by ethical standards and priorities focused on benefit to the organization or shareholder and may not align with the well-being of individual patients.[31] The incentive for large corporations to standardize and streamline medical management poses a particular challenge to supporting diverse patient preferences. The more recent development of ESRD Seamless Care Organizations, which take financial responsibility for the entire medical care of patients with ESRD, may offer the opportunity and financial incentive to incorporate a bigger picture and potentially more patient-centered approach to care including palliative options.[32] Continued advocacy by nephrology professional associations of this approach, including advocacy for monitoring of patient-centered quality metrics, may also encourage dialysis corporations to focus on quality of care.

Approach to Conflict Resolution in Decisions About Withholding and Withdrawing Dialysis

The Renal Physicians Association clinical practice guideline on withdrawing and withholding dialysis offers an orderly approach to ethical decision-making that facilitates the resolution of conflicts in values and preferences among patients, their surrogates, and clinicians (Box 23.1). In addition, there are a number of other bioethical frameworks available that offer a systematic approach to analyze ethical questions that arise in clinical practice. Casuistry is

---

BOX 23.1. Seven-Step Process of Ethical Decision-Making in Patient Care

1. What are the ethical questions?
2. What are the clinically relevant facts?
3. What are the values at stake?
4. List options. What could you do?
5. What should you do? Choose the best option from the ethical point of view.
6. Justify your choice. Refer back to the values and give reasons why some values are more important in this case than others.
7. How could this ethical issue have been prevented? Would any policies/guidelines/practices be useful in changing any problems with the system?

Reproduced from the Renal Physician's Association clinical practice guideline on withholding and withdrawing dialysis.[4]

TABLE 23.1. Casuistry or the "4-Box Method" for Approaching Ethical Concerns in Palliative Nephrology and Example Content[33]

Medical indications	Patient preferences
Is dialysis medically indicated? What other supportive treatments are indicated? What is the patient's prognosis given different treatment options?	What are the patients' goals? Does the patient have sufficient information and comprehend the clinical setting? If the patient lacks decision-making capacity, is there documentation indicating prior preferences? Who is a surrogate with decision-making authority?
Quality of life	Contextual features
What defines quality of life for the patient? What is the patient's life like now, and what can we predict it would be like under different treatment scenarios?	Do financial resource limitations play a role in decision-making? Are there conflicts of interest among stakeholders or institutions? What are the burdens and benefits of treatment to the patients' family and community? What cultural traditions, religious beliefs, and or legal considerations play a role in this scenario?

Source: Jonsen.[36]

one such framework in which 4 ethically relevant components of any clinical situation are described to support conflict resolution, and it may be particularly aligned with case-based reasoning already familiar to many medical providers (Table 23.1).

Practice Pointers

- Moral distress occurs when care providers are constrained from acting in accordance with their moral judgments because of situational or institutional pressures.[5] For nephrology providers, moral distress may occur both in situations of withdrawal of dialysis and other life-sustaining treatments and during provision of intensive therapies perceived to offer no discernable benefit.
- Patients and family members may also experience moral distress when struggling to reconcile competing priorities of concurrent values such as comfort, dignity, and independence.
- Moral concerns may arise if providers, patient, or family mistakenly perceive withholding dialysis as "no care" or withdrawing dialysis as actively causing death. Aligning care with patient-centered goals expressed by the patient or surrogate is an ethical approach in these situations.

Practice Improvement Opportunities

- Many instances of moral distress can be prevented by incorporating the supportive care practices described throughout this book, especially advance care planning, shared decision-making, and expansion of patient-centered care options such as medical management without dialysis.

- When faced with ethical dilemmas, 2 tools for finding a resolution are the 7-step process (Box 23.1) and the case-based casuistry 4-box method (Table 23.1).
- Consultation with palliative care colleagues may offer the opportunity to support complex and evolving patient values and goals including longevity, quality of life, and dignity.

References

1. Jonsen AR. *The Birth of Bioethics*. New York, NY: Oxford University Press; 1998.
2. Verberne WR, Geers AB, Jellema WT, Vincent HH, van Delden JJ, Bos WJ. Comparative survival among older adults with advanced kidney disease managed conservatively versus with dialysis. *Clin J Am Soc Nephrol*. 2016;11(4):633–640.
3. Carson RC, Juszczak M, Davenport A, Burns A. Is maximum conservative management an equivalent treatment option to dialysis for elderly patients with significant comorbid disease? *Clin J Am Soc Nephrol*. 2009;4(10):1611–1619.
4. Renal Physicians Association. *Shared Decision-Making in the Appropriate Initiation of and Withdrawal From Dialysis*. 2nd ed. Rockville, MD: Renal Physicians Association, American Society of Nephrology; 2010.
5. Lamiani G, Borghi L, Argentero P. When healthcare professionals cannot do the right thing: a systematic review of moral distress and its correlates. *J Health Psychol*. 2017;22(1):51–67.
6. Ladin K, Pandya R, Kannam A, et al. Discussing conservative management with older patients with CKD: an interview study of nephrologists. *Am J Kidney Dis*. 2018;71(5):627–635.
7. Davison SN, Jhangri GS, Holley JL, Moss AH. Nephrologists' reported preparedness for end-of-life decision-making. *Clin J Am Soc Nephrol*. 2006;1(6):1256–1262.
8. Russ AJ, Shim JK, Kaufman SR. The value of "life at any cost": talk about stopping kidney dialysis. *Soc Sci Med*. 2007;64(11):2236–2247.
9. Wong SP, Vig EK, Taylor JS, et al. Timing of initiation of maintenance dialysis: a qualitative analysis of the electronic medical records of a national cohort of patients from the Department of Veterans Affairs. *JAMA Intern Med*. 2016;176(2):228–235.
10. Song MK, Lin FC, Gilet CA, Arnold RM, Bridgman JC, Ward SE. Patient perspectives on informed decision-making surrounding dialysis initiation. *Nephrol Dial Transplant*. 2013;28(11):2815–2823.
11. Morton RL, Snelling P, Webster AC, et al. Dialysis modality preference of patients with CKD and family caregivers: a discrete-choice study. *Am J Kidney Dis*. 2012;60(1):102–111.
12. Moss AH. "At least we do not feel guilty": managing conflict with families over dialysis discontinuation. *Am J Kidney Dis*. 1998;31(5):868–883.
13. Kockler NJ. The principle of double effect and proportionate reason. *Virtual Mentor*. 2007;9(5):369–374.
14. Grubbs V, Moss AH, Cohen LM, et al. A palliative approach to dialysis care: a patient-centered transition to the end of life. *Clin J Am Soc Nephrol*. 2014;9(12):2203–2209.
15. Wong SP, Hebert PL, Laundry RJ, et al. Decisions about renal replacement therapy in patients with advanced kidney disease in the US Department of Veterans Affairs, 2000–2011. *Clin J Am Soc Nephrol*. 2016;11(10):1825–1833.
16. Kaufman S. *Ordinary Medicine: Extraordinary Treatments, Longer Lives, and Where to Draw the Line*. Durham, NC: Duke University Press; 2015.
17. Appelbaum PS. Clinical practice: assessment of patients' competence to consent to treatment. *N Engl J Med*. 2007;357(18):1834–1840.
18. Culver CM, Gert B. The inadequacy of incompetence. *Milbank Q*. 1990;68(4):619–643.
19. The SUPPORT Principal Investigators. A controlled trial to improve care for seriously ill hospitalized patients. The study to understand prognoses and preferences for outcomes and risks of treatments (SUPPORT). *JAMA*. 1995;274(20):1591–1598.
20. Kurella Tamura M, Montez-Rath ME, Hall YN, Katz R, O'Hare AM. Advance directives and end-of-life care among nursing home residents receiving maintenance dialysis. *Clin J Am Soc Nephrol*. 2017;12(3):435–442.

21. Hirschman KB, Kapo JM, Karlawish JH. Why doesn't a family member of a person with advanced dementia use a substituted judgment when making a decision for that person? *Am J Geriatr Psychiatry*. 2006;14(8):659–667.
22. Sehgal A, Galbraith A, Chesney M, Schoenfeld P, Charles G, Lo B. How strictly do dialysis patients want their advance directives followed? *JAMA*. 1992;267(1):59–63.
23. Gillick MR. Advance care planning. *N Engl J Med*. 2004;350(1):7–8.
24. Holley JL. Advance care planning in CKD/ESRD: an evolving process. *Clin J Am Soc Nephrol*. 2012;7(6):1033–1038.
25. O'Hare AM, Rodriguez RA, Hailpern SM, Larson EB, Kurella Tamura M. Regional variation in health care intensity and treatment practices for end-stage renal disease in older adults. *JAMA*. 2010;304(2):180–186.
26. Teno JM, Gozalo PL, Bynum JP, et al. Change in end-of-life care for Medicare beneficiaries: site of death, place of care, and health care transitions in 2000, 2005, and 2009. *JAMA*. 2013;309(5):470–477.
27. Davison SN. End-of-life care preferences and needs: perceptions of patients with chronic kidney disease. *Clin J Am Soc Nephrol*. 2010;5(2):195–204.
28. Holley JL, Carmody SS, Moss AH, et al. The need for end-of-life care training in nephrology: national survey results of nephrology fellows. *Am J Kidney Dis*. 2003;42(4):813–820.
29. Schwarze ML, Schueller K, Jhagroo RA. Hospice use and end-of-life care for patients with end-stage renal disease: too little, too late. *JAMA Intern Med*. 2018;178(6):799–801.
30. O'Hare AM, Hailpern SM, Wachterman M, et al. Hospice use and end-of-life spending trajectories in medicare beneficiaries on hemodialysis. *Health Aff (Millwood)*. 2018;37(6):980–987.
31. Ozar DT, Kristensen C, Fadem SZ, Blaser R, Singer D, Moss AH. Nephrologists' professional ethics in dialysis practices. *Clin J Am Soc Nephrol*. 2013;8(5):840–844.
32. Johnson DS, Meyer KB. Leading integrated kidney care entities of the future. *Adv Chronic Kidney Dis*. 2018;25(6):523–529.
33. Jonsen AR. *Clinical Ethics: A Practical Approach to Ethical Decisions in Medicine*. 6th ed. New York, NY: McGraw Hill; 2006.

24

Transforming Practice to Support Person-Centered Care for Patients With Advanced Kidney Disease

Ann M. O'Hare and Nancy C. Armistead

Contemporary patterns of care for patients with advanced kidney disease are far from person-centered. Large changes to health systems, payment structures, quality measurement, patient and provider education, and the culture in which care is delivered will be needed to support a more person-centered approach to care for members of this population. To uphold the essence of who our patients are, efforts are needed throughout the illness trajectory to foster the development of strong patient–provider relationships and extend the reach of these relationships across settings, to educate our patients about their treatment options and what to expect in the future, to offer opportunities for patients to involve their family members and close friends in their care, and ultimately to promote a culture in which providers are flexible, creative, and tireless in working with their colleagues and with their patients and their families to fulfill the mission of person-centered care of finding the "right treatment for the right person at the right time."

Introduction

The 2001 landmark report from the Institute of Medicine entitled "Crossing the Quality Chasm: A New Health System for the 21st Century" argued that modern health systems should strive to deliver care that is not just effective, timely, efficient, and equitable, but also patient-centered.[1] Patient-centered care was defined in the report as "care that is respectful of and responsive to individual patient preferences, needs, and values and ensuring that patient values guide all clinical decisions"[1] (p. 40).

There is now growing support within the nephrology community for a patient- or person-centered approach to caring for patients with advanced kidney disease in which care is squarely focused on supporting the values and goals of individual patients.[2-4] However, achieving this goal will not be easy because clinical practice guidelines, regulatory processes, and healthcare systems are still largely organized around diseases and organ systems and founded on a one-size-fits-all approach to care.[5] Not uncommonly and despite the best of intentions, system-level constraints conspire with the unpredictability of chronic illness to derail efforts to uphold what is most important to each person. And when health systems and providers fail to prioritize the goals of individual patients, this can engender feelings of mistrust, alienation, isolation, and even abandonment.[6]

In this chapter, we discuss the ways in which health systems can limit our ability to focus care on what is most important to patients with advanced kidney disease and offer suggestions for how these systems might be transformed to support a more person-centered approach to care throughout the course of illness (Table 24.1). The piece is organized around a series of scenarios intended to depict critical moments in the illness trajectories of patients with advanced kidney disease. These include outpatient care for patients with advanced kidney disease not on dialysis, care during episodes of acute illness, and decisions about dialysis initiation and care toward the end of life.

TABLE 24.1. Recommendations to Promote a Person-Centered Approach to Care throughout the Course of Advanced Kidney Disease

Goal	Recommendations
Promoting person-centered care for patients with advanced kidney disease not on dialysis	Development of care models to support a multidisciplinary team approach to caring for patients with advanced kidney disease not on dialysis including (but not limited to) those who wish to forgo dialysis; offer opportunities for patients to involve family members and close friends in their care; foster the development of strong patient–provider relationships; and equip providers to engage in conversations with patients and families about treatment options, prognosis, values, and goals.
Promoting a person-centered approach to dialysis decision-making and care during acute illness	Change the culture of inpatient care to promote continuity and coordination with the outpatient setting; find ways to leverage long-term patient–provider relationships to support inpatient care and decision-making; and offer professional education to strengthen providers ability to uphold patients' goals and values during medical crises (eg, training in communication skills, team building).
Promoting person-centered care for patients with advanced kidney disease who are seriously ill or dying	Ensure that patients are aware of relevant treatment options (eg, stopping dialysis, hospice and kidney supportive care), knowledgeable about health system defaults (ie., reflexive focus on life prolongation) and how to avoid these and have realistic expectations of what to expect in the future (eg, life expectancy, course of illness); offer opportunities for patients and families to participate in an ongoing process of advance care planning throughout the course of illness; increase flexibility in the provision of hospice and kidney supportive care; and find ways to leverage long-standing patient–provider relationships.

Outpatient Care for Patients With Advanced Kidney Disease Not on Dialysis

Case

Mr. Z is a 75-year old man who has been followed in renal clinic for the last 4 years. His serum creatinine has been relatively stable in the 4 to 5 mg/dL range over this time, and he feels well, with few signs or symptoms of chronic kidney disease. While he is not keen to start dialysis, he is also not ready to "throw in the towel." When educated about his treatment options, he didn't like the idea of doing dialysis himself at home. Thus, about a year ago, he underwent placement of an arteriovenous fistula to prepare for in-center hemodialysis, and this is now mature.

Discussion

The results of the Initiating Dialysis Early and Late (IDEAL) trial—an influential multicenter trial conducted in Australia and New Zealand that compared outcomes among patients randomized to start dialysis at higher (10–14 mL/min) and lower (5–7 mL/min) levels of estimated glomerular filtration rate (eGFR)—suggest that, on a population level, there is no benefit to a proactive approach to starting dialysis at higher levels of eGFR to avoid the complications of advanced kidney disease.[7] Rather, a strategy of close follow-up with a nephrologist until patients develop a clinical indication for dialysis (or reach lower levels of eGFR) appears to be just as safe as—and more cost effective than—starting dialysis earlier.

In the United States, relatively few patients with advanced kidney disease ultimately choose not to start dialysis when they are faced with this decision.[8] In fact, available evidence suggests that those patients who do express a desire to forgo dialysis often face immense pressure to the contrary.[9] However, many patients are uncertain whether they would want to start dialysis or are reluctant to do so until this treatment is truly needed.[10–13] Thus, having the infrastructure to manage patients with advanced kidney disease conservatively without dialysis is essential, not only for supporting those patients who have chosen to forgo dialysis, but also those who may be ambivalent or wish to delay starting dialysis for as long as possible.[14,15]

Caring for patients with advanced kidney disease involves managing disease complications such as anemia, volume overload, hyperparathyroidism, and acidosis, while preparing them for future treatment options including medical management without dialysis, hemodialysis, peritoneal dialysis, and transplant. Because patients with advanced kidney disease often have a range of other serious health conditions, caring for these patients also usually involves addressing concerns that may be unrelated to their underlying kidney disease and coordinating care with their other providers.[16] The inherent uncertainty about whether patients' kidney disease will progress and how quickly this might occur are pervasive concerns that can complicate, delay, or even paralyze clinical decision-making for members of this population.[17]

Fee-for-service reimbursement structures and the absence of well-developed care models for patients with advanced kidney disease not on dialysis add to the challenges of caring for members of this population. By providing excellent coverage for the select group of patients receiving renal replacement therapy, the Medicare ESRD entitlement program may have had the unintended effect of encouraging dialysis initiation in patients with advanced kidney disease.[14] The financial incentives favoring dialysis are evident when one compares physician current patterns of fee-for-service reimbursement for outpatient nephrology clinic care for patients with chronic kidney disease with that for outpatient dialysis care and inpatient nephrology consultation (Table 24.2).[18]

Documentation requirements to support billing can also work against a person-centered approach to care. These requirements—intended to provide accountability and guard against insurance and Medicare fraud—are grounded in an organ system-based approach to care. Under current fee-for-service billing arrangements, justification for visit complexity is tied to the completeness of the review of systems and physical exam.[19] Unfortunately, this approach may not align with patients' chief concerns at the time of the visit, especially if this includes social, functional, spiritual, and lifestyle matters that might be missed by a standard organ system review. Nor do current approaches to billing allow for the possibility that not all questions or issues need be addressed in a single visit, especially if the patient has more pressing concerns.

In many instances, open-ended listening is more important in centering care on the patient than completion of the physical exam or review of systems.[20,21] In this context, requirements for extensive documentation can take up precious time that could be spent addressing matters of importance to the patient, a concern that Centers for Medicare and Medicaid's (CMS) ongoing "Patients Over Paperwork" initiative seeks to address.[22] Although changes to billing requirements always carry potential for perverse incentives and unintended consequences, we expect that shifting reimbursement criteria away from a rigid procedure- and organ system-based checklist toward a more flexible approach of accounting for time spent and the extent to which patients' needs were met would go a long way to supporting a person-centered approach to care (Table 24.1).

The limited availability of multidisciplinary support for the care of patients with advanced kidney disease not on dialysis may also have the unintended effect of incentivizing

TABLE 24.2. Physician Reimbursement

Treatment Type	RVU for Service
Outpatient, not on dialysis	
High complexity new patient	3.17
Follow-up high complexity	2.11
Inpatient	
High complexity new patient	4.0
Follow-up high complexity (could be daily)	2.0
Outpatient, dialysis patient	
Outpatient home dialysis visit (encompassing one visit per month)	4.26
In-center hemodialysis care (encompassing 2–4 visits per month)	4.26

Abbreviation: RVU, relative value unit.

dialysis initiation. Once patients start dialysis in a Medicare-certified facility, access to a multidisciplinary care team—that includes, at minimum, a registered nurse, a physician treating the patient for end-stage kidney disease (ESKD), a social worker, and a dietitian—is mandated under CMS Conditions for Coverage.[23] The role of this team is to "develop and implement a written, individualized, comprehensive plan of care that specifies the services necessary to address the patient's needs, as identified by the comprehensive assessment and changes in the patient's condition, and must include measurable and expected outcomes and estimated timetables to achieve these outcomes."[23]

While it is generally agreed that patients with advanced kidney disease not on dialysis have much to gain from a multidisciplinary approach to care,[24] CMS (and most other payers) does not require this for members of this group. Consequently, it is often easier for providers to recommend dialysis initiation than continue to manage patients in outpatient nephrology clinic when their needs become more complex.[14] Because this shift may not coincide with the time the patient feels ready to start dialysis, care and incentive structures that slant the "playing field" in favor of dialysis initiation can work against a person-centered approach.

Another limitation of current models of outpatient nephrology care for patients with advanced kidney disease is their narrow focus on the patient–clinician dyad as the unit of interaction. This arrangement reflects the high premium placed on patients' autonomy and privacy in US healthcare systems. However, a narrow focus on the patient without consideration of their broader social context often means that involvement of family members and close friends in their care tends to be shaped more by system-level needs than those of patients and/or families.[25] Often family members don't become involved until late in the course of illness when there is a crisis and patients need assistance with decision-making. Offering opportunities for family involvement throughout the course of illness may be helpful for both patients and families. Similar concerns apply to the involvement of peer mentors, who can be an important source of support and guidance for patients with advanced kidney disease but are generally not integral to existing care structures and practices.[26,27]

A further impediment to person-centered care for patients with advanced kidney disease not on dialysis is that most of this care is delivered in medical settings (eg, hospital, clinic). This kind of "spoke-and-wheel" arrangement is convenient for medical providers but may not optimally serve the needs of patients and families. Outpatient clinic visits can also be difficult to individualize when time slots are standardized based on arbitrary criteria (new patient visit vs follow-up), there is a mismatch between the length of the visit and the complexity of care, and/or the visit complexity level is not known ahead of time (as is often the case). Other approaches to care delivery (eg, home visits, group visits, telehealth, virtual visits, hospital at home) may allow for more flexibility in care delivery, may be more likely to meet the needs of patients and families, and may make it easier for providers to get to know their patients as people.

Due to the relatively high frequency of outpatient visits among patients with advanced kidney disease and their prolonged course of illness, clinicians caring for these patients have an *extraordinary* opportunity to build meaningful relationships and shape patients' experiences of illness and care. Health system and reimbursement changes that sustain these relationships and allow them to flourish would go a long way to accomplishing what the physician and bioethicist Lydia Dugdale has described as "re-enchanting medicine."[21] She speaks not only of caring for the patient, but also of feeling "encouraged and energized" when establishing human connections with her patients. She argues persuasively that patient–provider relationships can and should be a cornerstone in sustaining patients, families, and clinicians through the course of illness.

Hospital Admission, Acute Illness, and Dialysis Initiation

Case

Approximately 1 month after his most recent renal clinic appointment, Mr. Z fell asleep while playing cards at his sister's home. He remembers almost nothing after his sister drove him home that night. When she came back 2 days later, she was alarmed to find him lying unconscious on the floor. Mr. Z was rushed via ambulance to the closest hospital whereupon he was found to have a profound respiratory and metabolic acidosis requiring intubation and prolonged mechanical ventilation for a presumed aspiration pneumonia. The patient's creatinine on admission was elevated to 7 mg/dL and remained elevated during his hospital stay, so he was started on dialysis and eventually discharged to begin outpatient treatment at a dialysis facility close to his home. When Mr. Z later reflected on this experience, he had no recollection of being asked whether he was willing to start dialysis. As he put it, the decision was made "for" rather than "by" him.

Discussion

Growing support for person-centered care—particularly for complex patients with limited life expectancy—has occurred against a backdrop of mounting regulatory efforts to lower healthcare costs, improve the quality of care, and reduce hospital admission and readmission. Because inpatient costs account for the bulk of healthcare spending in this country, efforts to limit hospital utilization have been at the core of CMS-led efforts to improve value in healthcare—that is, striving for similar or higher quality at lower cost. Consistent with this goal, initiation of dialysis in the hospital is viewed by many payers, health systems, and providers as a marker for low-quality care and something to be avoided. On the face of it, this approach seems aligned with patients' best interests. What patient would not want to avoid a hospital admission or readmission and minimize time spent in the hospital? Both Mr. Z and his sister would clearly have been better off if he had started dialysis in the outpatient setting before he became critically ill and had to start dialysis emergently. However, Mr. Z's experience is not that unusual: more than 50% of US patients with ESKD start dialysis in the hospital, including a subset like Mr. Z who are critically ill and have prolonged hospital stays.[28,29] Although some of these "crash starts" occur in patients with little or no prior nephrology care, the vast majority occur among patients under the care of a nephrologist, reflecting the complexity of caring for patients and the challenges of living with this often highly unpredictable disease. Like Mr. Z, patients can live with limited renal reserve for long periods of time with few signs and symptoms of illness. However, when these patients do become sick, they can deteriorate very rapidly and with little warning.

How could a "crash start" have been avoided in Mr. Z's case? Certainly, educating him and his family about the potential risks involved in waiting until he becomes sick to start dialysis (eg, perhaps by describing the kind of catastrophic event he eventually experienced) might have helped them to recognize that he was getting sick sooner than they did, perhaps when he fell asleep while playing cards. System changes that could support the feasibility of this approach might include accelerated access to nephrology services—perhaps leveraging the skills of physician extenders—to reduce reliance on the emergency medical system, better educational resources to support shared decision-making, and provide patients and their family members and close friends with a clear understanding of what to expect as their illness progresses and offering opportunities for patients to involve their family members and close friends in their care throughout the illness trajectory. Better communication between the clinicians caring for Mr. Z in the hospital and his outpatient nephrologist might also have helped to improve his experience of care and smooth his transition to dialysis. As it turned out, Mr. Z's outpatient nephrologist was not notified that he had been admitted to the hospital until after he had been discharged, nor did she even realize that he had a sister living nearby. For her part, Mr. Z's sister knew almost nothing about his condition because he had a habit of keeping things to himself.

Because of its potential role in supporting a person-centered approach to care in the outpatient setting, we believe that hospital admission should not necessarily be viewed as an unfavorable outcome for patients with advanced kidney disease. Indeed, by allowing patients to wait until they become sick enough that they feel ready to initiate dialysis, efforts to promote a person-centered approach to dialysis initiation in outpatient settings (ie, supporting patients to defer dialysis until they feel ready) will predictably lead to increased reliance on inpatient services. Conversely, reducing use of inpatient services around the time of dialysis initiation would probably require that providers encourage patients to begin dialysis before they become sick, perhaps before they feel ready. The difficulty with this approach, however, is that in a crisis, treatment decisions tend to be shaped more by provider practices and rescue defaults than by the preferences, goals, and values of individual patients.[8-10,30-32] Available evidence suggests that when patients with advanced kidney disease are admitted to the hospital there may be substantial momentum favoring dialysis initiation.[9,10,12] Unfortunately, just like Mr. Z, patients who initiate dialysis in the midst of a crisis may be left with little or no understanding of why dialysis was started and feeling like they had little say in the matter. To avoid this situation, efforts are sorely needed to change the culture of inpatient care to ensure that patients continue to have a strong voice in shaping their care while in the hospital, to find ways to leverage exiting patient–provider relationships that have evolved—often over many years—in the outpatient setting, and to prepare patients and their families for crisis situations.

End-of-Life Care

Case

About 2 years after starting dialysis, Mr. Z. confesses to his nephrologist that perhaps it would not have been the worst thing if his sister had not come by to check on him that day.

This prompts his nephrologist to start up a conversation about end-of-life care. During this conversation, she brings up the option of stopping dialysis were Mr. Z to get to the point where this treatment is too burdensome. Initially, Mr. Z did not quite understand what his nephrologist was talking about It was his understanding that he had to be on dialysis; could he really stop doing dialysis? His nephrologist then clarified that although he did not have to do dialysis, he would probably only live for a few weeks if he were to stop dialysis. She suggested that, were he to go this route, it would be important to be proactive in getting hospice involved to make sure that he and his family had the support and care they needed during his final weeks of life. Once Mr. Z understood what his nephrologist saying, he quickly responded that he was "not ready for that. Hospice is where they send you to die."

Discussion

Several studies have asked patients with advanced kidney disease about what kind of care they would want to receive if they were seriously ill or dying.[33,34] Most patients included in these studies said that they would want to receive care that focused on relief of suffering rather than life prolongation under these circumstances. Nevertheless, compared with other chronically ill populations, such as those with dementia and cancer, patients on dialysis are more likely to receive intensive inpatient-oriented patterns of care focused on life extension toward the end of their lives.[35-37] Conversely, they are less likely than patients with other serious illnesses to receive palliative care and hospice services.[38,39]

Available evidence suggests that many patients on dialysis have not completed an advance directive. Further, most advance directives make no mention of some of the unique treatment-specific decisions that these patients may face toward the end of life, including whether and when to stop dialysis treatment.[40] Although contemporary guidelines recommend that nephrologists engage in discussions about prognosis and treatment options with their patients, this is a neglected aspect of nephrology practice that is not addressed in most training and certification programs.[41] Consequently, most nephrologists do not feel equipped to engage in these kinds of conversations,[41,42] leaving many patients on dialysis with unrealistic or uncertain expectations about the future.[33] While dialysis facility staff often help patients to complete advance directives, CMS has only recently started to view this as a potential performance measure under the ESRD seamless care organization initiative. Unfortunately, a checklist approach to completion of advance directives may do little to promote a broader process of advance care planning in which patients, surrogates, and providers engage in an ongoing conversation about future care in the context of patients' goals and values.

Continued focus on life prolonging treatments in patients who are dying can result in missed opportunities to relieve suffering and preserve dignity. Not surprisingly, available evidence suggests that patients with advanced kidney disease receive lower quality end-of-life care than those with other life-limiting conditions like cancer and dementia, in part reflecting their more intensive patterns of end-of-life care. Significant system-level barriers to the delivery of hospice services likely also serve as a barrier to quality end-of-life care in this population. CMS rules restrict the provision of concurrent dialysis and hospice services to the small minority of patients for whom ESKD is not their primary life-limiting diagnosis with the result that most patients must discontinue dialysis before they can receive hospice services under Medicare.[38,39,43] It is thus not surprising that referral to hospice among patients on dialysis occurs less frequently and closer to the time of death than for other seriously ill populations.

To ensure that patients with advanced kidney disease receive end-of-life care that is congruent with their goals, values, and preferences, stronger efforts are needed to cultivate prognostic awareness, promote advance care planning, and educate about hospice and stopping dialysis among members of this population. Given that many patients with advanced kidney disease die in the hospital, as with dialysis initiation, efforts to improve the quality of end-of-life care for patients with advanced kidney disease will likely require considerable work to change the culture of inpatient care, build communication skills among nephrology providers, promote continuity and coordination between inpatient and outpatient settings and find ways to optimally leverage long-term patient–provider relationships.

Conclusion

Contemporary patterns of care for patients with advanced kidney disease are far from person-centered. Large changes to health systems, payment structures, quality measurement, patient and provider education, and the culture in which care is delivered will be needed to support a more a person-centered approach to care for members of this population. To uphold the essence of who our patients are, efforts are needed throughout the illness trajectory to foster the development of strong patient–provider relationships and extend the reach of these relationships across settings, to educate our patients about their treatment options and what to expect in the future, to offer opportunities for patients to involve their family members and close friends in their care, and ultimately to promote a culture in which providers are flexible, creative, and tireless in working with their colleagues and with their patients and their families to fulfill the mission of person-centered care of finding the "right treatment for the right person at the right time."

Practice Pointers

- Open-ended listing may be more important in centering care on the patient than traditional markers of quality care such as completion and documentation of the physical exam or review of systems.
- Engage in person-centered education and communication with patients and family so that they have a good understanding of what to expect in the future not only in terms of their illness trajectory but also about the way the health system works, including common defaults.
- Adopt a person-centered approach to dialysis initiation that is guided by patient readiness. A strategy of close follow-up with a nephrologist until patients develop a clinical indication for dialysis appears to be just as safe as, and more cost effective than, starting dialysis.

Practice Improvement Opportunities

- Shift reimbursement criteria away from a rigid procedure- and organ system-based approach toward a more flexible approach that accounts for time spent and the extent to which patients' needs are met.
- Foster an infrastructure that supports a multidisciplinary approach to caring for patients with advanced kidney disease that embraces a range of treatment options including, but not limited to, dialysis and offers opportunities for involvement of family members/close friends and peer mentorship.
- Ensure that patients with ESKD receive end-of-life care that is congruent with goals, values, and preferences through stronger efforts to cultivate prognostic awareness, promote advance care planning, and collaborate with patients and their loved ones.

Acknowledgment

We would like to than Dr. Jeff Perlmutter for valuable input on this chapter.

References

1. Institute of Medicine, Committee on Quality of Health Care in America. *Crossing the Quality Chasm: A New Health System for the 21st Century.* Washington, DC: National Academy Press; 2001.
2. Harris DCH, Davies SJ, Finkelstein FO, et al. Increasing access to integrated ESKD care as part of universal health coverage. *Kidney Int.* 2019;95(4S):S1–S33.
3. Davison SN, Levin A, Moss AH, et al. Executive summary of the KDIGO Controversies Conference on Supportive Care in Chronic Kidney Disease: developing a roadmap to improving quality care. *Kidney Int.* 2015;88(3):447–459.
4. Chan CT, Blankestijn PJ, Dember LM, et al. Dialysis initiation, modality choice, access, and prescription: conclusions from a Kidney Disease: Improving Global Outcomes (KDIGO) Controversies Conference. *Kidney Int.* 2019;96(1):37–47.
5. O'Hare AM, Rodriguez RA, Bowling CB. Caring for patients with kidney disease: shifting the paradigm from evidence-based medicine to patient-centered care. *Nephrol Dial Transplant.* 2016;31(3):368–375.
6. O'Hare AM, Richards C, Szarka J, et al. Emotional impact of illness and care on patients with advanced kidney disease. *Clin J Am Soc Nephrol.* 2018;13(7):1022–1029.
7. Cooper BA, Branley P, Bulfone L, et al. The Initiating Dialysis Early and Late (IDEAL) study: study rationale and design. *Perit Dial Int.* 2004;24(2):176–181.
8. Wong SP, Hebert PL, Laundry RJ, et al. Decisions about renal replacement therapy in patients with advanced kidney disease in the US Department of Veterans Affairs, 2000–2011. *Clin J Am Soc Nephrol.* 2016;11(10):1825–1833.
9. Wong SPY, McFarland LV, Liu CF, Laundry RJ, Hebert PL, O'Hare AM. Care practices for patients with advanced kidney disease who forgo maintenance dialysis. *JAMA Intern Med.* 2019;179(3):305–313.
10. Wong SP, Vig EK, Taylor JS, et al. Timing of initiation of maintenance dialysis: a qualitative analysis of the electronic medical records of a national cohort of patients from the Department of Veterans Affairs. *JAMA Intern Med.* 2016;176(2):228–235.
11. Russ AJ, Shim JK, Kaufman SR. The value of "life at any cost": talk about stopping kidney dialysis. *Soc Sci Med.* 2007;64(11):2236–2247.
12. Kaufman SR, Shim JK, Russ AJ. Old age, life extension, and the character of medical choice. *J Gerontol B Psychol Sci Soc Sci.* 2006;61(4):S175–184.

13. Kaufman SR. *Ordinary Medicine: Extraordinary Treatments, Longer Lives, and Where to Draw the Line.* Durham, NC: Duke University Press; 2015.
14. Ladin K, Smith AK. Active medical management for patients with advanced kidney disease. *JAMA Intern Med.* 2019;179(3):313–315.
15. Wong SPY, O'Hare AM. Making sense of prognostic information about maintenance dialysis versus conservative care for treatment of advanced kidney disease. *Nephron.* 2017;137(3):169–171.
16. Tonelli M, Wiebe N, Manns BJ, et al. Comparison of the complexity of patients seen by different medical subspecialists in a universal health care system. *JAMA Netw Open.* 2018;1(7):e184852.
17. Schell JO, Patel UD, Steinhauser KE, Ammarell N, Tulsky JA. Discussions of the kidney disease trajectory by elderly patients and nephrologists: a qualitative study. *Am J Kidney Dis.* 2012;59(4):495–503.
18. Centers for Medicare and Medicaid Services. Physician fee schedule: overview. https://www.cms.gov/apps/physician-fee-schedule/overview.aspx. Updated October 4, 2019.
19. Hendrickson MA, Melton GB, Pitt MB. The review of systems, the electronic health record, and billing. *JAMA.* 2019;322(2):115–116.
20. O'Hare AM. Patient-centered care in renal medicine: five strategies to meet the challenge. *Am J Kidney Dis.* 2018;71(5):732–736.
21. Dugdale LS. Re-enchanting medicine. *JAMA Intern Med.* 2017;177(8):1075–1076.
22. Center for Medicare and Medicaid Services. Patients over paperwork. https://www.cms.gov/About-CMS/story-page/patients-over-paperwork.html. Accessed April 13, 2020.
23. Department of Health and Human Services, Centers for Medicare & Medicaid Services. Medicare and Medicaid programs: conditions for coverage for end-stage renal disease facilities. CMS-3818-F. https://www.cms.gov/Regulations-and-Guidance/Legislation/CFCsAndCoPs/Downloads/ESRDfinalrule0415.pdf. Published April 15, 2008.
24. Hemmelgarn BR, Manns BJ, Zhang J, et al. Association between multidisciplinary care and survival for elderly patients with chronic kidney disease. *J Am Soc Nephrol.* 2007;18(3):993–999.
25. O'Hare AM, Szarka J, McFarland LV, et al. "Maybe they don't even know that I exist": challenges faced by family members and friends of patients with advanced kidney disease. *Clin J Am Soc Nephrol.* 2017;12(6):930–938.
26. Ghahramani N. Potential impact of peer mentoring on treatment choice in patients with chronic kidney disease: a review. *Arch Iran Med.* 2015;18(4):239–243.
27. Hughes J, Wood E, Smith G. Exploring kidney patients' experiences of receiving individual peer support. *Health Expect.* 2009;12(4):396–406.
28. Wong SP, Kreuter W, O'Hare AM. Healthcare intensity at initiation of chronic dialysis among older adults. *J Am Soc Nephrol.* 2014;25(1):143–149.
29. O'Hare AM, Wong SP, Yu MK, et al. Trends in the timing and clinical context of maintenance dialysis initiation. *J Am Soc Nephrol.* 2015;26(8):1975–1981.
30. Hetzler PT 3rd, Dugdale LS. How do medicalization and rescue fantasy prevent healthy dying? *AMA J Ethics.* 2018;20(8):E766–E773.
31. Kaufman SR. *And a Time to Die: How American Hospitals Shape the End of Life.* New York, NY: Scribner; 2005.
32. Kruser JM, Cox CE, Schwarze ML. Clinical momentum in the intensive care unit: a latent contributor to unwanted care. *Ann Am Thorac Soc.* 2017;14(3):426–431.
33. Wachterman MW, Marcantonio ER, Davis RB, et al. Relationship between the prognostic expectations of seriously ill patients undergoing hemodialysis and their nephrologists. *JAMA Intern Med.* 2013;173(13):1206–1214.
34. Davison SN. End-of-life care preferences and needs: perceptions of patients with chronic kidney disease. *Clin J Am Soc Nephrol.* 2010;5(2):195–204.
35. Wachterman MW, Lipsitz SR, Lorenz KA, Marcantonio ER, Li Z, Keating NL. End-of-life experience of older adults dying of end-stage renal disease: a comparison with cancer. *J Pain Symptom Manage.* 2017;54(6):789–797.
36. Wachterman MW, Pilver C, Smith D, Ersek M, Lipsitz SR, Keating NL. Quality of end-of-life care provided to patients with different serious illnesses. *JAMA Intern Med.* 2016;176(8):1095–1102.

37. Wong SP, Kreuter W, O'Hare AM. Treatment intensity at the end of life in older adults receiving long-term dialysis. *Arch Intern Med.* 2012;172(8):661–663; discussion 663–664.
38. Wachterman MW, Hailpern SM, Keating NL, Kurella Tamura M, O'Hare AM. Association between hospice length of stay, health care utilization, and Medicare costs at the end of life among patients who received maintenance hemodialysis. *JAMA Intern Med.* 2018;178(6):792–799.
39. Murray AM, Arko C, Chen SC, Gilbertson DT, Moss AH. Use of hospice in the United States dialysis population. *Clin J Am Soc Nephrol.* 2006;1(6):1248–1255.
40. Feely MA, Hildebrandt D, Edakkanambeth Varayil J, Mueller PS. Prevalence and contents of advance directives of patients with ESRD receiving dialysis. *Clin J Am Soc Nephrol.* 2016;11(12):2204–2209.
41. Davison SN, Jhangri GS, Holley JL, Moss AH. Nephrologists' reported preparedness for end-of-life decision-making. *Clin J Am Soc Nephrol.* 2006;1(6):1256–1262.
42. Holley JL, Davison SN, Moss AH. Nephrologists' changing practices in reported end-of-life decision-making. *Clin J Am Soc Nephrol.* 2007;2(1):107–111.
43. Grubbs V, Moss AH, Cohen LM, et al. A palliative approach to dialysis care: a patient-centered transition to the end of life. *Clin J Am Soc Nephrol.* 2014;9(12):2203–2209.

Index

Tables, figures and boxes are indicated by *t*, *f* and *b* following the page number

For the benefit of digital users, indexed terms that span two pages (e.g., 52–53) may, on occasion, appear on only one of those pages.

Accreditation Council for Graduate Medical Education, 60
acetaminophen, 155–58
acetylcholinesterase inhibitors, 193
active medical management without dialysis. *See* medical management without dialysis
activities of daily living, 188–89, 227
acupuncture, 149*t*, 173–74
acute illness, 253–54
acute kidney injuries
    advance care planning and, 201
    case study, 197–98, 204, 206–7
    communication about, 205–6, 206*f*
    dialysis time-limited trials for, 202–4, 203*f*
    disagreements on management of, 204
    foregoing dialysis with, 201–2
    functional status and outcomes, 199–200
    incidence rate of, 198
    informing patients about, 199
    long-term outcomes with, 199, 200–1
    mortality rates with, 198, 199–200
    prognoses with, 199–201
    recommended approach to, 198
    shared decision-making with, 89, 198–99
    specialty palliative care for, 204–5
acute pain, 149–50, 149*t*
advance care planning, 7
    acute kidney injuries and, 201
    barriers to adoption of, 101
    case studies, 98–99, 116–17, 121
    clinician's role in, 103–4
    current use of, 101
    definitions, 99
    description of, 28
    on dialysis preferences, 101, 104–5, 117–18
    with dialysis withdrawal, 228–29, 229*f*, 233
    documentation in, 100–1, 100*t*, 117, 121
    education on, 103
    effectiveness of, 99–100, 120–21
    elicitation of patient preferences, 105
    goal of, 28, 99
    guidelines for, 102*t*, 103
    lack of, 28
    outputs of, 100–1, 100*t*
    patient capacity and, 101, 104, 242–43
    for patients on nondialysis pathway, 142–43
    people involved in, 99, 101
    POLST, 100*t*, 101, 104–6, 116–17, 118–22, 234*f*
    process steps, 103*f*, 103–4, 117
    questions to facilitate, 104*b*, 105
    registries for, 118, 119, 120
    systems for, 99, 117, 118*f*, 118–21, 119*b*
    timing of, 50, 101
    tools for implementation, 102*t*
    West Virginia's system, 118–21, 118*f*, 119*b*
    workflow incorporation, 103
advance directives
    completion rates, 28, 101, 120
    description of, 100, 100*t*
    failure to address dialysis with, 117–18, 255
    limitations to, 242–43
    living wills, 98–99, 100
    substituted judgment and, 242–43
affective-cognitive domain, 88

Agency for Healthcare Research and Quality, 89
Alexander, Shana, 13
Alzheimer's dementia, 192, 193
American Academy of Hospice and Palliative Medicine, 4, 69–70, 79
American Society of Internal Artificial Organs, 16
American Society of Nephrology, 4, 16, 19, 78–79
amionbutyric acid analogs, 172–73
amitriptyline, 155–58, 156t
anemia management, 141–42
angiotensin-converting enzymes inhibitors, 140–41
angiotensin receptor blockers, 140–41
antidepressants, 70, 71, 155, 181–82
anxiety, 181t, 182–83
Artificial Kidney Center, 13
"Ask-Tell-Ask," 93–94, 94t
assessments
  of cognitive functioning, 192
  of family caregivers, 112, 112b
  of frailty, 189, 190b
  outcomes with medical management without dialysis, 143b, 143
  of pain (see pain assessment)
  of patient needs (see needs assessment)
  psychosocial concerns, 179, 180f, 181t
  for risk of falls, 190, 191
  of symptoms, 28, 50, 53–54, 151–53, 152f, 169
Australian models, 41, 143

Beck Depression Inventory, 53–54
behavioral changes, 109
behavioral domain, 88, 185
behavioral therapies, 153t, 182, 182t
benzodiazepines, 183
bereavement services, 71, 113
best practices recommendations, 7
bioethics, 18, 240. See also Ethical issues
blood pressure management, 140–41
Brief Pain Inventory, 153
British Columbia Renal Agency, 41
Brophy v New England Sinai Hospital Inc., 232
buprenorphine, 160, 161t
burnout
  causes of, 78–79, 81
  correlates of, 77, 77b
  defined, 77
  of family caregivers, 110
  in nephrology, 78–79, 81
  in palliative care, 79, 81
  prevalence, 77, 78, 79
  solutions to, 79–81

Canada, 41
cancer
  as comorbidity, 70
  comparisons to kidney disease, 25, 28–29
  survival rates, 138t
  treatments, 70–71
carbamazepine, 155–58, 156t
cardiovascular comorbidities, 140–41
care continuum, 25–26, 36
care coordination. *See* coordinated care
Caregiving Stress Appraisal Tool, 112
CARES Program, 37–38
care transitions
  care coordination practices for, 217
  case, 211–12
  to end-of-life care, 215–16
  strategies to address challenges, 216, 216t
case managers, 72–73
casuistry, 244–45, 245t
Center to Advance Palliative Care, 72–73
cerebrovascular disease, 192
Certificate of Public Need, 17
change, 43
chaplains, 68
Chapters Health System Open Access hospice, 40
Charlson Comorbidity Index (CCI), 130, 131
Choosing Wisely (AAHPM), 69–70, 88
Chronic Kidney Disease Antidepressant Sertraline Trial (CAST), 181–82
chronic kidney disease (CKD)
  care by stage of disease, 7f
  care coordination management programs for, 37, 39
  improved pathway for elderly patients, 24f
  needs assessment, timing of, 50
  shared decision-making with, 89
  stages 1 to 3, 213
  stage 4, 50, 58–59, 67, 87–88, 214–15
  stage 5, 50, 138–39, 142, 214–15
CKD. *See* chronic kidney disease
Clinical Frailty Scale, 189
Clinical Practice Guideline on Shared Decision-Making, 19
Clinical Practice Guidelines for Quality Palliative Care, 4, 68
clinicians. *See* Nephrologists; Physicians
CMS (Centers for Medicare & Medicaid Services). *See* medicare
Coalition for Supportive Care of Kidney Patients, 4, 7, 19, 104–5. See also Kidney End-of-Life Care Coalition
codeine, 159–60
cognition, 191
cognitive assessment, 192
cognitive behavioral therapy (CBT), 182, 182t
cognitive impairment, 191
  adverse outcomes with, 192
  case studies, 67, 188–89
  cerebrovascular disease and, 192

decision-making capacity and, 101, 104, 198–99, 201, 229, 241–43
  interventions in suspected cases of, 192, 193*t*
  management strategies for, 193–94, 194*t*
  prevalence of, 191–92
  research focus on, 194
  risk factors for, 191–92, 193*f*
  screening for, 192
Cohen prognostic model, 130, 131–32
collaboration, 41, 43, 71–72, 214
communication
  Ask-Tell-Ask, 90*t*, 93–94, 94*t*, 97
  barriers to, 91, 215
  breaking bad news, 205, 206*f*
  conflict resolution and, 204
  conversation guide, 91–93, 92*t*
  discussion between patient and physician, 27, 60–61, 120, 122, 129–30
  elicitation of patient preferences, 105, 228–29
  frameworks for conversations, 91–93, 92*t*, 93*t*, 94*t*, 205–6, 206*f*
  on goals of care, 205
  between physicians, 254
  responses to emotion, 95
  silence, allowing for, 94*t*, 95
  with teams, 73–74, 214
communication skills, 62, 63*t*, 80–81
communication tools, 93–95, 94*t*, 95*t*
community resources, 72–73
comorbidities, 25, 26–27, 70–71, 137
Completing the Continuum of Nephrology Care, 4
comprehensive conservative care. *See* medical management without dialysis
Comprehensive Geriatric Assessment (CGA), 189
comprehensive regional programs, 37, 40–41
concurrent hospice/dialysis programs, 37, 40
conflict resolution, 204, 244–45
conflicts of interest, 244
conservative kidney management, 41. See also medical management without dialysis
continuity of care, 71–72, 119–20, 214
coordinated care, 71–72, 212
  around care transitions, 217
  case, 211–12
  in early stages of CKD, 213
  in later stages of CKD, 214–15
  models, 6, 71–72, 212, 217
  roles in, 213*f*, 214–15
  treatment decision point, 214
costs
  of hospice care, 30–32, 32*f*
  in last month of life, 32*f*, 32
  of treatment, 14–15, 17–18
  with and without hospice, 32
"Crossing the Quality Chasm" (Institute of Medicine), 248

cultural attitudes, 43, 240–41
cultural humility, 111
cultural norms, 111, 142
culture change, 43
culture of "death denial," 4
CYP3A4 gene, 159
CYP2D6 gene, 159–60

deaths. *See* mortality rates
decision aids, 96
decision making. *See also* Shared decision-making
  with ambivalence, 70
  "best interest" standard, 242
  case study in, 67–68
  clinical practice guidelines for, 60–61
  cognitive impairment and, 28, 192
  conflict resolution in, 204, 244–45
  critical juncture for, 214
  on dialysis initiation, 70, 127–28, 137–38, 250
  ethical process of, 244*b*
  goal conflicts and, 70
  as part of advance care planning, 104–5
  patient capacity for, 101, 104, 198–99, 201, 229, 241–43
  substituted judgment in, 28, 100, 104, 198–99, 232, 242–43
  unrealistic expectations and, 27
dementia, 191, 192, 193, 221. *See also* Cognitive impairment
depression, 230
  case study, 70, 178–79, 182
  diagnosis of, 179, 181*t*
  prevalence, 53–54, 179
  screening instruments for, 53–54, 179
  treatment options, 181–82, 182*t*
dialysis
  for acute care injuries in ICU settings, 201–4, 207
  advance care planning and, 101, 104–5, 117–18
  burdens of, 221–22, 228
  concurrent hospice/dialysis programs, 37, 40
  decision making on (*see* decision making; Shared decision-making)
  as default option, 29, 88, 138
  dependence after acute kidney injury, 200–1
  discontinuation of (*see* dialysis withdrawal)
  economic incentives for, 43
  equipoise in benefits of, 127–28, 136–37, 137*b*
  foregoing of, 29, 58–59, 201–2, 250 (*see also* medical management without dialysis)
  history of, 13–14, 17–18, 18*f*
  hospice care and, 30–32, 31*f*
  incremental, 224
  initiation, 27, 241–42, 250–54
  modalities, 89, 221–22
  palliative (*see* Palliative dialysis)

dialysis (cont.)
   patient prognosis and, 127–29
   patient selection for, 13
   quality of life and, 25, 136–37, 138–39, 221
   scheduling frequency, 224
   standard treatment of, 29
   statistics, historical, 17–18
   survival benefit with, 25, 138, 138*t*, 139–40, 221
   trials of, 138, 202–4, 203*f*
   and uremic pruritus, 171–72
   withdrawal (*see* Dialysis withdrawal)
dialysis centers, 17–18, 40, 60–61, 68, 224, 244
Dialysis Clinics, Inc. (DCI), 39, 40
Dialysis Falls Risk Index, 191
Dialysis Morbidity Study, 17
Dialysis Outcomes and Practice Patterns Study (DOPPS), 169
dialysis providers, 17–18, 18*f*
Dialysis Symptom Index, 221
dialysis withdrawal, 7, 228
   advance care planning and, 101, 228–29, 229*f*, 233
   associated factors, 228
   case studies, 71, 227–28, 235, 254–55
   discussions about, 212, 215, 232, 233, 254–55
   education about, 231–32
   ethical issues with, 68, 232, 240–41, 243
   mortality from, 221–22, 228
   option to reconsider, 232
   patient autonomy and, 128
   patient decisional capacity and, 241–43
   patient preferences about, 118
   prognoses with, 231
   rates of, 29, 138, 139*t*
   rationale for, 229–31
   reasons for, 29, 229–31, 230*f*
   religious beliefs about, 68
   shared decision-making on, 127–28
   steps for, 233–35, 234*f*
   as suicide, 232
   supportive care recommendations, 232–33, 232*b*
   symptom management during, 233–35, 234*t*
   system-level barriers, 243
   in time-limited trials of dialysis, 138
dietary management, 142
disease-oriented approach, 19, 32
disease progression
   focus of care and, 213*f*
   informing patients on, 128–29
   provider roles and, 213*f*
   risk equation for, 132
   uncertainty about, 250
do not attempt resuscitation (DNAR) orders, 101
do not resuscitate (DNR) orders, 101, 120
double effect principle, 241
durable power of attorney, 21–22, 100*t*, 105, 198–99

Dutrochet, Rene J.H., 13–14
Dying in America, 6, 119
dying process, 113, 223, 231, 233

e-Directive Registry (West Virginia), 119–20
Edmonton Symptom Assessment System, 51, 53–54, 151–53, 152*f*, 221
education
   on dialysis withdrawal, 231–32
   for family members, 113
   nephrology fellowship, 60, 130, 207
   on pain management, 149*t*
   in palliative care, 59, 60–64
elderly patients. *See* Older patients
embedded programs, 37–38
emotional support, 112–13, 112*b See also* psychosocial concerns
emotions, 95
end of life. *See also* Hospice
   care transition at, 215–16
   case studies, 71, 254–55
   coordination of care, 71
   cost in last month, 32
   discussion of between physician and patient, 27, 60–61, 120, 122, 129–30
   dying process, 113, 223, 231, 233
   education on, 113
   experiences of, 22, 32–33
   high-intensity care at, 29–30, 31*f*, 255
   hospitalizations at, 215–16
   ICU admissions by state, 30*f*
   lack of documentation for, 22
   lack of planning, 29–30
   for medical management without dialysis pathway, 142–43
   pain management at, 162*f*, 162–63
   patient-centered care during, 254–56
   patient preferences for, 118, 255, 256
   quality of care, 255–56
   race- and ethnicity-based disparities, 29–30
   symptom management algorithm for, 163*f*
end-stage kidney disease (ESKD), 14–15
   case studies, 49, 116–17, 188–89
   cost in last month, 32
   decision aids on, 96
   epidemiology of, 26–27
   family care during, 109
   ICU admissions by state, 30*f*
   incidence rates, 26–27
   palliative care resources in, 62*t*
   shared decision-making with, 89
   symptom burden with, 25
   timeline of key events in development of care system, 15*t*
   trajectory of, 30, 221

End-Stage Renal Disease Peer Work Group, 4
entitlement legislation, 17
epidemiology, 26–27
EQ-5D (European quality-of-life
    instrument), 52–53
ESAS-R (Edmonton Symptom Assessment
    System), 51, 53–54
ESKD Seamless Care Organization (ESCO)
    program, 38–39, 244
ESRD Concurrent Care Program, 40
ESRD program
    champions of, 15–16
    entitlement legislation, 17
    financial implications of, 17–18, 250–51
    government support, 15
    history of, 13–15, 15t
    quality improvement studies, 17
    statistics on, 17–18
    timeline of key events, 15t
ESRD Quality Incentive Program, 19, 223, 224
Ethics consultation, 204
ethical issues, 18, 240
    case, 239–40
    casuistry framework for, 244–45, 245t
    conflict resolution in decision making, 244–45
    conflicts of interest as, 244
    disparities in care access, 243
    moral uncertainty, 240–41
    patient autonomy and, 88, 117–18, 232
    patient decisional capacity and, 241–43
    seven-step process of ethical
        decision-making, 244b
    system-level concerns, 243
    value conflicts, 240–41
    in withdrawing dialysis, 68, 232, 240–41, 243
    in withholding dialysis, 240–43
ethnicity disparities, 29–30
European quality-of-life instrument (EQ- 5D),
    51, 52–53
European Renal Best Practice Working Group, 189
evidence base, 43
exercise, 149t

falls
    assessment of risk, 190, 191
    interventions to prevent, 190
    outcomes of, 190
    prevalence of, 190
    risk factors for, 190, 190b
family caregivers
    assessment of, 112, 112b
    burnout of, 110
    case study, 108, 109, 110
    conflicts with, 112–13
    coping techniques for, 112–13

cultural humility and, 111
education on end of life, 113
emotional support for, 112–13, 112b
meetings with, 111–12
recommendations for, 111–12
referrals to support, 113, 113b
stress on, 110
supportive care discussions, 110, 111–12
support systems of, 113
unmet needs of, 113
family-centered care, 111–12, 114
family involvement, 91–93, 109, 114
    in advance care planning, 22, 99, 104
    case study, 108, 109, 110
    challenges with, 110–11
    current evidence on, 109–11
    in discussions, 110–11
    in doctor visits, 110
    positive outcomes with, 109–10
    stress and, 110
family systems theory, 109
fatigue, 22, 28, 149, 168, 172, 174, 185, 221
fee-for-service billing, 250–51, 251t
fentanyl, 70–71, 160, 161t, 162–63
financial issues, 18, 224, 243, 250–51. *See also* Costs
for-profit treatment centers, 17–18
Frail Elderly Patient Outcomes on Dialysis, 189
frailty
    approach to, 190b
    assessments for, 189, 190b
    case study, 188–89
    conceptual definition of, 189
    features of, 189
    patient outcomes and, 189
    survival rate and, 221

gabapentin, 70–71, 155, 156t, 172–73
generalist palliative care, 5–6, 68
geriatric nephrology. *See also* Cognitive
        impairment
    case study, 188–89
    fall risk in, 190–91
    frailty issues in, 189
Glazer, Shep, 16
global summits, 1–4, 25
goals of care, 22, 88–89, 104b, 105, 205,
        214, 230–31
Gordon and Betty Moore Foundation, 4
Gottschalk, Carl, 15
government support, 15
Graham, Thomas, 13–14

haloperidol, 162–63
Hartke, Vance, 16
Hass, George, 13–14

healthcare agents, 100, 104
healthcare system, 18, 243–44, 248–49, 252
healthcare utilization, 212, 221
health-related quality of life. *See* Quality of life
heart failure patients, 28–29
hemodialysis, 14, 21–22, 28–29
hemoglobin, 141–42
holistic approach, 61, 114
Holland Home (Michigan), 40
home-based care
    hospice services for, 30–32, 231, 235
    specialty palliative care in, 38–39, 72
"hope and worry" statements, 205–6
hospice, 28–29, 234–35
    barriers to service delivery, 255–56
    concurrent hospice/dialysis programs, 37, 40
    costs of, 30–32, 32*f*
    defined, 5*b*
    disparities in care access, 243
    focus of, 6, 73
    home care with, 30–32, 231, 235
    referrals to, 71, 73, 255–56
    regulations regarding, 30–32, 40, 255–56
    utilization of, 30–32, 31*f*, 215–16, 222, 255
hospitalizations
    admissions, 30*f*, 253–54
    of dialysis patients *versus* other conditions, 221
    at end of life, 29–30, 215–16
    length of stay and, 109, 121
    palliative care consultations during, 28–29
    patient-centered care during, 253–54
    readmissions, 222
hydromorphone, 70–71, 159–60, 161*t*
hypertension management, 140–41

ICU. *See* intensive care units
IDEAL (Initiating Dialysis Early and Late) trial, 250
Independent Kidney Care Alliance, 40
individualized care plans, 69
inflammation, 171
informed consent, 27, 88
Inglehart, John, 18
Initiating Dialysis Early and Late (IDEAL) trial, 250
Integrated Palliative Care Outcome Scale- Renal, 151–53, 223
Integrated Palliative Outcome Scale- Renal (IPOS-R), 49, 51, 53–54
integrated supportive care, 24*f*, 212, 213*f*, 214–15, 217
intensive care units. *See also* acute kidney injuries
    admissions of ESKD by state, 30*f*
    length of stay, 109
    mortality risk in, 199–200

interdisciplinary teams. *See* multidisciplinary teams
International Society of Nephrology's Global Kidney Health Summits, 1–4, 25
IPOS-R, 49, 51, 53–54
iron deficiency. *See* anemia management
itch. *See* pruritus; uremic pruritus

Jackson, Henry "Scoop," 15
Johnson, Lyndon, 15
Joint Commission, 72

Karnofsky Performance Scale, 199–200, 200*t*
KDQOL (Kidney Disease Quality of Life), 51–52, 53
ketamine, 155–58, 156*t*
Khan-Wright (K-W) Index, 130, 131
Kidney Clinic, 37–38
Kidney Comprehensive Advanced Renal Disease and ESKD Support (CARES) Program, 37–38
kidney disease. *See* chronic kidney disease; End-stage kidney disease
Kidney Disease: Improving Global Outcomes (KDIGO), 1–4, 7, 55
Kidney Disease Outcomes Initiative, 17
Kidney Disease Quality of Life (KDQOL), 51–52, 53
Kidney End-of-Life Care Coalition, 4 see coalition for Supportive Care of Kidney Patients
Kidney Failure Risk Equation, 132
Kidney Supportive Care Implementation Quotient, 33
knowledge, lack of palliative care, 4
Kolff, Willem, 14

leadership, 43, 139–40
lidocaine, 162–63
life expectancy, 25, 129, 130–32. *See also* prognoses
Life magazine, 13
life prolongation, 68, 235, 240, 255–56
living wills, 98–99, 100. *See also* advance directives
Long, Russell, 15

maintenance hemodialysis, 28, 171, 190*b*, 221, 222–23
Mayo Clinic, 28–29
mechanical ventilation support, 30, 116–17, 202–4, 239, 253
medical management without dialysis, 7, 25, 144
    advance care planning and, 142–43
    anemia management in, 141–42
    appropriate messages about, 43
    availability of option, 22, 25, 39–40
    barriers to, 29, 139–40, 243
    case, 136–37, 143–44
    challenges with, 139–40

components of, 6, 140, 141b
defined, 5t
end-of-life care and, 142–43
equating to "no care," 29, 39–40, 240–41
hypertension management in, 140–41
nutritional management in, 142
online resources for, 141b
outcomes assessments for, 143b, 143
patient care during, 140–43
patient indications for, 127–28, 136–37, 137b
programs, 37, 39–40
quality assurance in, 143
quality of life and, 136–37, 138–40
quick guide to, 144b
standard of care for, 40
supportive care and, 6
survival rates with, 139–40
symptom management in, 142
symptom prevalence, 168f
timing of, 138–40
medical orders, 100, 100t, 101, 119–20, 233. See also Advance care planning and POLST
Medical Outcomes Study, 51
Medical Review Boards, 17
Medicare, 17
    Conditions for Coverage, 251–52
    hospice regulations, 30–32, 40, 255–56
    origins of, 15, 16
medications. *See also* specific condition
    adjuvant therapies, 154–58, 156t
    anticonvulsants, 155
    antidepressants, 70, 71, 155, 181–82
    drug interactions, 159–60
    for pain (*see* Pain management)
    topical therapies for UP, 172
    toxicity, 150, 155, 159–60
Medscape surveys, 78
memantine, 193
mental health, 178–79
methadone, 70–71, 160, 161t
mild cognitive impairment. *See* cognitive impairment
mobile specialty care teams, 37, 38–39
models of care. *See* supportive care models
Montreal Cognitive Assessment, 192
morality, 68
morphine, 160
mortality rates
    with acute kidney injuries, 198, 199–200
    age factors in, 26–27, 26t, 199–200
    with comorbidities, 26–27, 26t, 27f
    of ESKD population, 26–27
    in intensive care units, 199–200
    population comparisons, 26–27, 26t, 199–200, 215–16

multidisciplinary teams
    access to, 251–52
    in integrated supportive care model, 212, 213f, 217
    lack of formal structure, 70
    members of, 204–5
    with nondialysis option, 140
    palliative care education for, 61
    role of, 251–52

nalbuphine ER, 173
nalfurafine, 173
naltrexone, 173
National Association of Patients on Hemodialysis, 16
National Consensus Project, 68
National Cooperative Dialysis Study, 17
national guidelines, 43
National Kidney Foundation (NKF), 16, 104–5
needs assessment, 50
    case study, 49
    current evidence, 49–55
    program level-Kidney Supportive Care Implementation Quotient (KSC-IQ), 33
    timing of, 50
needs gap, 22–25, 23f. *See also* unmet needs
nephrologists
    board certifications of, 37
    burnout in, 78–79, 81
    case management by, 6
    expertise of, 6, 44, 137–38
    referrals to, 213
    role in shared decision-making, 137–38, 214
    second opinions from, 137–38
    supportive care provision by, 59
nephrology
    as career choice, 78–79
    case complexity in, 78
    culture of, 43
    global summits on, 1–4, 25
    job satisfaction in, 78–79
    training programs, 6, 59, 60–61
nephrology nurse practitioners, 37
NephroTalk curriculum, 205
network organizations, 17
neuropathic pain, 149t, 150, 154–58
neuropathy, 171
New South Wales, Australia, 38, 41
nociceptive pain, 149t, 150, 158
nonabandonment principle, 139–40
nonsteroidal anti-inflammatory drugs (NSAIDs), 150, 158
Northwest Kidney Centers, 38–39
NSAIDs, 150, 158
NURSE approach, 95, 95t

nurse care coordinators, 39
nurse practitioners, 37, 40
nursing facilities, 221, 235
nutritional management, 142

older patients, 25, 29, 30, 127–28. *See also* geriatric nephrology
open-ended questions, 94–95, 94*t*
opiate receptor modulators, 173
opioids
    adverse effects of, 160, 162–63
    considerations for use of, 158
    metabolism of, 158–60
    pharmacokinetics of, 161*t*
    recommendations on, 160
outcomes
    with acute kidney injury, 199, 200–1
    assessment tools for nondialysis pathway, 143*b*, 143
    with cognitive impairment, 192
    disparities in, 243
    falls, associated with, 190
    with family involvement, 109–10
    frailty and, 189
    with palliative dialysis, 222
    referrals and, 213, 214–15
    shared decision making and, 88
    spirituality, impact of, 184
outpatient care
    case, 250
    person-centered approach in, 254
    specialty palliative care in, 72
oxycodone, 159–60

pain
    categorization, 149–50, 149*t*
    chronicity of, 149–51
    defined, 149
    intensity of, 150
    nature of, 151
    prevalence of, 148
    quality of life and, 148, 151, 153
    recurrent, 149–50
    types of, 149–50, 149*t*
pain assessment, 148
    PQRST approach, 151, 151*t*
    screening tools for, 151–53, 152*f*
    systemic approach to, 150–51
    treatment goals and, 151
pain management, 70–71, 148
    adjuvant therapies, 154–58, 156*t*
    drug–drug interactions, 159–60
    at end of life, 162*f*, 162–63
    nonpharmacological approaches to, 153, 153*t*
    opioids for, 158–60, 161*t*, 162–63
    principles of, 154*t*
    stepwise selection of analgesics, 154–55, 155*f*
    systematic pharmacological approach, 154–63
palliative care. *See also* primary palliative care; specialty palliative care; supportive care
    benefits of, 79, 81, 222
    burnout in, 79, 81
    conflicts of interest, 244
    consultation, 6, 28–29, 69–70, 72, 73*t*, 73–74, 75, 121, 122, 207, 214–15, 222, 246
    cornerstone of, 69
    defined, 5–6, 5*b*, 49–50
    disparities in care access, 243
    domains of, 68
    expertise in, 41, 44
    generalist vs specialist 5–6, 68
    lack of knowledge, 4
    lack of, 255
    skills, 59, 60*t*, 81
    in U.S., 4
    workforce shortage in, 59
palliative care education
    communication skills development in, 62, 63*t*
    guidelines for, 64
    of multidisciplinary teams, 61
    of nephrology trainees, 59, 60–61
    resources, 62*t*, 63*t*
Palliative Care Provider Directory, 72–73
Palliative Care Quality Network, 222
palliative dialysis, 40, 224–25, 241
    assessment and, 223
    balance of, 222*f*
    barriers to, 224
    case, 220, 224
    current evidence on, 222–24
    outcomes with, 222
    patient indicators for, 222–23
    reasons for, 221–22
    role for, 221–22
    versus standard dialysis, 223, 223*t*
Palmetto Kidney Care Alliance ESCO, 39
panic disorder, 68
Parkinson's disease, 193
Pathways Project, 4, 7–8, 40, 64, 111
    best practices, 7, 64
patient-centered care, 8, 19, 256
    billing approaches and, 251, 251*t*
    case study, 250, 253, 254–55
    defined, 248
    dialysis initiation and, 252, 254
    documentation requirements and, 251
    during hospitalizations, 253–54
    ideal *versus* current state of care, 22–25, 23*f*, 24*f*
    in outpatient settings, 250–53
    recommendations to promote, 249*t*
    system-level constraints to, 248–49

patient decision aids, 96
patient education, 36
Patient Health Questionnaire, 178–79
patient information, 128–29, 199–201, 214
patient outcomes. *See* Outcomes
patient preferences
    on dialysis, 101, 104–5, 117–18
    documentation of (*see* advance care planning)
    elicitation of, 8, 19, 22, 27–28, 91, 96, 105
    for end of life, 118, 255, 256
patient-reported outcome measures (PROMs), 50, 52*t*
    administration, 54–55
    benefits of using, 50
    descriptions of, 51–54, 52*t*
    guidelines for use, 55
    implementation strategy, 54*f*, 54–55
    Oxford review of, 51
    types of, 51, 51*t*
patients
    acceptable level of better, 230–31
    adherence, 88
    age factors, 25, 26–27, 29, 30
    autonomy, 88, 117–18, 128, 232
    care experiences of, 19
    comorbidities in, 25, 26–27, 70–71, 137
    coping mechanisms, 184
    decision-making capacity, 101, 104, 198–99, 201, 229, 241–43
    fears, 91–93, 183, 223
    goals of care, 22, 88–89, 104*b*, 105, 205, 214
    hopes of, 130, 138–39, 223
    independence of, 29, 221
    nonabandonment of, 139–40
    priorities of, 27, 28, 221, 228
    religious beliefs of, 68
    self-determination, 88, 232
    sleep hygiene, 49
    sources of strength, 91–93
    swallowing difficulties, 162–63
    trust in clinician, 88, 224
    understanding of illness, 88, 91–94, 201
    values of, 91, 104*b*, 105, 202, 228
patient satisfaction, 88
Patient Self-Determination Act, 101, 242–43
peritoneal dialysis, 188–89, 213, 221–22, 224
person-centered care. *See* patient-centered care
PERSON mnemonic, 205
phototherapy, 173
physical therapies, 153*t*
physician reimbursement, 251*t*
physicians. *See also* nephrologists; primary care providers
    biases, 111
    case study on care approach, 58–59
    communication between, 254
    discussions with patients, 27, 60–61, 120, 122, 129–30
    elicitation of patient preferences, 22, 27
    intuition of, 131
    priorities for patient outcomes, 27
    prognostic accuracy of, 130, 131
    skill sets by level of care, 1*f*
physician wellness. *See also* burnout
    case study, 76–77
    crisis of, 77–78
    resilience and, 80–81
    solutions to, 79–81
    work demands and, 78–79, 80–81
Plan-Do-Study-Act (PDSA) cycle, 54*f*, 54
Plante, Charles, 16
POLST, 98–99, 101, 118–20, 121. *See also* advance care planning
power of attorney, 21–22, 105
pregabalin, 155, 172–73
primary care providers, 5–6, 101, 213, 214–15
primary palliative care. *See also* palliative care education
    appropriate involvement of, 69*t*
    conceptual model of, 59*f*
    defined, 5–6, 59
    need for, 59
    skills in, 59, 60*t*, 68
professional practice, 244
prognosis, 7. *See also* cohen prognostic model
    in acute kidney injury cases, 199–201
    barriers to sharing information on, 129–30
    calculators for, 96, 129*t*
    case study, 127, 128, 129, 130
    with dialysis withdrawal, 231
    discordance about, 128
    discussion between patient and physician, 27, 91–93, 128, 129–30
    hope and, 130, 138–39
    indices, 130–32
    overestimation of, 127–28
    patient awareness of, 22, 27, 128
    patients desire for information on, 128–29
    predictive models for, 60–61
    quality of life and, 130
    uncertainty of, 128–29, 130, 137–38, 202–4
Promoting Excellence in End-of-Life Care, 4
PROMS. *See* patient-reported outcome measures
provider orders, 101
provider orders for life-sustaining treatment (POLST), 98–99, 101, 119–20, 121. *See also* advance care planning
provider roles, 213*f*
proxies, 100, 104, 198–99

pruritus. See also Uremic pruritus
    defined, 169
    nonuremic causes of, 170b
    uremic (see uremic pruritus)
psychonephrology, 185
psychosocial concerns
    assessment of, 179, 180f, 181t
    case study, 178–79, 182, 183, 184
    inattention to, 28
    management of, 179, 180f
    research on, 185
    support for, 232, 233
psychotherapy, 149t, 178–79, 182, 182t, 183
Public Law 92-603, 17
PubMed searches, 1, 14–15

quality assurance, 143
quality improvement activities, 17
Quality Incentive Program, 19
quality metrics, 223, 224
quality of care, 17
quality of life, 21–22
    among maintenance dialysis patients, 221
    dialysis benefit and, 136–37
    discontinuation of dialysis and, 29
    least acceptable levels, 230–31
    with medical management without dialysis pathway, 136–37, 138–40
    pain and, 148, 151, 153
    in post-acute kidney injury cases, 199, 200–1
    prognoses and, 130
    spirituality and, 184
    symptom burden and, 50
Quinton, Wayne, 14

racial disparities, 29–30, 111, 191–92, 224
Real Engagement Achieving Complete Health (REACH), 39
Reasons for Geographic and Racial Differences in Stroke, 191–92
referrals
    for family caregiver support, 113, 113b
    to hospice, 71, 73, 255–56
    from primary care to nephrologists, 213
    to specialty care, 38–39, 214–15
refractory symptoms, 71
reimbursements, 19, 251t
REIN index, 130, 131
religious beliefs, 68, 70, 142, 184
REMAP approach, 91, 93, 93t
Renal Physicians Association, 4, 19, 103–5, 243
Renal Supportive Care Clinic (Northwest Kidney Centers), 38–39

Renal Supportive Care Clinic (University of Pittsburgh), 37–38, 40
Renal Supportive Care Model (Australia), 41
resilience, 80–81
Rettig, Richard, 16
Robert Wood Johnson Foundation, 4

Saunder, Cicely, 71
Schafstat, Sophia, 14
Schreiner, George, 16
Scribner, Belding, 14
Scribner shunt, 14
Seattle Artificial Kidney Center, 240
selective serotonin reuptake inhibitors, 155–58, 181–82, 183
sepsis, 22, 98, 239
serious illness, defined, 68
Serious Illness Conversation Guide, 91–93, 92t
SF-36 (Short-Form Health Survey), 51
Shared Decision in the Appropriate Initiation of and Withdrawal from Dialysis, 4, 198
shared decision-making, 7, 88, 96
    with acute kidney injury, 89, 198–99
    case study, 87–88
    with CKD patients, 89
    clinical guidelines for, 19
    communication tools for, 93–95, 94t
    components of, 89
    decision aids for, 96
    defined, 27
    on dialysis initiation, 127–28
    on dialysis withdrawal, 127–28
    with ESKD patients, 89
    evidence favoring, 88
    frameworks for, 90t, 91–93, 92t, 93t, 94t
    lack of, 27
    nephrologists' role in, 137–38, 214
    recommendations for use, 88
    second opinions, getting, 137–38
    settings for, 88–89
    timing considerations, 88–89, 214
SHARE model, 89, 90t
Short-Form Health Survey (SF-36), 51
skilled nursing facilities, 221, 235
skills
    communication skills development, 62, 63t, 80–81
    of practitioners by level of care, 1f
    in primary palliative care, 59, 60t, 81
    in resilience, 80–81
Social Security Act, 16, 240
Social Security Amendments, 17
social workers, 72–73, 223
specialty palliative care
    access to, 72–73, 74

for acute kidney injury patients, 204–5
case study in, 67–68
collaboration in, 71–72
communication with, 73–74
coordinated care model of, 6, 71–72, 214
defined, 5–6
inpatient *versus* outpatient, 29
lack of consultation, 28–29
relationship building with, 74
requests for, 73–74
resource locating, 72–73
skills in, 60*t*
standard for, 72
supply and demand mismatch, 68
team members in, 72
type of consultation by, 72, 73–74
in various care settings, 71–72
when to consult, 69–70, 69*t*, 73, 73*b*, 214–15
SPIKES communication strategy, 205, 206*f*
SPIRES Framework, 91, 93, 94*t*
spirituality, 68, 70, 181*t*, 184
spiritual needs, 184, 185
staffing models, 41
substituted judgments, 242–43. *See also* surrogates
suicide, 232
supportive care
along care continuum, 25–26, 36
barriers to provision of, 60–61
components of, 7–8, 25*f*
contribution by stage of disease, 7*f*
definition of, 4–6, 5*b*, 68
for dialysis withdrawal, 232–33, 232*b*
field of, 1
gap in U.S., 25–32
lack of, 28–29
versus medical management without dialysis, 6–7
need for, 1
providers of, 212
service availability, 217
in U.S., 4
utilization of, 215–16
supportive care clinics, 140
supportive care models, 36–37
barriers to success, 43
comparisons between, 37, 41, 42*t*
examples of, 37–41
integrated models, 24*f*, 212, 213*f*, 214–15, 217
literature review on, 37
program development, 36–37
program types, 37
selection considerations, 41–43, 44
success facilitators, 43
Supreme Court ruling, 232
surprise question, 101, 130, 131

surrogates, 100, 104, 198–99, 232, 242–43
survival
benefit with dialysis, 25, 138, 138*t*, 139–40, 221
frailty and, 221
versus quality of life prioritization, 221, 255
spirituality and, 184
symptom management, 7, 168–69. *See also* pain management
case studies, 70–71, 167–68
for CKD managed without dialysis, 142
with dialysis withdrawal, 233–35
dietary interventions, 142
in different patient populations, 168
at end of life, 163*f*
lack of, 28
of refractory symptoms, 71
symptoms
assessment of, 28, 50, 53–54, 151–53, 152*f*, 169
burden of, 25, 50, 53, 168
common in CKD, 28, 169, 221
impact of, 168
prevalence, 168*f*, 221
quality of life and, 50
underrecognition of, 28, 169
systemic inflammation, 171

Technical Expert Panel, 8
technology, 13–14, 43, 240
Teflon, 14
terminal care. *See* Hospice
terminal diagnoses, 30–32
terminal illness (nonrenal), 71, 202, 211–12
terminology, 5*b*
time-limited trials, 67, 70, 89, 138, 202–4, 203*f*, 205, 207
total pain concept, 71, 150
trade-offs, 29, 70, 91–93
training. *See also* palliative care education
in communication skills, 62, 63*t*, 80–81
as facilitator of program success, 43
in resilience, 80–81
tramadol, 159–60
Transactions of the American Society of Artificial Internal Organs, 14
transplantation, 17–18, 69–70, 89, 128, 214, 230–31
treatment. *See also* Decision making
adherence, 168
costs, 14–15, 17–18
entitlement and, 18
goals of, 18, 70, 151
modalities, 19, 26*t*
options, 22, 29, 50, 67, 87–88, 214
Truman Medical Centers (Kansas City, Missouri), 40
trust issues, 111, 224

UK National Institute for Health and Care
    Excellence, 190
ultraviolet B light (UVB), 173
United States Renal Disease Service, 17
University of Pittsburgh program, 37–38, 40
unmet needs, 1, 26–32
    addressing, 32, 54–55
    assessment of (*see* needs assessment)
    case studies of, 21–22, 49
    current state of, 22–25, 23*f*, 184, 214–15
    of family caregivers, 113
    identification of, 50, 53
UPMC Family Hospice, 40
UPMC Palliative and Supportive Institute, 38
uremia, 14–15, 181*t*
uremic pruritus
    case study, 167–68
    clinical presentation, 169–70
    dialysis adequacy and, 171–72
    epidemiology of, 169
    pathophysiology, 171
    prevalence of, 169
    step-wise approach to management of, 174
    treatments for, 171–74

value conflicts, 240–41
values, 91, 104*b*, 105, 202, 228
ventilation support, 30, 116–17, 202–4, 239, 253
visiting specialty care teams, 37, 38–39
vividiffusion, 13–14

weight reduction, 149*t*
wellness. *See* Physician wellness
West Virginia advance care planning program,
    118–21, 119*b*
West Virginia Center for End-of-Life
    Care, 120
wish-worry-wonder statements, 94*t*, 95
World Health Organization, 4, 154–55, 189

xerosis, 171, 172

yoga, 149*t*
Yorkshire Dialysis Decision Aide (YoDDA), 96